ULCERATIVE COLITIS FROM GENETICS TO COMPLICATIONS

Edited by **Mustafa M. Shennak**

Ulcerative Colitis from Genetics to Complications
Edited by Mustafa M. Shennak

Published by InTech
Janeza Trdine 9, 51000 Rijeka, Croatia

Publishing Process Manager Danijela Duric

Technical Editor Teodora Smiljanic

Cover Designer InTech Design Team

Additional hard copies can be obtained from orders@intechopen.com

Ulcerative Colitis from Genetics to Complications, Edited by Mustafa M. Shennak
p. cm.
ISBN 978-953-307-853-3

For EU product safety concerns:
IN TECH d.o.o., Prolaz Marije Krucifikse Kozulić 3, 51000 Rijeka, Croatia,
info@intechopen.com or visit our website at intechopen.com.

Meet the editor

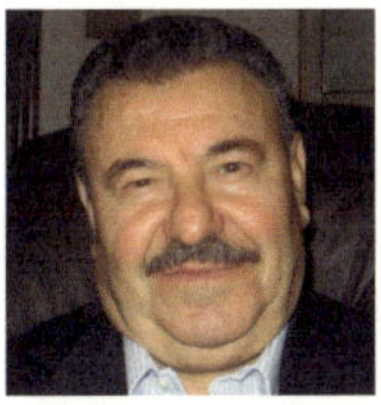

Professor Mustafa M. Shennak received his MD 1967 from Istanbul University, Faculty of Medicine, his Doctorate in Internal Medicine, and gained his Fellowship in Gastroenterology and Liver diseases, 1972. Professor Shennak was the first Jordanian certified gastroenterologist who initiated upper and lower fiberoptic endoscopy, in Jordan, in 1973. In 1979 he went to University College Hospital of London where he worked with consultant Dr. Paul Salmon. Thereafter he returned to Jordan to initiate Therapeutic Endoscopic procedures including Retrograde Chlangio-Pancreatography (ERCP) diagnostic and therapeutic. He was appointed full time teaching staff member, at University of Jordan followed by Chairman of the Internal Medicine department and then chief GI & Liver Division and Endoscopy Unit where he currently resides. Professor Shennak has served as President of the Jordanian Gastroenterology Society since 2008 and is a member at the editorial board of the medical journal, Hepatogastroenterology - the official journal of IASGO. He has more than 45 national and international publications to his credit.

Contents

Preface

Ulcerative Colitis (UC) is a rapidly evolving medical field and will continue to be very exiting for the foreseable future. Although the underlaying cause of this disease is still unknown, great scientific research dealing with various issues related to different aspects of this disease are published every day.

Chapters included in this book review the most recent literature on related advancements on this chronic, controllable yet incurable disease. Aspects like epidemiology, pathophysiology, genetics, incriminated etiologies, clinical aspects, complications, disease management including advancements in the diagnostic and therapeutic options, have been documented within this book by well known clinicians, researchers and world-wide authorities in their fields.

Subjects that have been tackled in this book include:

Evolutionary Insights into the "Population-Specificity" of the Genetic Factors Associated with Inflammatory Bowel Diseases by Dr Shigeki Nakagome and Hiroki Oota

Research of Immunology Markers of UC by Dr. David Díaz-Jiménez, Dr Katya Carrillo, Dr Rodrigo Quera and Dr Marcela A. Hermoso

Ulcerative Colitis and Microorganisms by Dr. José Miguel Sahuquillo Arce and Dr Agustín Iranzo Tatay

Primary Sclerosing Cholangitis by Dr Sophia Jagroop and Prof. Ramona Rajapakse

Colorectal Cancer in Ulcerative Colitis Patients by Dr Joseph D. Feuerstein and Dr Sharmeel K. Wasan

Ulcerative Colitis and Colorectal Cancer: Aneuploidy and Implications for Improved Screening by Dr Jens K. Habermann, Dr Gert Auer, Dr Thomas Ried and Dr Uwe J. Roblick

Carcinogenesis in Ulcerative Colitis by Dr Adam Humphries, Dr Noor Jawad, Dr Ana Ignjatovic, Dr James East and Dr. Simon Leedham

Ulcerative Colitis-Associated Colorectal Cancer Prevention by 5-Aminosalicylates: Current Status and Perspectives by Dr Jean-Marie Reimund et al.

Drug therapy for UC by Dr. Yousef Ajlouni and Prof. Mustafa Shennak.

Novel treatments for Ulcerative Colitis by Dr Tran Cuong, Dr. Rosa Katsikeros, Dr Suzanne M. Abimosleh

All authors have done a great job documenting the most up to date literature on each subject.

I am confident that this book on UC will be a valuable addition to each doctor's library interested in this subject or for physicians dealing with patients suffering from this disease. Authors have also included figures and diagrams to depict their point and to reach easily to the minds of the readers in the simplest way.

Mustafa M. Shennak
Faculty of Medicine, University of Jordan,
Jordan

1

Evolutionary Insights into the "Population-Specificity" of the Genetic Factors Associated with Inflammatory Bowel Diseases

Shigeki Nakagome[1] and Hiroki Oota[2]
[1]*The Institute of Statistical Mathematics,*
[2]*Kitasato University School of Medicine*
Japan

1. Introduction

Inflammatory bowel disease (IBD) – a generic term for Crohn's disease (CD) and ulcerative colitis (UC) – represents great risks for inheritance, such as high sibling recurrent risks (λs in CD and UC: 20-35 and 8-15) and high monozygotic concordance rates (50% to 60%). Recent genome-wide association studies (GWAS) have successfully identified many causative genes (risk variants) for IBD. These discoveries highlight the importance of autophagy and innate immunity as determinants of dysregulated host-commensal bacteria interactions in the intestine. Some of the risk-variants are shared between CD and UC, indicating both similarities and differences in their etiologies. Most of the IBD risk-variants, however, have been reported in European-ancestry populations, and these associations are not always reproduced in non-European ancestry populations, suggesting a population-specific susceptibility to IBD. In fact, some of the IBD risk variants showed no association with CD and UC in East Asians. Hence, IBD's causative factors should be defined as genetically different between Europeans and East Asians; it is essential that we expand GWAS into non-European populations so as to unravel the causes of its population-specific susceptibility and identify IBD risk variants in each geographic population. It is widely an accepted idea that the risk variants of complex diseases, including IBD, are retained not only in patients, but also in healthy controls. Because the risk variants spread prevalently into geographically diverse populations, it is plausible that their origins could be dated before *Homo sapiens'* expansion out of Africa; that is, the fate of risk variants must be affected by human population history, such as demography, migration and natural selection. Here, we suggest that an evolutionary perspective of IBD genomics could provide essential clues for resolving significant questions: (1) Do the risk-variants have similar allele frequencies in different populations? (2) How are the risk-variants prevalent in human populations? (3) What factors can cause the inconsistency of GWAS-results across geographic populations? In this chapter, we first provide an overview of the evolutionary characteristics of disease-causative variants in Mendelian diseases and complex diseases. Secondly, we review the recent progress of IBD genetic/genomic studies among both European and East Asian populations. Finally, we discuss the evolutionary consequences of population-specific susceptibility to IBD and the importance of its use for diverse human populations in the future of GWAS.

2. Genetic studies of IBD and population-specific susceptibility

IBDs are complex diseases in which multiple genetic and environmental factors are likely to contribute to pathogenesis. Human genomics studies have concentrated their attention on the identification of the genetic variants underlying these diseases over the past decade, since none of the complex diseases are inherited in a simple Mendelian fashion. The genetic characteristics of variants are significantly different between Mendelian (monogenic) diseases and complex (multi-factorial) diseases, both of which constitute the basis of genetic mapping strategies (e.g., linkage analysis and case-control association studies) for the revelation of their role in the aetiology of clinically defined phenotypes. Disease alleles are a specific subset of all the genetic variants present in human populations, and the origin of diseases can be addressed by population genetics modelling from the geographic distribution of disease variants. We first summarize some general approaches to identify disease alleles and the evolutionary characteristics of the variants, and we then introduce the recent genetic studies of IBD.

2.1 Genetic and evolutionary characteristics of diseases variants

Genetic mapping provides a powerful approach to identify genes and the biological processes underlying human diseases. From a vast amount of human genetic variations, a number of efforts have been made to identify those responsible for Mendelian diseases through linkage analysis. This method looks for a correlation between segregation (i.e. linkage) and phenotype within family pedigrees by using DNA sequence variants as genetic markers, without the need for prior an assumption about biological function. Since the causative variants for Mendelian diseases show high penetrance (proportion of individuals with a particular genotype who manifest a given phenotype), they tend to be transmitted into familial members in the Mendelian fashion. Thus, Mendelian diseases often feature a low frequency of causative mutations (< 1%: rare variants) (Fig. 1a).

In contrast to Mendelian diseases, much less success has been achieved using linkage-based approaches for complex diseases (Risch and Merikangas 1996; Risch 2000; Altmuller et al. 2001). A single copy of the risk allele is sufficient to cause a Mendelian disease in the autosomal dominant pedigree, whereas the risk allele is neither sufficient nor necessary for complex diseases to occur (Knight 2009). The lack of Mendelian segregation of a complex disease in most families argues against the sufficiency of a mutation in any one gene (Chakravarti 1999). As alternative approaches to tracing transmission in families, one might localize disease's genes through association studies that compare the frequencies of genetic variants among affected and unaffected individuals. Based on a set of single nucleotide polymorphisms (SNPs) - which usually consists of several hundred thousand markers - a number of efforts have been made in GWAS. These scans show that the susceptibility variants involved in complex diseases have low or medium penetrance (i.e. incomplete penetrance) so that the disease variants are carried by healthy individuals, as well as by patients (Fig. 1a).

Based on these genetic properties of alleles, we can address the origins of disease variants in terms of evolutionary genetics. Mendelian diseases - which are usually due to highly penetrant and deleterious alleles that segregate in specific families - fit relatively simple *equilibrium* models of mutation-selection balance, in which disease alleles are removed by purifying selection and continually appearing through the mutation process (Di Rienzo 2006). These disease mutations are likely to have occurred relatively recently in human

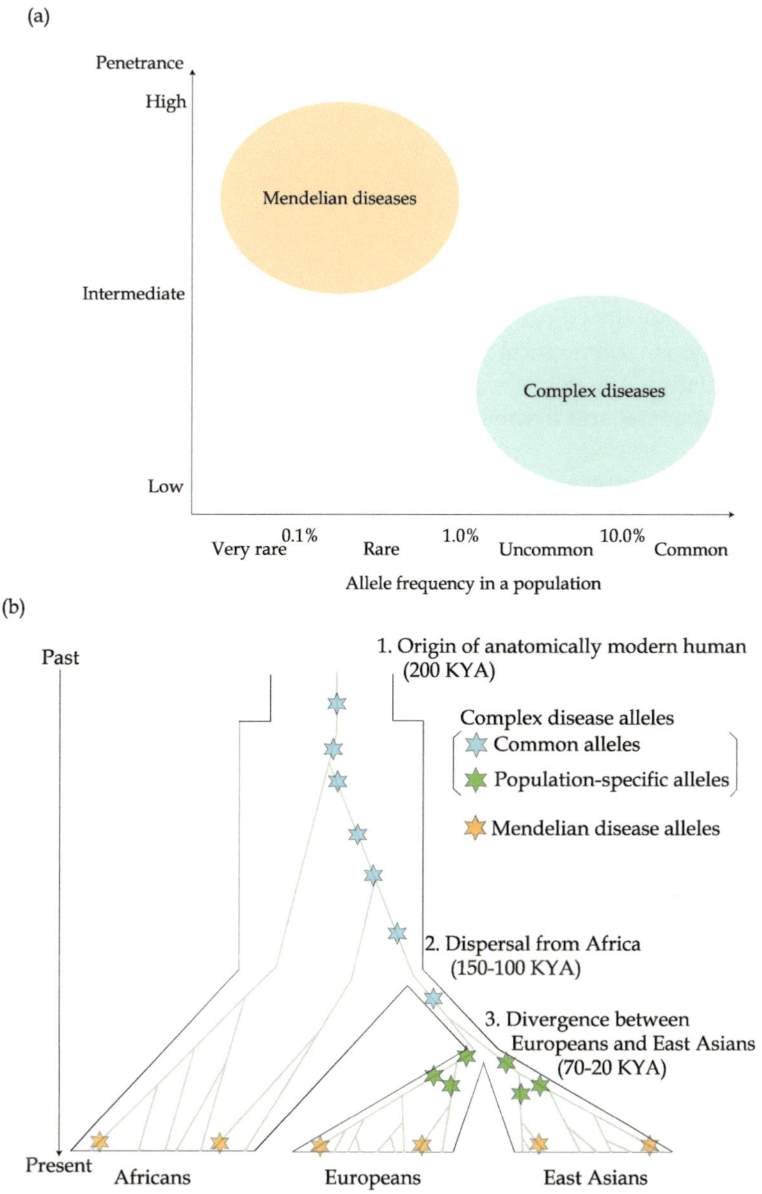

Fig. 1. The genetic properties of Mendelian disease and complex disease alleles. (a) Mendelian disease alleles have a high penetrance and their frequencies are very rare. In contrast, complex disease alleles are present both in patients and healthy controls in a population. This figure is modified from Box 7 in McCarthy et al. (2008). (b) The schematic diagram of human evolutionary history shows that anatomically modern humans originated in Africa around 200 thousand years ago (KYA). A small subset of ancestral populations dispersed from Africa around 150 to 100 KYA and then separated into Europeans and East Asians around 70 to 20 KYA. Mendelian disease alleles are likely to be recent mutations, while complex disease alleles - including common alleles and population-specific alleles - appeared before human population divergences

history (Fig. 1b). However, this *equilibrium* model is not applied to complex diseases, because of incomplete penetrance, gene-to-environmental interactions and polygenic inheritance. Most of the complex disease alleles spread across human populations, and these variants appeared before the divergence of populations. The complex disease alleles identified from GWAS are most common among geographically separated populations (e.g. Africans, Europeans and East Asians) (light-blue stars in Fig. 1b). Another phase of GWAS would be needed to focus on population-specific alleles (green stars in Fig. 1b) because of missing heritability (i.e. many of the genetic factors thought to be responsible for complex diseases can only explain between 5% and 50% of the diseases' heritability) and population-specific susceptibility. Specifically, these alleles have been jointly exposed to selective pressures and human demography, both of which are specific events to a particular geographic population. We describe population differences in susceptibility to IBD between Europeans and Japanese, and discuss evolutionary insights into the susceptibility to IBD.

2.2 Genetic studies of IBD in "European-ancestry populations"

Several studies have shown that an individual with IBD is more likely to have a relative with the disease (Budarf et al. 2009). Population-based studies find that 5-10% of patients have a first-degree family member with IBD, with the calculated sibling recurrence risk (λ_s: the ratio of the risk for the siblings of a patient to develop the disease compared to the risk for a general member of the same population) estimated to be 30-40 fold for CD and 10-20 fold for UC. The concomitant rate is significantly greater for monozygotic individuals than for dizygotic twins, for both CD (50-58% versus 0-12%) and UC (6-14% versus 0-5%) (Binder 1998). Hence, there are strong genetic contributions towards the risk of IBD, and especially for CD.

2.2.1 Genetic studies of CD

Generally, most of family-based studies have had limited success in finding genes for complex diseases, because of the non-Mendelian inheritance for the disease phenotypes. Nevertheless, linkage and positional cloning approaches have identified a nucleotide-binding oligomerization domain containing 2 (*NOD2*, also designated *CARD15* and IBD1) as the first susceptible gene for CD (Hugot et al. 2001; Ogura et al. 2001a). Moreover, the IBD5 risk haplotype was identified from the linkage disequilibrium (LD) mapping of trios, and the risk haplotype included functionally interesting candidate genes: prolyl 4-hydroxylase (*P4HA2*), the interferon regulatory factor 1 (*IRF1*), and the organic cation transporter (OCTN) gene cluster (*SLC22A4* and *SLC22A5*, encoding OCTN1 and OCTN2, respectively) (Rioux et al. 2001; Peltekova et al. 2004). Since then, GWAS have been substantially improving our understanding of the biological pathways underlying the pathogenesis of CD, since the genetic contribution to CD is greater than to UC. A recent meta-analysis of the pooled data for six independent GWAS comprising 6,333 individuals with CD and 15,056 controls has reported 71 susceptibility loci (30 new susceptibility loci) to CD (Franke et al. 2010), and replicated the previously validated associations, including *NOD2* and IBD5, as well as other CD genes identified from several independent GWAS (Yamazaki et al. 2005; Duerr et al. 2006; Hampe et al. 2007; Libioulle et al. 2007; Parkes et al. 2007; Raelson et al. 2007; Rioux et al. 2007; The Wellcom Trust Case Control Consortium 2007; Barrett et al. 2008; Kugathasan et al. 2008). Therefore, the advent of GWAS has dramatically increased the number of susceptibility loci to CD in people of European descent.

2.2.2 Genetic studies of UC

CD and UC share many diagnostic features, and relatives with CD or UC are likely to be at an increased risk of developing either form of IBD, indicating the existence of both phenotype-specific and shared susceptibility loci for CD and UC. Before GWAS in UC, candidate gene approaches to the susceptibility loci identified in CD were conducted in UC. It was shown that several genes - including the interleukin-23 receptor (*IL23R*), the NK2 transcription-factor-related, locus 3 (*NKX2-3*) and the macrophage stimulating 1 (*MST1*) - were also significantly associated with UC, whereas the other representative genes in CD, such as *NOD2*, showed no susceptibility to UC (Fisher et al. 2008; Franke et al. 2008). Subsequently, GWAS - as well as these candidate gene association studies - have identified 18 susceptibility loci for UC, including established risk loci specific to UC, such as the hepatocyte nuclear factor 4α (*HNF4A*), the cadherin 1 (*CDH1*) and the laminin β1 subunit (*LAMB1*) that are highlighted with the role of defective barrier function in UC pathogenesis (Barrett et al. 2009). A meta-analysis of six GWAS datasets of UC, comprising 6,687 cases and 19,718 controls, has identified 29 additional risk loci, increasing the number of UC loci to 47 (Anderson et al. 2011). The total number of confirmed IBD risk loci is about 99, and a minimum of 28 show shared association signals between CD and UC. Thus, recent GWAS successes have accelerated our knowledge about the commonalities and unique features of the aetiology between CD and UC.

2.3 Genetic studies of IBD in Japanese ("non-European-ancestry") populations

Many GWAS's efforts to identify susceptibility genes of IBD have been successful in European-ancestry populations, and recent advances have provided substantial insights into the maintenance of mucosal immunity and the pathogenesis of IBD (Xavier and Podolsky 2007). Furthermore, some of the IBD variants have also had their pathogenic roles demonstrated by *in vivo* and *in vitro* functional studies. *NOD2*, one of the established susceptibility genes to CD (Hugot et al. 2001; Ogura et al. 2001b), encodes a protein that recognizes pathogen-associated molecular patterns: common motifs of the peptidoglycan product muramyl dipeptide (MDP), which modulates both innate and adaptive immune responses (Shaw et al. 2011). The cytosine insertion in *NOD2* exon 11 (3,020C) results in a frameshift and generates a truncated NOD2 protein (1,007 of 1,040 amino acid residues), which induces impaired activation of the transcriptional factor NF-κB (Chamaillard et al. 2003). For *ATG16L* encoding a key autophagy molecule, the patients with a homozygote of alanine at 300 amino acid residues (T300A) display disorganised or diminished granules in Paneth cells, which are specialised epithelial cells for controlling the intestinal environment by the release of granules (Cadwell et al. 2008). Several additional lines of evidence, including transgenic mouse experiments for the susceptibility genes (Cadwell et al. 2008; Cadwell et al. 2010; Travassos et al. 2010), show a functional deficiency of CD variants. However, significant associations between these genomic regions and IBD have not been detected in non-European populations, suggesting that there is a population-specific susceptibility to IBD.

The incidence of IBD has been increasing substantially within the Japanese population. The prevalence rate has risen seven times between 1,985 and 2,006 (Hilmi et al. 2006). The disease-mapping strategy of early association studies in Japan was to test the susceptibilities of genes reported from European-ancestry populations using Japanese IBD patients and controls. The candidate gene study shows that the *NOD2* variants statistically and functionally confirmed in Europeans are completely absent - both in patients and controls - in the Japanese population (Yamazaki et al. 2002). This result is consistent with the other

East Asian populations, such as Korean (Croucher et al. 2003) and Chinese (Guo et al. 2004). To elucidate the similarities and differences of susceptibility to IBD between Europeans and the Japanese, associations with CD and UC have been tested for seven susceptible genomic regions, including *NOD2, IL23R, ATG16L1, TNFSF15, SLC22A4, IRGM,* and 10q21 (Nakagome et al. 2010). Each of these genomic regions, which have been confirmed by multiple independent GWAS and the meta-analysis described above, is known to be associated with CD in European-ancestry populations. Moreover, Nakagome et al. (2010) have focused on a local differences in susceptibility to IBD within Japanese populations, because the population stratification (differences in allele frequencies between sub-populations due to different ancestry) is observed between Honshu (the eastern area of Japan's main-island) and Kyushu-Okinawa (the southwestern islands of the Japanese archipelago) (Yamaguchi-Kabata et al. 2008). Afterwards, the association of nine SNPs located in the seven genomic regions was examined in the Kyushu population, consisting of 130 individuals with CD, 82 individuals with UC, and 168 controls (Table 1), and which was also compared with the genotype data from the European and Honshu Japanese populations.

2.3.1 Differences in susceptibility to IBD between Europeans and Japanese

The samples acquired from each of the Kyushu Japanese subjects are first analysed to determine the genotypes of the nine SNPs, which are previously identified from the CD-associated genomic regions (Table 1). These samples are also examined in order to determine any association of CD or UC with the risk alleles that had been identified in European-ancestry populations. Table 2 illustrates the genotype frequencies as well as allele frequencies between cases and controls. The *p*-values of the χ^2 test corrected by the permutation test are shown in Table 3. In the Kyushu Japanese subjects, the risk alleles for *NOD2* (rs2066844, rs2066845, rs2066847) and *SLC22A4* (rs1050152) are not found to be present. The analysis of the *IL23R* (rs11209026) gene shows that the risk allele is fixed in the CD cases, the UC cases and the control. Thus, these SNPs are not polymorphic in the Japanese population, which confirms previous studies (Yamazaki et al. 2002; Yamazaki et al. 2004; Yamazaki et al. 2007). In contrast, the remaining four SNP sites (i.e. rs2241880, rs3810936, rs10065172, and rs10761659) are shown to be polymorphic (Table 2). Furthermore, three of the SNPs, including rs2241880 in *ATG16L1*, rs10065172 in *IRGM*, and rs10761659 in 10q21, do not show any significant association with either CD or UC (Table 3). Only one SNP site was found to be significantly associated with CD (p-value = 0.047) and UC (p-value = 0.050) is in the *TNFSF15* gene (rs3810936). The odds ratio (OR) of the risk allele ("G" allele in rs3810936) is 1.551 (95% CI: 1.090-2.207) for CD and 1.692 (95% CI: 1.117-2.562) for UC (Table 3).

The differences in allele frequency between the Kyushu and Honshu subjects are further compared by an χ^2 test that included the Kyushu (K-) CD, the Honshu (H-) CD and each control (2-by-2 pairs: K-CD and H-CD, K-controls and H-controls, K-CD and H-controls, K-controls and H-CD) (Fig. 2). A significant association between *TNFSF15* (rs3810936) and CD is detected in all pairs of CD-controls from both the Kyushu and Honshu subjects. Previous studies of Honshu Japanese subjects have examined a greater number of SNPs in the other six genome regions, compared to Nakagome et al. (2010), but do not detect a significant association between CD and these SNPs (Yamazaki et al. 2002; Yamazaki et al. 2004; Yamazaki et al. 2007; Yamazaki et al. 2009). As an exception, Yamazaki et al. (2005) identified *TNFSF15* as a CD susceptibility gene in the Honshu subjects, due to a significant association ($p < 0.0001$) between 20 SNP sites and CD. Using the Kyushu subjects, Nakagome et al. (2010) supports the previous results which demonstrated that the CD

Table 1. Susceptibility genes of IBD

Susceptibility genes	No. of previous studies[a]	SNP IDs genotyped in this study	SNP type	Amino acid changes
NOD2	1, 2, 5, 6, 9, 10, 11, and 12	rs2066844 rs2066845 rs2066847	Nonsynonymous Nonsynonymous Insetion (C allele)	Arg > Trp Gly > Arg frame shift
IL23R	5, 7, 9, 10, 11, and 12	rs11209026	Nonsynonymous	Alg > Gln
ATG16L1	6, 9, 11, and 12	rs2241880	Nonsynonymous	Thr > Ala
TNFSF15	4, 11, and 12	rs3810936	Synonymous	-
SLC22A4	3, 6, 8, 10, and 11	rs1050152	Nonsynonymous	Leu > Phe
IRGM	8 and 11	rs10065172	Synonymous	-
10q21	9 and 11	rs10761659	Non-coding	-

[a] The numbers are corresponding to previous GWAS: 1. Hugot et al. (2001); 2. Ogura et al. (2001); 3. Peltekova et al. (2004); 4. Yamazaki et al. (2005); 5. Duerr et al. (2006); 6. Hampe et al. (2007); 7. Libioulle et al. (2007); 8. Parkes et al. (2007); 9. Raelson et al. (2007); 10. Rioux et al. (2007); 11. The Wellcom Trust Case Control Consortium (2007); 12. Kugathasan et al. (2008).

Susceptibility genes	SNP IDs	Alleles	Risk allele *A* [a]	Genotype frequency [b]									Allele frequency		
				CD			UC			Controls			CD	UC	Controls
				AA	*Aa*	*aa*	*AA*	*Aa*	*aa*	*AA*	*Aa*	*aa*	*A* / *a*	*A* / *a*	*A* / *a*
NOD2	rs2066844	C/T	T	0	0	100	0	0	100	0	0	100	0/100	0/100	0/100
	rs2066845	G/C	C	0	0	100	0	0	100	0	0	100	0/100	0/100	0/100
	rs2066847	-/C	C insertion	0	0	100	0	0	100	0	0	100	0/100	0/100	0/100
IL23R	rs11209026	A/G	G	100	0	0	100	0	0	100	0	0	100/0	100/0	100/0
ATG16L1	rs2241880	A/G	G	8	40	53	7	32	61	7	39	55	28/72	23/77	26/74
TNFSF15	rs3810936	A/G	G	49	47	4	57	34	9	39	49	12	73/27	74/26	63/37
SLC22A4	rs1050152	C/T	T	0	0	100	0	0	100	0	0	100	0/100	0/100	0/100
IRGM	rs10065172	T/C	C	36	47	16	40	44	16	37	51	12	60/40	62/38	63/38
10q21	rs10761659	A/G	G	54	36	10	46	44	10	47	42	10	72/28	68/32	68/32

[a] Associated alleles were referred from the previous studies and annotated as "*A* ".

[b] The genotypes were shown as "*AA* " homozygote of risk alleles, "*Aa* " heterozygote of risk and non-risk alleles, and "*aa* " homozygote of non-risk alleles.

Table 2. Number of genotypes and alleles in the Kyushu subjects

susceptibility genes identified in Europeans are not significantly associated with CD in the Japanese population. The data on the *TNFSF15* gene using the Kyushu subjects also indicated a significant positive association with CD. Therefore, these results strongly support *TNFSF15* as a CD susceptibility gene in the Japanese population.

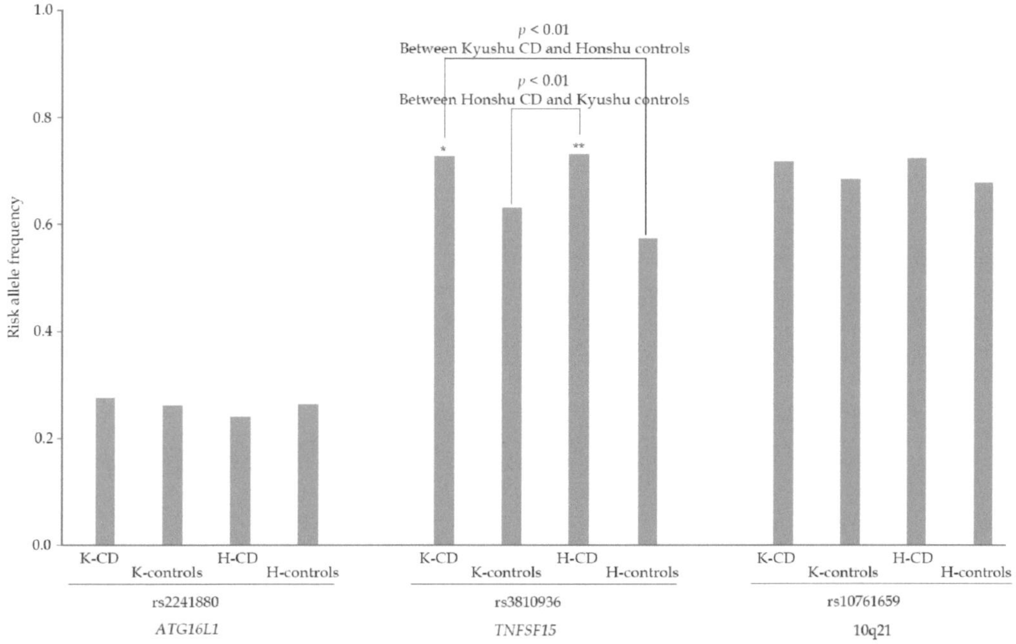

Fig. 2. The distributions of risk allele frequency for three SNPs (rs2241880, rs3810936, rs10761659) in the Kyushu and Honshu subjects. The abbreviations, K-CD, K-controls, H-CD and H-controls indicate Kyushu CD, Kyushu-controls, Honshu CD, and Honshu-controls. The asterisks above the columns indicate a significant allele frequency difference between cases and controls in the same region (*p*-values for the Kyushu subject are referred from Table 3 and those for the Honshu subject are referred from Yamazaki et al. (2005)). A single asterisk denotes $p < 0.05$, and double asterisks denote $p < 0.01$

2.3.2 Genotype association with CD and UC

Disease alleles on autosomes are present as heterozygote or homozygote in an individual, and their effects can be categorised as dominant, recessive or additive. The genotype association of the four polymorphic SNP sites is tested in CD or UC, respectively. No significant association of *ATG16L1* (rs2241880), *IRGM* (rs10065172), or 10q21 (rs10761659) is observed with either CD or UC. The different significances of *TNFSF15* (rs3810936) between CD and UC are shown in the recessive model (i.e. *AA* vs. *Aa* + *aa*) and the dominant model (i.e. *AA* + *Aa* vs. *aa*) (Table 3). In the recessive model, the test shows a significant association between the homozygote for the risk allele and UC (*p*-value = 0.019). The OR of the risk allele homozygote is determined to be 2.132 (95% CI: 1.247 - 3.644). In the dominant model, both the heterozygote and the homozygote for the risk allele are found to be significantly associated with CD (*p*-value = 0.025 and OR = 3.497, 95% CI: 1.341 - 9.117). Thus, the effect of susceptibility in the *TNSF15* risk allele (rs3810936) is likely to be different between CD and UC of the Kyushu Japanese.

Susceptibility genes	SNP IDs	Allele (*A* / *a*)				Genotype (*AA* / *Aa* / *aa*) Recessive model (*AA* vs others)				Dominant model (*AA* + *Aa* vs others)			
		p-values		Odds ratio (95% CI)		*p*-values		Odds ratio (95% CI)		*p*-values		Odds ratio (95% CI)	
		CD	UC	CD	UC	CD	UC	CD	UC	CD	UC	CD	UC
ATG16L1	rs2241880	0.986	0.948	1.077 (0.744 - 1.557)	0.855 (0.551 - 1.327)	0.997	0.767	1.161 (0.477 - 2.828)	1.091 (0.388 - 3.068)	1.000	0.994	1.079 (0.678 - 1.716)	0.770 (0.448 - 1.322)
TNFSF15	rs3810936	0.047*	0.050*	1.551 (1.090 - 2.207)	1.692 (1.117 - 2.562)	0.232	0.019*	1.539 (0.966 - 2.454)	2.132 (1.247 - 3.644)	0.025*	0.744	3.497 (1.341 - 9.117)	1.499 (0.608 - 3.693)
IRGM	rs10065172	0.921	1.000	0.886 (0.634 - 1.237)	0.987 (0.670 - 1.454)	0.999	0.974	0.956 (0.592 - 1.543)	1.137 (0.660 - 1.960)	0.710	0.826	0.682 (0.355 - 1.311)	0.737 (0.347 - 1.568)
10q21	rs10761659	0.849	1.000	1.171 (0.818 - 1.674)	0.995 (0.664 - 1.490)	0.741	0.999	1.284 (0.808 - 2.041)	0.965 (0.566 - 1.644)	1.000	0.994	1.039 (0.484 - 2.229)	1.077 (0.443 - 2.616)

* p-values < 0.05.

Table 3. Associations of alleles and genotypes with Crohn's disease or ulcerative colitis in the Kyushu subjects

2.3.3 Differences in the Genotype Relative Risk between CD and UC

The genotype relative risk (GRR) test (Schaid and Sommer 1993) is conducted for the SNP site of rs3810936 (*TNFSF15*) that is found to be significantly associated with CD or UC. This test is adopted so as to determine whether the dominant, recessive or additive model best fit the observed genotype frequency using the likelihood ratio test. Based on the likelihood method, the GRR test is modified to include unrelated individuals and also low penetrance variants.

Let A be the disease-associated allele, and let a be the non disease-associated allele. The probability of disease is defined, conditional on the genotype at the particular SNP site, as:

$$f_{2case} = P(D \mid AA),\ f_{1case} = P(D \mid Aa),\ f_{0case} = P(D \mid aa)\,, \tag{1}$$

where D is the event that an individual has the disease. The complex disease allele is retained not only in cases but also in healthy controls. Next, the probability of non-disease is defined, conditional on the genotype at the particular SNP site, as:

$$f_{icontrol} = 1 - f_{icase}(i = 0,1,2)\,, \tag{2}$$

Assuming that a population is in the Hardy-Weinberg equilibrium, then by Bayes' rule we have:

$$P(AA \mid D) = \frac{\psi_{2case} p^2}{R_{case}},\ P(Aa \mid D) = \frac{\psi_{1case} 2pq}{R_{case}},\ P(aa \mid D) = \frac{q^2}{R_{case}}\,, \tag{3}$$

$$P(AA \mid N) = \frac{\psi_{2cotrol} p^2}{R_{control}},\ P(Aa \mid N) = \frac{\psi_{1cotrol} 2pq}{R_{control}},\ P(aa \mid N) = \frac{q^2}{R_{control}}\,, \tag{4}$$

where,

$$\psi_{2case} = \frac{f_{2case}}{f_{0case}},\ \psi_{1case} = \frac{f_{1case}}{f_{0case}},\ R_{case} = \psi_{2case} p^2 + \psi_{1case} 2pq + q^2\,, \tag{5}$$

$$\psi_{2control} = \frac{f_{2control}}{f_{0control}},\ \psi_{1control} = \frac{f_{1control}}{f_{0control}},\ R_{control} = \psi_{2control} p^2 + \psi_{1control} 2pq + q^2\,, \tag{6}$$

p is the population frequency of A, q is the frequency of a, and N is the non-disease state. Note that the likelihood depends on four independent parameters, ψ_{2case}, ψ_{1case}, p_{case}, and f_{0case}. A standard numerical maximisation procedure can then be used to find the maximum-likelihood estimates of ψ_{2case}, ψ_{1case}, p_{case}, and f_{0case} with the likelihood

$$\begin{aligned} &L(\psi_{2case}, \psi_{1case}, p, f_{0case}) = P(AA \mid D)^{n_{AAcase}} P(Aa \mid D)^{n_{Aacase}} P(aa \mid D)^{n_{aacase}} \\ &P(AA \mid N)^{n_{AAcontrol}} P(Aa \mid N)^{n_{Aacontrol}} P(aa \mid N)^{n_{aacontrol}}\,, \end{aligned} \tag{7}$$

where n_{AAcase}, n_{Aacase}, n_{aacase} or $n_{AAcontrol}$, $n_{Aacontrol}$, $n_{aacontrol}$ are the observed numbers of cases or controls exhibiting each genotype.

We considered the following four hypotheses:

i. No association of the marker with disease, H_0: $\psi_{1case} = \psi_{2case} = 1$,
ii. Dominant disease expression, H_D: $\psi_{1case} = \psi_{2case} = \psi$,
iii. Recessive disease expression, H_R: $\psi_{1case} = 1$,
iv. Additive disease expression, H_A: $\psi_{1case} = \psi$, $\psi_{2case} = 2\psi$.

The maximum likelihood estimate can be found by maximising the likelihood function under each hypothesis with the condition: $0 < p < 1$, $1 < \psi_{1case}$, $1 < \psi_{2case}$, and $0 < f_{0case} < 1$. As described by Scaid and Sommer (1993), we next adopted the likelihood-ratio test (LRT). The LRT statistics for testing the hypothesis of no association is:

$$\chi_2^2 = 2log[L(\hat{p}, \hat{\psi}_{2case}, \hat{\psi}_{1case}, \hat{f}_{0case})/L(p,1,1, f_{0case})], \tag{8}$$

The statistics for testing the hypothesis of a dominant model are:

$$\chi_1^2 = 2log[L(\hat{p}, \hat{\psi}_{2case}, \hat{\psi}_{1case}, \hat{f}_{0case})/L(p, \psi, \psi, f_{0case})], \tag{9}$$

The statistics for testing the hypothesis of a recessive model are:

$$\chi_1^2 = 2log[L(\hat{p}, \hat{\psi}_{2case}, \hat{\psi}_{1case}, \hat{f}_{0case})/L(p,1, \psi_{2case}, f_{0case})], \tag{10}$$

Finally, the statistics for testing the hypothesis of an additive model are:

$$\chi_1^2 = 2log[L(\hat{p}, \hat{\psi}_{2case}, \hat{\psi}_{1case}, \hat{f}_{0case})/L(p, \psi, 2\psi, f_{0case})]. \tag{11}$$

For the SNP site (rs3810936) in *TNFSF15*, four parameters – including ψ_{2case}, ψ_{1case}, p_{case}, and f_{0case} – are inferred from the general likelihood equation so that the likelihood ratio test can be applied to (7). Based on these hypotheses, the CD likelihood ratio test rejects the null (LRT p-value = 0.005), recessive (LRT p-value = 0.024) and additive models (LRT p-value = 0.021) (Table 4). However, the dominant model was not rejected (LRT p-value = 0.361). In contrast, the UC likelihood ratio test was not found to reject any of the models, most likely due to a lack of power. Nevertheless, the recessive model demonstrates a better fit with the observed genotype frequency than do the dominant and additive models (LRT p-values are not assessed because the same Log*L* value is in both the recessive and the full model). These results are also supported by Akaike information criterion (AIC) values, which show the minimum values of the CD dominant model (AIC = 540.562) and of the UC recessive model (AIC = 470.516) (Table 4). Thus, the statistical test for the genotype risk of rs3810936-G showed that the CD mGRR data best fits the dominant model, while the UC mGRR data best fits the recessive model.

The similarities and differences between CD and UC are thought to be important in understanding the pathogenesis of each disease (Dubois and van Heel 2008). The results from the mGRR tests clearly show that the genotype of the rs3810936-G allele in *TNFSF15* exhibits a different effect in CD compared to UC. The risk of the rs3810936-G allele was determined to be comparable between CD and UC (OR: 1.551 fold in CD and 1.692 fold in UC) (Table 3). However, the genotype relative risk between CD and UC was found to be greatly different (the risk of "GA" or "GG": 3.604 fold or 4.310 fold in C; no risk or 1.679 fold in UC) (Table 4). Thus, it is likely that the risk variant of *TNFSF15* functions as a "dominant" allele in CD, whereas it functions as a "recessive" allele in UC.

Model	Crohn's disease							Ulcerative colitis						
	Log$L$	ψ_{1case}	ψ_{2case}	p	f_{0case}	AIC[a]	LRT p-values	Log$L$	ψ_{1case}	ψ_{2case}	p	f_{0case}	AIC[a]	LRT p-values
Full	-266.863	3.604	4.310	0.635	0.006	541.726	-	-232.258	1.000	1.679	0.667	0.238	472.516	-
Null (no association)	-272.188	-	-	0.674	0.881	548.376	0.005**	-236.100	-	-	0.831	0.669	476.200	0.146
Dominant	-267.281	3.580	3.580	0.646	0.000	540.562	0.361	-235.704	1.310	1.310	0.668	0.233	477.408	0.063
Recessive	-269.425	-	1.000	0.714	1.000	544.850	0.024*	-232.258	-	1.679	0.667	0.238	470.516	*N.A.*[b]
Additive	-269.512	3.383	6.766	0.598	0.000	545.024	0.021*	-232.390	1.000	2.000	0.648	0.115	470.780	0.716

[a] The AIC is $-2\log L + 2k$, where k is the number of estimated parameters.
[b] *N. A.* means "not assessed" (there is no LRT p-values, because Log$L$ value in Recessive model is equal to that in Full model).
* p-values < 0.05
** p-values < 0.01

Table 4. Modified genotype relative risk (mGRR) test of rs3810936 for CD and UC in the Kyushu subjects

2.3.4 Population-specific susceptibility to IBD

Given that CD and UC inheritance do not follow the typical Mendelian fashion, it is possible that the dominant/recessive effect of the risk allele (i.e. the biological roles of the disease etiology), as suggested by the mGRR test above, is shaped by the multiple genetic and environmental factors that are involved in each disease's mechanism. Recently, it has been argued that the reciprocal interaction between multiple genetic and environmental factors is important for complex diseases (Emison et al. 2005). The CD risk alleles identified in Europeans are absent - or not associated with CD - in the Japanese population, except for *TNFSF15*. Ethnic group-specific susceptibility is not a novel idea, and has generally been observed in complex diseases (Altshuler et al. 2008; Rosenberg et al. 2010; Bustamante et al. 2011). Furthermore, the CD risk allele in *TNFSF15* is also associated with UC in the Kyushu population. However, a previous study has found no association with UC at the same SNP in *TNFSF15,* using non-Kyushu Japanese subjects (Kakuta et al. 2006). These results imply that UC, as well as CD, may exhibit a population-specific susceptibility within the various Japanese subjects, similar to the susceptibility shown to exist between Japanese and European subjects. Using world-wide population samples, Myles et al. (2008) have examined the allele frequencies of complex diseases, including CD, and indicated the importance of geographic variation in disease-associated alleles (Myles et al. 2008). Specifically, allele frequencies have commonly been observed to be gradients among human populations (Tishkoff et al. 1996; Oota et al. 2004; Tishkoff and Kidd 2004; The International HapMap Consortium 2005; The International HapMap Consortium 2007), including the Japanese population (Yamaguchi-Kabata et al. 2008). Hence, allele frequencies fluctuate in each geographic region where environmental factors are different, and the population-specific susceptibility of complex diseases might be reflected by subdivisions (i.e. subpopulations) among human populations. Population-specific genetic and environmental factors are likely to cause dominant or recessive genotype risks in each subpopulation. Therefore, it is necessary to investigate a greater number of local cases and controls in order to reveal the mechanisms of complex diseases.

2.4 Evolutionary Insights into the geographic variation of IBD risk alleles

Most of the genetic variants susceptible to complex diseases, including IBD, appeared before the divergences of human populations (Fig. 1b), and geographic gradients in allele frequencies are attributed to differences in evolutionary history, such as migration, changes in population size and natural selection among the populations. A representative example of a disease-causative allele maintained by environmental adaptation is that associated with sickle-cell anaemia, which causes severe anaemia, but its frequency is highly maintained in particular geographical regions because it confers resistance to malaria (Pasvol et al. 1978). Another example is the thrifty genotype hypothesis (Neel 1962) that the genetic predisposition to type II diabetes is the consequence of metabolic adaptations to an ancient lifestyle characterised by a fluctuating and unpredictable food supply and high levels of physical activity. With the switch to a sedentary lifestyle and energy-dense diets in civilised countries, the thrifty genotype is no longer advantageous and gives rise to disease phenotypes. The genetic variants that have been found to confer IBD risks point to the importance of innate immunity, autophagy and phagocytosis in IBD pathogenesis. Hence, we attribute population-specific IBD susceptibility to natural selection on the IBD variants, or the other variation(s) closely linked to the IBD risk alleles (i.e. genetic hitchhiking) which might be an adaptation to pathogen infections in ancestral human populations. Indeed, CD risk alleles in *NOD2* (rs2066844, rs2066845, and rs2066847) and in *SLC22A4* (rs1050152) - all of them involve amino acid changes or frameshift - are completely absent in Japanese populations (Table 2), and possibly specific to European populations. These alleles might have been maintained only in European-ancestry populations by natural selection. To reveal the mechanisms of how IBD risk alleles are spread throughout human populations, in the near future we would like to collect detailed polymorphism data from geographically diverse populations so as to conduct evolutionary and population genetics analysis to detect the signal(s) of natural selection.

Evolutionary insights into the genetic properties of individual risk alleles are useful for understanding how we can translate the results from GWAS in one population to other diverse populations so as to understand the similarities and differences among GWAS results in geographically separated populations. Hence, population genetic data and modelling efforts have had important roles in the characterization of disease alleles and in the planning of GWAS, respectively. More importantly, the current disease allele frequency and heterogeneity in IBD susceptible alleles among populations are the products of a long-term human evolutionary history, and population-specific variants are likely to confer substantial risks of IBD in a particular population. Therefore, population-genetic modelling of the IBD risk alleles will highlight quantitative differences in population-specific mutations and provide a comprehensive catalogue of the intermediate variants, which are neither rare (< 1% in a population) nor common (> 5% in any populations), specific to a geographic region (Fig. 1b).

3. Conclusion

Among complex diseases, GWAS have produced numerous successes in identifying genes and genetic loci that contribute to IBD susceptibility. Despite distinct clinical features, approximately 30% of IBD-associated loci (28/99) are shared between UC and CD, indicating that these diseases engage common pathways and may be part of a mechanistic continuum (Khor et al. 2011). However, findings from GWAS in European-ancestry populations are not always easily translated into the rest of the world, which implies that the IBD-relevant biological pathways are different among geographic populations. Medical and evolutionary approaches are essential in the next phase of researches on human complex diseases. As to the medical studies, GWAS and whole-genome sequence approaches should incorporate geographically diverse populations and provide a comprehensive catalogue of candidate risk alleles. The important idea is that the worldwide human population and its distribution of disease-risk variation represent a singular outcome of human evolutionary history which will underlie future disease-mapping studies. Population-genetic modelling for disease alleles has become important in unravelling the reasons why the risk of IBD has remained within human populations. Evolutionary research should translate the outputs from large-scale medical studies to biological interpretations for the genetic backgrounds of IBD. As the technological barriers to the production of genomic data continue to fall, it can be hoped that the human genomics community will accept the challenge of capitalising on the full range of human diversity in the next wave of investigations of the variants that underlie IBD, since the expansion of our understanding for human diversity is significant in the examination of any new aspects of genetic variation associated with IBD's pathogenesis. Therefore, evolutionary insights into IBD genetics will give a way to a paradigm of understanding inter-population and inter-individual differences in these diseases mechanisms and of developing personalised medicine for the prevention of and care for IBD sufferers.

4. Acknowledgement

This was supported by a Grant-in-Aid for Scientific Research (C) from JSPS (19570226) to HO, by a Grant-in-Aid for Scientific Research (B) from JSPS (21370108) to HO, and by a Grant-in-Aid for JSPS Research fellow (21-7453) to SN.

5. References

Altmuller, J., L. J. Palmer, G. Fischer, H. Scherb, and M. Wjst. 2001. Genomewide scans of complex human diseases: true linkage is hard to find. Am J Hum Genet 69:936-950.

Altshuler, D., M. J. Daly, and E. S. Lander. 2008. Genetic mapping in human disease. Science 322:881-888.

Anderson, C. A.G. BoucherC. W. LeesA. FrankeM. D'AmatoK. D. Taylor et al. 2011. Meta-analysis identifies 29 additional ulcerative colitis risk loci, increasing the number of confirmed associations to 47. Nat Genet 43:246-252.

Barrett, J. C., S. Hansoul, D. L. Nicolae, J. H. Cho, R. H. Duerr, J. D. Rioux et al. 2008. Genome-wide association defines more than 30 distinct susceptibility loci for Crohn's disease. Nat Genet 40:955-962.

Barrett, J. C., J. C. Lee, C. W. Lees, N. J. Prescott, C. A. Anderson, A. Phillips et al. 2009. Genome-wide association study of ulcerative colitis identifies three new susceptibility loci, including the HNF4A region. Nat Genet 41:1330-1334.

Binder, V. 1998. Genetic epidemiology in inflammatory bowel disease. Dig Dis 16:351-355.

Budarf, M. L., C. Labbe, G. David, and J. D. Rioux. 2009. GWA studies: rewriting the story of IBD. Trends Genet 25:137-146.

Bustamante, C. D., E. G. Burchard, and F. M. De la Vega. 2011. Genomics for the world. Nature 475:163-165.

Cadwell, K., J. Y. Liu, S. L. Brown, H. Miyoshi, J. Loh, J. K. Lennerz et al. 2008. A key role for autophagy and the autophagy gene Atg16l1 in mouse and human intestinal Paneth cells. Nature 456:259-263.

Cadwell, K., K. K. Patel, N. S. Maloney, T. C. Liu, A. C. Ng, C. E. Storer, R. D. Head, R. Xavier, T. S. Stappenbeck, and H. W. Virgin. 2010. Virus-plus-susceptibility gene interaction determines Crohn's disease gene Atg16L1 phenotypes in intestine. Cell 141:1135-1145.

Chakravarti, A. 1999. Population genetics--making sense out of sequence. Nat Genet 21:56-60.

Chamaillard, M., D. Philpott, S. E. Girardin, H. Zouali, S. Lesage, F. Chareyre, T. H. Bui, M. Giovannini, U. Zaehringer, V. Penard-Lacronique, P. J. Sansonetti, J. P. Hugot, and G. Thomas. 2003. Gene-environment interaction modulated by allelic heterogeneity in inflammatory diseases. Proc Natl Acad Sci U S A 100:3455-3460.

Croucher, P. J., S. Mascheretti, J. Hampe, K. Huse, H. Frenzel, M. Stoll, T. Lu, S. Nikolaus, S. K. Yang, M. Krawczak, W. H. Kim, and S. Schreiber. 2003. Haplotype structure and association to Crohn's disease of CARD15 mutations in two ethnically divergent populations. Eur J Hum Genet 11:6-16.

Di Rienzo, A. 2006. Population genetics models of common diseases. Curr Opin Genet Dev 16:630-636.

Dubois, P. C., and D. A. van Heel. 2008. New susceptibility genes for ulcerative colitis. Nat Genet 40:686-688.

Duerr, R. H., K. D. Taylor, S. R. Brant, J. D. Rioux, M. S. Silverberg, M. J. Daly et al. 2006. A genome-wide association study identifies IL23R as an inflammatory bowel disease gene. Science 314:1461-1463.

Emison, E. S., A. S. McCallion, C. S. Kashuk, R. T. Bush, E. Grice, S. Lin, M. E. Portnoy, D. J. Cutler, E. D. Green, and A. Chakravarti. 2005. A common sex-dependent mutation in a RET enhancer underlies Hirschsprung disease risk. Nature 434:857-863.

Fisher, S. A., M. Tremelling, C. A. Anderson, R. Gwilliam, S. Bumpstead, N. J. Prescott et al. 2008. Genetic determinants of ulcerative colitis include the ECM1 locus and five loci implicated in Crohn's disease. Nat Genet 40:710-712.

Franke, A., T. Balschun, T. H. Karlsen, J. Hedderich, S. May, T. Lu, D. Schuldt, S. Nikolaus, P. Rosenstiel, M. Krawczak, and S. Schreiber. 2008. Replication of signals from recent studies of Crohn's disease identifies previously unknown disease loci for ulcerative colitis. Nat Genet 40:713-715.

Franke, A., D. P. McGovern, J. C. Barrett, K. Wang, G. L. Radford-Smith, T. Ahmad et al. 2010. Genome-wide meta-analysis increases to 71 the number of confirmed Crohn's disease susceptibility loci. Nat Genet 42:1118-1125.

Guo, Q. S., B. Xia, Y. Jiang, Y. Qu, and J. Li. 2004. NOD2 3020insC frameshift mutation is not associated with inflammatory bowel disease in Chinese patients of Han nationality. World J Gastroenterol 10:1069-1071.

Hampe, J., A. Franke, P. Rosenstiel, A. Till, M. Teuber, K. Huse et al. 2007. A genome-wide association scan of nonsynonymous SNPs identifies a susceptibility variant for Crohn disease in ATG16L1. Nat Genet 39:207-211.

Hilmi, I., Y. M. Tan, and K. L. Goh. 2006. Crohn's disease in adults: observations in a multiracial Asian population. World J Gastroenterol 12:1435-1438.

Hugot, J. P., M. Chamaillard, H. Zouali, S. Lesage, J. P. Cezard, J. Belaiche et al. 2001. Association of NOD2 leucine-rich repeat variants with susceptibility to Crohn's disease. Nature 411:599-603.

Kakuta, Y., Y. Kinouchi, K. Negoro, S. Takahashi, and T. Shimosegawa. 2006. Association study of TNFSF15 polymorphisms in Japanese patients with inflammatory bowel disease. Gut 55:1527-1528.

Khor, B., A. Gardet, and R. J. Xavier. 2011. Genetics and pathogenesis of inflammatory bowel disease. Nature 474:307-317.

Knight, C. J. 2009. Human Genetic Diversity: Functional consequences for health and disease. Oxford University Press Inc, New York, NY.

Kugathasan, S., R. N. Baldassano, J. P. Bradfield, P. M. Sleiman, M. Imielinski, S. L. Guthery et al. 2008. Loci on 20q13 and 21q22 are associated with pediatric-onset inflammatory bowel disease. Nat Genet 40:1211-1215.

Libioulle, C., E. Louis, S. Hansoul, C. Sandor, F. Farnir, D. Franchimont et al. 2007. Novel Crohn disease locus identified by genome-wide association maps to a gene desert on 5p13.1 and modulates expression of PTGER4. PLoS Genet 3:e58.

McCarthy, M. I., G. R. Abecasis, L. R. Cardon, D. B. Goldstein, J. Little, J. P. Ioannidis, and J. N. Hirschhorn. 2008. Genome-wide association studies for complex traits: consensus, uncertainty and challenges. Nat Rev Genet 9:356-369.

Myles, S., D. Davison, J. Barrett, M. Stoneking, and N. Timpson. 2008. Worldwide population differentiation at disease-associated SNPs. BMC Med Genomics 1:22.

Nakagome, S., Y. Takeyama, S. Mano, S. Sakisaka, T. Matsui, S. Kawamura, and H. Oota. 2010. Population-specific susceptibility to Crohn's disease and ulcerative colitis; dominant and recessive relative risks in the Japanese population. Ann Hum Genet 74:126-136.

Neel, J. V. 1962. Diabetes mellitus: a "thrifty" genotype rendered detrimental by "progress"? Am J Hum Genet 14:353-362.

Ogura, Y., D. K. Bonen, N. Inohara, D. L. Nicolae, F. F. Chen, R. Ramos et al. 2001a. A frameshift mutation in NOD2 associated with susceptibility to Crohn's disease. Nature 411:603-606.

Ogura, Y., N. Inohara, A. Benito, F. F. Chen, S. Yamaoka, and G. Nunez. 2001b. Nod2, a Nod1/Apaf-1 family member that is restricted to monocytes and activates NF-kappaB. J Biol Chem 276:4812-4818.

Oota, H., A. J. Pakstis, B. Bonne-Tamir, D. Goldman, E. Grigorenko, S. L. Kajuna, N. J. Karoma, S. Kungulilo, R. B. Lu, K. Odunsi, F. Okonofua, O. V. Zhukova, J. R. Kidd, and K. K. Kidd. 2004. The evolution and population genetics of the ALDH2 locus: random genetic drift, selection, and low levels of recombination. Ann Hum Genet 68:93-109.

Parkes, M., J. C. Barrett, N. J. Prescott, M. Tremelling, C. A. Anderson, S. A. Fisher et al. 2007. Sequence variants in the autophagy gene IRGM and multiple other replicating loci contribute to Crohn's disease susceptibility. Nat Genet 39:830-832.

Pasvol, G., D. J. Weatherall, and R. J. Wilson. 1978. Cellular mechanism for the protective effect of haemoglobin S against P. falciparum malaria. Nature 274:701-703.

Peltekova, V. D., R. F. Wintle, L. A. Rubin, C. I. Amos, Q. Huang, X. Gu, B. Newman, M. Van Oene, D. Cescon, G. Greenberg, A. M. Griffiths, P. H. St George-Hyslop, and K. A. Siminovitch. 2004. Functional variants of OCTN cation transporter genes are associated with Crohn disease. Nat Genet 36:471-475.

Raelson, J. V., R. D. Little, A. Ruether, H. Fournier, B. Paquin, P. Van Eerdewegh et al. 2007. Genome-wide association study for Crohn's disease in the Quebec Founder Population identifies multiple validated disease loci. Proc Natl Acad Sci U S A 104:14747-14752.

Rioux, J. D., M. J. Daly, M. S. Silverberg, K. Lindblad, H. Steinhart, Z. Cohen et al. 2001. Genetic variation in the 5q31 cytokine gene cluster confers susceptibility to Crohn disease. Nat Genet 29:223-228.

Rioux, J. D., R. J. Xavier, K. D. Taylor, M. S. Silverberg, P. Goyette, A. Huett et al. 2007. Genome-wide association study identifies new susceptibility loci for Crohn disease and implicates autophagy in disease pathogenesis. Nat Genet 39:596-604.

Risch, N., and K. Merikangas. 1996. The future of genetic studies of complex human diseases. Science 273:1516-1517.

Risch, N. J. 2000. Searching for genetic determinants in the new millennium. Nature 405:847-856.

Rosenberg, N. A., L. Huang, E. M. Jewett, Z. A. Szpiech, I. Jankovic, and M. Boehnke. 2010. Genome-wide association studies in diverse populations. Nat Rev Genet 11:356-366.

Schaid, D. J., and S. S. Sommer. 1993. Genotype relative risks: methods for design and analysis of candidate-gene association studies. Am J Hum Genet 53:1114-1126.

Shaw, M. H., N. Kamada, N. Warner, Y. G. Kim, and G. Nunez. 2011. The ever-expanding function of NOD2: autophagy, viral recognition, and T cell activation. Trends Immunol 32:73-79.

The International HapMap Consortium. 2005. A haplotype map of the human genome. Nature 437:1299-1320.

The International HapMap Consortium. 2007. A second generation human haplotype map of over 3.1 million SNPs. Nature 449:851-861.

The Wellcom Trust Case Control Consortium. 2007. Genome-wide association study of 14,000 cases of seven common diseases and 3,000 shared controls. Nature 447:661-678.

Tishkoff, S. A., E. Dietzsch, W. Speed, A. J. Pakstis, J. R. Kidd, K. Cheung, B. Bonne-Tamir, A. S. Santachiara-Benerecetti, P. Moral, M. Krings, S. Paabo, N. Risch, T. Jenkins, and K. K. Kidd. 1996. Global patterns of linkage disequilibrium at the CD4 locus and modern human origins. Science 271:1380-1387.

Tishkoff, S. A., and K. K. Kidd. 2004. Implications of biogeography of human populations for 'race' and medicine. Nat Genet 36:S21-27.

Travassos, L. H., L. A. Carneiro, M. Ramjeet, S. Hussey, Y. G. Kim, J. G. Magalhaes et al. 2010. Nod1 and Nod2 direct autophagy by recruiting ATG16L1 to the plasma membrane at the site of bacterial entry. Nat Immunol 11:55-62.

Xavier, R. J., and D. K. Podolsky. 2007. Unravelling the pathogenesis of inflammatory bowel disease. Nature 448:427-434.

Yamaguchi-Kabata, Y., K. Nakazono, A. Takahashi, S. Saito, N. Hosono, M. Kubo, Y. Nakamura, and N. Kamatani. 2008. Japanese population structure, based on SNP genotypes from 7003 individuals compared to other ethnic groups: effects on population-based association studies. Am J Hum Genet 83:445-456.

Yamazaki, K., D. McGovern, J. Ragoussis, M. Paolucci, H. Butler, D. Jewell et al. 2005. Single nucleotide polymorphisms in TNFSF15 confer susceptibility to Crohn's disease. Hum Mol Genet 14:3499-3506.

Yamazaki, K., Y. Onouchi, M. Takazoe, M. Kubo, Y. Nakamura, and A. Hata. 2007. Association analysis of genetic variants in IL23R, ATG16L1 and 5p13.1 loci with Crohn's disease in Japanese patients. J Hum Genet 52:575-583.

Yamazaki, K., A. Takahashi, M. Takazoe, M. Kubo, Y. Onouchi, A. Fujino, N. Kamatani, Y. Nakamura, and A. Hata. 2009. Positive association of genetic variants in the upstream region of NKX2-3 with Crohn's disease in Japanese patients. Gut 58:228-232.

Yamazaki, K., M. Takazoe, T. Tanaka, T. Ichimori, S. Saito, A. Iida, Y. Onouchi, A. Hata, and Y. Nakamura. 2004. Association analysis of SLC22A4, SLC22A5 and DLG5 in Japanese patients with Crohn disease. J Hum Genet 49:664-668.
Yamazaki, K., M. Takazoe, T. Tanaka, T. Kazumori, and Y. Nakamura. 2002. Absence of mutation in the NOD2/CARD15 gene among 483 Japanese patients with Crohn's disease. J Hum Genet 47:469-472.

2

Research of Immunology Markers of UC

David Díaz-Jiménez[1], Katya Carrillo[2],
Rodrigo Quera[2] and Marcela A. Hermoso[1]
[1]*Disciplinary Program of Immunology, Institute of Biomedical Sciences, Faculty of Medicine, Universidad de Chile,*
[2]*Gastroenterology Unit, Clínica Las Condes*
Chile

1. Introduction

Several risk factors are recognized to increase an individual's susceptibility to develop inflammatory bowel disease (IBD) that are related to molecules that play a role in intestinal homeostasis and mucosal immune response to luminal antigens. The hallmark of IBD is a chronic, recurrent inflammation of a particular segment of the gastrointestinal tract, which is presented as a loss and damage of the intestinal epithelial barrier, exposing immune cells to luminal antigens, that might finally trigger the recruitment and activation of other immune cells and unleashing an exaggerated immune response (Abraham and Cho, 2009; Kaser et al., 2010).

Mucosa immune response in general includes different mechanisms of induction, regulation and resolution (Medzhitov, 2010). Different factors participating in these mechanisms will act as inductors, initiating an inflammatory response that will be detected by specialized sensors or sentinel cells. This process will subsequently lead to the production of inflammatory mediators that will affect different tissues; eliciting changes in their functional state that will optimize an adaptation process to the harmful condition associated to the inflammatory response (Medzhitov, 2010).

Due to the chronicity of the inflammatory response, in IBD the mechanisms that regulate and resolve the induction of the inflammatory process are defective. Although the constant induction of the inflammatory process prevents an effective regulation and resolution, making difficult to estimate the key processes involved in the development of IBD.

Since that immune system and cytokines has been linked with the pathogenia of inflammatory disorders, including IBD, the clinical and pathological significance of IL-33/ST2L system in UC, is consistently supported by *in vitro* and *in vivo* studies. The involvement of the inflammatory mediator IL-33 in the activation the other immune cells might result in a chronic inflammatory response in the colonic mucosa that is reflected at the systemic level. To avoid an exaggerated immune response, the host has developed mechanisms to counteract the resulting inflammation through the release of soluble receptors, such as sST2. These decoy molecules are potential surrogate of immunological markers for UC.

2. Intestinal inflammatory process in ulcerative colitis

IBD is a chronic, relapsing-remitting condition that affects the gastrointestinal tract. The aetiology of IBD has not been fully elucidated, although, it has been described as a multifactorial disease, in which genetics, environmental factors and immune system have a leading role (Abraham and Cho, 2009; Xavier and Podolsky, 2007). IBD is a complex polygenic disease in which many genes, related or not, through their contribution and interaction with environmental factors are involved in the final disease manifestation (Bouma and Strober, 2003; McGovern et al., 2010; Risch and Merikangas, 1996; Thompson and Lees, 2011).

The two major types of IBD are Crohn's disease (CD) and ulcerative colitis (UC), both with unique characteristics that make them different at the clinical, cellular and molecular level (Thompson and Lees, 2011). CD may affect a portion of the intestine in a segmental fashion and present a transmural inflammation that extends the entire intestinal wall; whereas in UC a diffuse and continuous inflammation is confined to the mucosa of the colon (Baumgart and Carding, 2007). Histopathologic features of UC confirm that the inflammatory process is limited to the mucosa and typically consists in an increase of inflammatory cells, such as polymorphonuclear granulocytes (Nishida et al., 2002), that extends through the crypt wall (cryptitis) or inside glands with subsequent formation of cryptic abscesses. Moreover, UC is also characterized by crypt architectural distortion due to epithelial injury, shortening or branching of the glands, goblet cells depletion; and presence of lymphoid aggregates associated to oedematous and congestive lamina propria (Silverberg et al., 2005). According to the features previously described, UC pathogenesis can be explained by a deregulation of the inflammatory response of the intestinal mucosa due to epithelial barrier defects to luminal antigens in genetically susceptible individuals. Thus, those diseases characterized by the presence of a defective epithelial barrier show a deregulation of inflammatory processes (Kaser et al., 2010).

Inflammation in UC is restricted to the most superficial layer of the colonic mucosa. Mechanisms that possible may lead to the epithelial injury are reflected by architectural crypt distortion, an increase in the distance between crypts or a decrease in the crypt number; however they are not fully understood. Nonetheless, these mechanisms are likely responsible for the induction of the distinctive inflammatory process of the disease.

Recently, considerable evidence (murine models, genetic studies, *in vitro* assays, etc) has demonstrated that UC and CD involve an uncontrolled primary response of the innate immune system against intestinal luminal compounds, mainly mediated by macrophages, mast cells and neutrophils (Kaser et al., 2010). This uncontrolled inflammation will redound in a scarcely resolutive T and B cells-mediated adaptive immune response. However, in spite of all this information the mechanism involved in the activation of the cellular response is still unknown. This enquiry has highlighted several line of research focused in the study role of the innate immune system in IBD pathogenesis.

2.1 Innate immune receptors in ulcerative colitis pathogenesis

Innate immune response is the first line of defence that protects the host from invasive pathogens and is responsible for their rapid recognition, detection, and elimination. This response initiates and defines the adaptive immunity that is executed by B and T cells. The strategies of recognition in the innate immune system are based on identification of pathogen-associated molecular patterns (PAMPs) through pattern recognition receptors

(PRRs) located on the cell surface or in intracellular compartments, such as endosomes. PRRs are also responsible of the initial recognition of damage-associated molecular pattern (DAMPs) and participate in phagocytosis, activation of pro-inflammatory intracellular pathways, opsonization, complement activation and induction of apoptosis (Medzhitov, 2001). PRRs include Toll-like receptors (TLRs), Nod like receptors (NLRs), RIG-I-like receptor (RLRs), and C-type lectin receptors (CLR) (Kawai and Akira, 2010; Kumagai and Akira, 2010). TLRs are the best characterized family of PRRs that are involved in immune response mechanisms to protect epithelial barrier integrity and invasive microorganisms elimination, contributing to the tolerance and the homeostatic balance of the intestinal mucosa (Podolsky, 2002). TLRs belong to the IL-1 receptor/Toll-like receptor (TLR-IL-1R) superfamily and contain several leucine reach repeats in their extracellular domain and intracellular toll/IL-1 receptor (TIR) domain. TLRs are expressed in both innate immune cells, including macrophages and dendritic cells (DCs) and epithelial cells. The major TLR signalling pathways is the activation of the transcription factors, such as nuclear factor-κB (NFκB) and activating protein-1 (AP-1) that direct to the production of pro-inflammatory cytokines, chemokines, and adhesion molecules (Wang et al., 2001). In pathological conditions, such as in IBD, over-activation of TLRs may induce defective signalling, allowing the induction, amplification and perpetuation of harmful immune responses and the development of a chronic inflammation reflected by an impaired function of the epithelial barrier (Cario, 2010; Kamada et al., 2008).

2.1.1 Pathogenic role of TLR2 in ulcerative colitis

In murine models of colitis, Rakoff-Nahoum et al demonstrated that in TLR2 and adaptor MyD88- deficient mice, microflora-dependent TLR2 signalling is required for the homeostasis of the intestinal epithelium and protects gut epithelia (Rakoff-Nahoum et al., 2004). Clinical evidence supports the close relationship between TLR2 over-expression and UC (Cario et al., 2000). Genetic factor involved in UC, some TLR2 polymorphisms have been described, such as SNP Arg753Gly, which affects the recruitment of signalling pathway molecules and influences over inflammation and disease severity in UC patients with no impact on its susceptibility (Pierik et al., 2006). The nucleotide deletion of TLR2 gene at position -196 to −174 might be associated to a higher risk of severe corticoid-dependence in UC (Wang et al., 2007). Intestinal mucosa isolated lamina propria mononuclear cells show a higher expression of TLR2 in IBD patients than in healthy controls (Cario et al., 2000) and submitted data). In addition, peripheral blood monocytes obtained from IBD patients have a high content of TLR2 on the cell surface, which correlate to a high production of TNF-α in response to receptor agonists (Canto et al., 2006). On the other hand, we have recently shown high levels of TLR2 in colonic mucosa of UC patients and that these finding might be related to a higher expression of TLR2 in $CD33^+CX3CR1^+$ macrophage surface in comparison to controls (submitted results). UC patients also presented elevated levels of soluble TLR2 (sTLR2), which has been shown to sequester TLR2 ligands thus, reversing TLR2 pathway activation (LeBouder et al., 2003). At the moment, evidence indicates that sTLR2 generation might be related to post-transduction mechanisms, suggesting that high levels of transmembrane TLR2 in UC intestinal macrophages might be the main cellular source of this decoy receptor. The generation of sTLR2 might be explaining a compensatory mechanism to restrain the exaggerated inflammation triggered by over-activation of TLR2 in intestinal mucosa of UC patients. This inflammatory condition might explain the participation of sTLR2 to counteract the epithelial damage generated as a consequence of activation of pro-inflammatory signalling pathways, without restabilising the mucosa homeostasis.

2.2 Epithelium in innate immune response

The intestinal epithelial cells (ECs) are continually exposed to bacteria (microbiota and enteric pathogens); however, this interaction does not usually generate a pathological inflammatory response. To maintain integrity and normal function of the intestinal tract, ECs not only constitute a physical barrier that keeps a balance between local homeostatic response and host defence against microbiota and pathogens, but also, provides important functions in the regulation of the mucosal immunity. Recent studies indicate that in response to challenges, intestinal ECs through PRRs drives the expression of critical Th2-driving cytokines, such as IL-25, TSLP and IL-33, which mediate the initiation and interplay between innate and adaptive immunity (Bulek et al., 2010; Schleimer et al., 2007).

IL-33 expression is induced in the intestinal epithelium by exogenous stimuli, including allergens, microbiota, pathogens and pro-inflammatory cytokines (IL-1 and TNF-α), coordinating the immune regulation to maintain homeostasis and drive a protective Th2 phenotype (Schmitz et al., 2005). However, elevated production of these cytokines will be associated with inflammatory Th2 condition in lesions of the mucosa producing pathological changes in the tissue (Schmitz et al., 2005). The IL-33 signalling pathways might exert distinct impact on other inflammatory cells that amplified and perpetuated the immune responses permitting the development of a chronic inflammation (Figure 1).

During inflammatory episodes, different cells, such as lymphocytes, macrophages, neutrophils and mast cells infiltrate the intestinal mucosa, promoting increased production of pro-inflammatory cytokines associated with different immune profiles. In patients diagnosed with UC, Th2 cytokines such as IL-4, IL-5 and IL-13 have been associated (Beltran et al., 2009; Bernstein et al., 2005). In relation to Th2 response that characterized UC, IL-33 is also able to polarize naive T cells into Th2 cells and induce production of IL-4, IL-5 and IL-13 that resulted in pathological changes in the intestinal architecture that includes eosinophilic infiltrates, increased mucus production and epithelial cells hyperplasia and hypertrophy (Figure 1).

2.3 Pathogenic role of the IL-33/ST2 system in ulcerative colitis

Recently, we and others have reported that IL-33 expression is increased in colonic mucosa of UC patients, particularly in those with moderate to severe activity of the disease (Beltran et al., 2010; Kobori et al., 2010; Pastorelli et al., 2010; Seidelin et al., 2010). It has been proposed that in UC, IL-33 may be released by injured epithelial cells to induce pro-inflammatory cytokines production (i.e. IL-1, IL-6, TNF-α, IL-5 and IL-13) through activation of ST2L in mast cells, macrophages, eosinophils and neutrophils (Luthi et al., 2009). Moreover, IL-33 expression is restricted to the epithelial layer of the intestine (Beltran et al., 2010; Pastorelli et al., 2010). In addition, activation of ST2L in dendritic cells may contribute to the polarization to IL-5 and IL-13-producing Th2 cells (Rank et al., 2009) and in basophiles the induction of IL-13-dependent fibrosis (Pecaric-Petkovic et al., 2009). Those cytokines induced by IL-33, mostly IL-13, may have detrimental effects on epithelial barrier function (Heller et al., 2005). Together, the effects induced by IL-33 might amplify the local inflammatory response, and therefore, contributing to perpetuation of pathogenic inflammatory process that is characteristic of the disease (Palmer and Gabay, 2011).

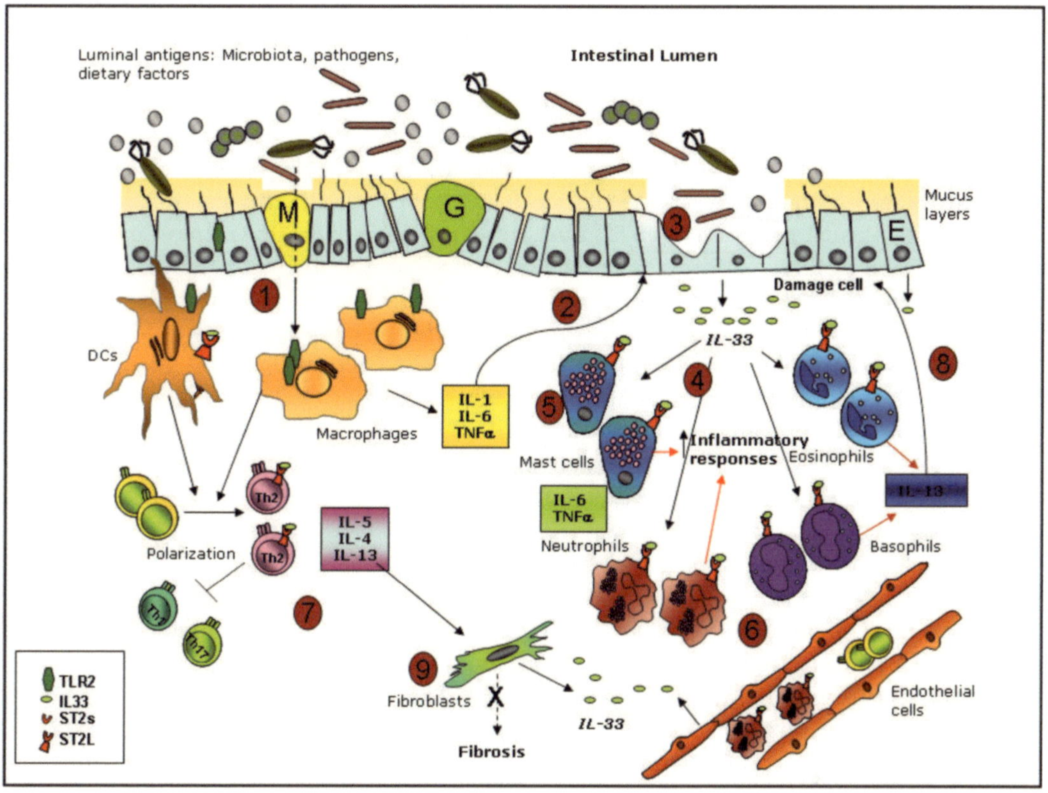

Fig. 1. Role of IL-33/ST2 receptor system in UC. In ulcerative colitis (UC) epithelia is more exposed to pathogens, as mucus layer is deficient to prevent their access to the barrier, with persistent inflammation that also promote epithelial disruption. The tissue injury can be a consequence of infections or the access of the microbiota, which are linked to the development of IBD. The over-activation of TLR2 present in the macrophage cell surface (1) will produce inflammatory cytokines, as well as, tumor necrosis factor (TNF-α) and IL-1 (2), that promote the epithelial injury (3). Tissue damage leads to the release of interleukin-33 (IL-33) from epithelial cells (4), which acts as an early inducer of inflammation. IL-33 induce the expression of pro-inflammatory cytokines in cells that express ST2 receptor (mast cells (5), neutophils activated, eosinophils and basophils (6)). Moreover, IL-33 may drive antigen sensitization and polarization to T helper 2 (Th2) -mediated inflammation (7) during the development of UC owing to its ability to activate dendritic cells (DCs) and to recruit, polarize and activate Th2 cells that also express ST2 receptor. IL-33 can induce eosinophilia by mast cells through the induction of IL-13 secretion. IL-13 exerts detrimental effects on epithelial barrier function, favoring the effects of IL-33 (8). Mast cell-mediated inflammation may drive a robust proliferation of fibroblast toward fibrosis formation, however high levels of sST2 might counteract this cellular effect of IL-33. (M: M cells; G: Goblet cells and E: Epithelial cells)

2.3.1 Components of the IL-33/ST2 system

Clinical and experimental data have shown that activation of IL-33/ST2 pathway is primarily occurring in diseases that affect epithelial barriers, such as asthma, arthritis and UC (Palmer and Gabay, 2011). ST2 protein (IL1RL1) is encoded by a single gene located on chromosome 2q12 (Tominaga et al., 1991), that is part of the TLR-IL-1R superfamily. Three types of *st2* gene products are generated by alternative splicing: ST2L, which is the complete form of protein, the receptor itself, that has a TIR intracellular domain (similar to Toll/Interleukin-1 receptors domain), a transmembrane and an extracellular domain formed by three immunoglobulin-like domains that binds IL-33; a soluble form of ST2 (sST2) that lacks the transmembrane and intracellular domains, but can also recognize IL-33; and a form bound to the plasma membrane (vST2) that ,similar to sST2, lacks the intracellular domain. The production of these isoforms is under the control of two distinct promoters (proximal and distal) which have a differential activity depending on the cell type (Gachter et al., 1996; Iwahana et al., 1999). The differential function of the promoters allows a 3′ differential processing of st2 mRNA to generate the STL2 and sST2 isoforms (Bergers et al., 1994). To date, the cellular and molecular context that might activate a defined promoter it is still uncertain, and the signalling pathways required to produce one protein over the other, is even less clear. Many studies recognized pro-inflammatory properties to ST2L receptor activation and anti-inflammatory effects to the soluble form sST2. However, since there is no an experimental model available where characteristics of one of the protein isoforms are conserved, the attribution of these functional effects to ST2 remains under speculation.
Since IL-33 cytokine was described as the ligand of ST2L receptor, its effect has been associated to a Th2 immune profile (Schmitz et al., 2005). The signalling pathway activated upon ligand binding to ST2L is common to all members of the TLR-IL-1R superfamily, involving recruitment of MyD88, IRAKs and TRAF6 adaptor molecule which leads to phosphorylation of Mitogen-Activated Protein Kinases (MAPK) such as ERK1, ERK2 and p38 pathways and the consequent activation of NFκB and AP-1 to induce pro-inflammatory gene expression (Palmer et al., 2008; Schmitz et al., 2005).

2.3.2 Cellular sources of IL-33/ST2 system

ST2L receptor expression has been mainly associated to immune cells, such as mast cells, macrophages, dendritic cells, NK cells, eosinophils, basophils, Th2 lymphocytes and activated neutrophils (Allakhverdi et al., 2007; Ho et al., 2007; Komai-Koma et al., 2007; Rank et al., 2009; Suzukawa et al., 2008a) (Figure 1). Polymorphonuclear leukocytes have been also demonstrated to produce the soluble form sST2. However, sST2 has been primarily associated to fibroblasts, epithelial and endothelial cells (Hayakawa et al., 2007). The ligand of ST2, IL-33, was initially described as a nuclear protein, and is constitutively expressed by cells in contact with external surfaces, such as epithelial and endothelial cells (Baekkevold et al., 2003), and is potentially released in response to tissue damage, to rapidly activate the innate immune system (Palmer and Gabay, 2011). Induced expression of IL-33 has been reported in different cell types, in resident as well as in infiltrating inflammatory cells (Oboki et al., 2011). IL-33 is the most recently described member of the IL-1 cytokine family (Schmitz et al., 2005), has been attributed to have similar functions to IL-1α exerting dual effects as a nuclear factor as well as a pro-inflammatory cytokine (Carriere et al., 2007; Cayrol and Girard, 2009; Roussel et al., 2008; Talabot-Ayer et al., 2009). IL-33 gene does not encode a secretion signal peptide, such as other cytokines, so that its secretion is not

produced by conventional mechanisms (Lamkanfi and Dixit, 2009; Zhao and Hu, 2010). It has been suggested that IL-33 is released during cell necrosis, similar to what was previously described for the alarmins, as an inflammatory response that will produce early activation of innate immune system cells (Haraldsen et al., 2009; Lamkanfi and Dixit, 2009).
One of the major cellular sources of the receptor ST2L in the intestinal mucosa is mast cells (Figure 1) which have been demonstrated to have important roles in the distinctive inflammatory process of UC (Allakhverdi et al., 2007; Iikura et al., 2007; Lee et al., 2002; Moritz et al., 1998). Mast cells are considered true sensors of cell injury in tissue exposed to the exterior (Enoksson et al., 2011). These cells might be responsible of orchestrating and enhancing the innate immune response induced by IL-33 in the intestinal mucosa in UC patients, since mast granulatory products have been detected in inflamed areas of the intestine (Bischoff et al., 1996).

2.3.3 Regulation of IL-33/ST2 inflammatory pathway: Role of sST2

One of the hallmarks of UC is chronicity, and periods of active inflammation (flare-ups) and remission. This special feature of UC opens different questions about inflammation regulation. The clinical practice can demonstrate classic endoscopic and histologic patterns of active inflammation in patients, where, mild mucosa inflammation is generally characterized by vascular congestion, erythema, oedema and granularity (Pineton de Chambrun et al., 2010). When inflammation becomes severe in UC, friability, spontaneous bleeding and macroscopic ulcers of different sizes are mainly observed (D'Haens et al., 2007; Fefferman and Farrell, 2005). Therefore, a patient in remission, after a period with lesions, the mucosa might have a reduced inflammatory process, reflected by mucosal healing (MH) and a decrease in cellular infiltrates (Lichtenstein and Rutgeerts, 2010; Rutgeerts et al., 2007). The MH is characterized by restoration of a normal vascular pattern, absence of friability, bleeding, erosions and ulcers in all intestinal segments of the mucosa visualized in the intestine from UC patients (Lichtenstein and Rutgeerts, 2010; Rutgeerts et al., 2007). However, at a cellular level, there is no consensus on the processes leading to MH. Only restoration, proliferation and differentiation of epithelial cells adjacent to the injured area will allow intestinal wound healing (Iizuka and Konno, 2011). Many reports support the evidence that activation of IL-10 signalling pathway may have a leading role in regulation of the inflammatory process (Li and He, 2004; Shih and Targan, 2008). IL-10-deficient mice (IL-$10^{-/-}$) spontaneously reproduce a colitis phenotype similar to human colitis (Bristol et al., 2000; Kuhn et al., 1993; Rennick et al., 1997). In this mice model, the intestine damage is characterized by the presence of large and thick crypts, and low number of goblet cells, allowing the development of spontaneous colitis (Thompson and Lees, 2011). However, since IL-10 participation might be primarily associated to cellular processes that regulate and resolve the inflammatory response, in chronic inflammation condition, such as UC, its contribution might be relevant to achieve a homeostatic balance (Mosser and Zhang, 2008). Clinical and experimental data have shown sST2 counteractive effect over the activation of IL-33/ST2L pathway and resolution of inflammation (Takezako et al., 2006). Soluble ST2 inhibits IL-33 activity in *in vitro* assays of mast cells stimulated with the cytokine thus blocking the signalling pathway and the release of pro-inflammatory cytokines (Hayakawa et al., 2007; Ho et al., 2007; Palmer et al., 2008; Sanada et al., 2007; Weinberg, 2009). In murine asthma models, pre-treatment with recombinant ST2 reduced IL-13 content in bronchoalveolar lavage fluid induced by intranasal administration of IL-33 (Hayakawa et al., 2007). Similarly, intraperitoneal administration of sST2 reduced the severity, extent of inflammation and number of affected joints, as well as plasma concentration of pro-inflammatory cytokines in collagen-induced arthritis in mice (Leung et al., 2004). Also, in methylated-BSA induced-rheumatoid arthritis mice model, therapeutic effect of sST2 was also manifested in decrease of neutrophils recruitment to affected joints (Verri et al., 2010). In UC, recent reports have demonstrated that sST2 levels correlate with the severity of the disease (Beltran et al., 2010; Diaz-Jimenez et al., 2011); hence a reduction in protein levels could be used as a biomarker to determine clinical remission. However, although information points to an anti-inflammatory role of sST2, evidence also shows a direct relationship to the disease. Given that UC patients cursing with severe activity have evidently increased plasma levels of sST2, this condition was shown to directly correlate with increased intestinal levels (Diaz-Jimenez et al., 2011). A possible and appealing explanation to this issue is that intestinal increase of sST2 levels reflected in plasma evident a mechanism to prevent an exaggerated immune response; however it might be insufficient to resolve the pathological inflammation distinctive to severe UC (Akhabir and Sandford, 2010).

2.4 IBD genetics

As previously mentioned, IBDs have an important genetic background. Relationship between certain genes and susceptibility to a particular disease has been possible due to molecular characterization made in the past decades (Hardy and Singleton, 2009; Manolio, 2010). Genetic factors relevant in IBD have been demonstrated, through the identification of risk polymorphisms, their loci and genes involved (Barrett et al., 2008; Vermeire et al., 2010). Nevertheless, genetic contributing to disease risk is more profoundly documented in CD than in UC. Many of these risk factors might be related to molecules that participate in the immune response directed to preserve intestinal homeostasis (Carter et al., 2001; Henckaerts et al., 2007). For example, mutations in NOD2/CARD15 gene have acquired great importance as a susceptibility gene for CD. Association between NOD2/CARD15 gene variants and susceptibility and severity of the disease suggest that these mutant alleles may have a prognostic value of an unfavourable outcome and high requirement of surgery (Alvarez-Lobos et al., 2005; Annese et al., 2005; Seiderer et al., 2006). In UC, genes encoding glycoprotein e-cadherin and laminins, such as ECM1, CDH1 and Lamb1, involved in epithelial barrier function and in regulation of inflammatory process, have emerged as significant determinants of susceptibility (Thompson and Lees, 2011). High levels of ST2L protein expression have been described in polygenic and multifactorial diseases recognized to be caused by inflammatory response and with a compromise of the epithelial barrier, such as asthma, atopic dermatitis and systemic lupus erythematosus (Ali et al., 2009; Kuroiwa et al., 2001; Mok et al., 2010; Oshikawa et al., 2001a; Shimizu et al., 2005). These pathologies are also characterized by a high number of local inflammatory infiltrates (mast cells, basophils, neutrophils and eosinophils) and high plasma concentration of sST2, as was also described for UC. Since the physiopathologic role of this protein has been already described, genetic studies have been searching for single nucleotide polymorphism (SNP) in the *st2* gene locus. To date, two case-control studies, one in atopic dermatitis (Shimizu et al., 2005) and another in asthma (Ali et al., 2009), have analyzed the presence of SNPs located in the distal promoter of the *st2* gene. Among these, only the A allele of SNP -26999G/A (rs6543116), could be related to an increase in gene transcription, higher serum levels of sST2, and a higher risk to develop the disease (Shimizu et al., 2005). Whereas in asthma the presence of the AA genotype was only found in a small fraction of the studied population, it seems to be more often in severe corticoid-dependent asthma patients associated to a worsen course of the disease (Ali et al., 2009).

At the moment, there are no studies to demonstrate a possible association between SNPs present in the *st2* gene and IBD susceptibility. However, our preliminary results seem to not support this association. Recently, two publications related to Genome-Wide Association (GWA) have made possible the detection of risk genes and *loci* associated with complex diseases, such as IBD (Barrett et al., 2008; Hampe et al., 2007; Rioux et al., 2007). In these studies, the *loci* that contains the *st2* gene has not been directly implicated in UC susceptibility. However, the *locus* containing genes for IL1R, IL18R1 and IL18RAP, previously related to UC and with a high linkage disequilibrium (LD) represents an interesting candidate that might be involved in the development and course of the disease (Akhabir and Sandford, 2010). In line with this, a new SNP located in the non-codifying region of *st2* gene (rs1420101), has been associated with eosinophilia in asthma and other inflammatory diseases, such as chronic obstructive pulmonary disease (COPD) and myocardial infarction. Gudbjartsoon et al. (Gudbjartsson et al., 2009) showed that there is no correlation between this genetic variant and the increased number in eosinophils, or with previously described genetic variants associated to CD (rs917997) (Zhernakova et al., 2008) and celiac disease (rs13015714) (Hunt et al., 2008). Since the IL-33/ST2 signalling pathway has a role in maturation, survival and activation of eosinophils, also in recruitment and regulation of Th2 cell function, the available information is consistent with a greater contribution of this system in eosinophil-mediated inflammation (Stolarski et al., 2010; Suzukawa et al., 2008b). The role of eosinophils in the aetiology and pathogenesis of UC is not completely clear. However, evidence shows a 10-fold higher content of eosinophils in patients with active UC compared to healthy individuals (Kristjansson et al., 2004). In these patients, tissue eosinophilia induced by IL-33 might have a detrimental effect on intestinal structural integrity. As previously mentioned, polymorphonuclear cells constitute an important source of ST2, making an interesting issue the analysis of the presence of these new SNPs in samples of UC patients.

2.5 Soluble ST2 as a biomarker of activity in ulcerative colitis

Many symptoms of UC and CD are similar, but there are some subtle differences. Clinical presentation are rather unspecific, thus further studies are necessary to achieve a differential diagnosis of the diseases. Colonoscopy through biopsy analysis remains the foundation for IBD diagnosis. However, several studies have shown a considerable variability in endoscopic and histological changes of intestinal mucosa (higher inter- and intra-observer variability in determination of the disease activity; low precision and reproducibility of the observations and scarce correlation between endoscopic appearance and clinical indices with treatment response) (D'Haens et al., 2007; Osada et al., 2010; Regueiro et al., 2011). This discrepancy has led physicians and immunologists to search for clinically relevant molecules as biomarkers, non-invasive indicators that objectively assess the damage that is taking place at the intestinal mucosa (Gisbert et al., 2007; Tibble and Bjarnason, 2001; Vermeire et al., 2006). The ideal marker not only might allow for differential diagnosis but also establish prognosis, activity and severity of the disease, risks or complications, relapses, recurrence and clinical remission, besides evaluation of treatment response (Gisbert and Gomollon, 2007; Gisbert et al., 2007; Tibble and Bjarnason, 2001; Vermeire et al., 2006).

Since intestinal inflammation in IBD patients is associated with acute-phase response and recruitment of immune cells to the site of inflammation, a high production of protein in the mucosa might be detected in serum and/or stool. Among the most commonly used molecules associated with IBD in clinical practice are serological biomarkers, including anti-microbial antibodies (ASCA, ANCA, anti-OmpC, anti-Cbir, anti-I2 and anti-glycans), other plasma proteins (albumin, C-reactive protein (CRP), cytokines, adhesion molecules, among others) and stool proteins (calprotectin, lactoferrin, and neutrophil-elastase) (Li et al., 2008). Most of former serological biomarkers, (mainly ASCA and ANCA) individually have the disadvantage of moderate sensitivity and specificity to predict intestinal inflammation and do not correlate with clinical and disease activity (Papp et al., 2007). C-reactive protein is an objective inflammatory marker and correlates with severe disease activity (Karoui et al., 2007; Rodgers and Cummins, 2007; Solem et al., 2005), however, it is a systemic inflammatory marker elevated in several other inflammatory diseases and with low specificity by diagnosing patients with mild disease activity (Karoui et al., 2007; Rodgers and Cummins, 2007; Solem et al., 2005; Vermeire et al., 2004).

Faecal calprotectin is another biomarker; it is a calcium-binding protein mainly present in neutrophil granules and has the theoretical benefit of having greater specificity for the diagnosis of gastrointestinal diseases. Calprotectin concentration is directly proportional to the migration of neutrophil to the gastrointestinal tract and is not altered by extra-intestinal diseases (Gisbert and McNicholl, 2009; Langhorst et al., 2008; Schoepfer et al., 2010; Sipponen et al., 2008). In addition, calprotectin levels most directly correlate to histological features rather than with endoscopic indexes, suggesting that this marker has a better sensitivity for the evaluation of disease activity than endoscopic procedures (Burns et al., 2003; Poullis et al., 2002). Calprotectin is generally detected in a small sample using simple and low cost methods and is relatively stable in the stool. Although calprotectin has many advantages as a biomarker and is highly sensitive to detect intestinal inflammation (Langhorst et al., 2008), it is not specific for IBD since other gastrointestinal diseases, such as colorectal cancer (Roseth et al., 1993; Tibble et al., 2001) or gastrointestinal infections, were shown to present high levels of this protein (Summerton et al., 2002; Tibble et al., 2002; Pezzilli et al., 2008).

Several clinical studies have reported an increase in plasma levels of sST2 in patients with inflammatory processes, including asthma (Oshikawa et al., 2001b), autoimmune diseases (rheumatoid arthritis, erythematosus systemic lupus and progressive systemic scleroderma) (Kuroiwa et al., 2001), cardiovascular diseases (Weinberg et al., 2003), trauma and sepsis (Brunner et al., 2004). Currently, plasma level of sST2 might work as a biomarker for diagnosis and /or prognosis of several cardiac function conditions directly related to myocardial injury (Diez, 2008; Rehman et al., 2008; Weinberg, 2009; Weinberg et al., 2003). In the context of IBD, we have reported high levels of sST2 that has been proposed as a reliable biomarker of UC activity (Diaz-Jimenez et al., 2011). In UC, serum levels of sST2 grouped by active and inactive, according to endoscopic disease activity index (inactive defined as a Mayo endoscopic score $\geq$ 1 point), were 33.19 pg/mL and 235.80 pg/mL, respectively. Differences observed in serum concentration were statistically significant ($p<0.0001$) to discriminate between active and inactive condition. Also, the correlation ROC curve shown a cut-off for sST2 level at 74.87 pg/mL that allow the discrimination between the grade of disease activity (AUC = 0.92) with a sensitivity and specificity of 83.33%. Additionally, serum sST2 levels directly correlated with the degree of endoscopic activity (r = 0.76) according to Mayo endoscopic sub-score classification (0 = normal or inactive state, 1 = mild, 2 = moderate, and 3 = severe disease). According to histopathologic findings (Gomes et al., 1986), levels of sST2 also correlated to the specific index (r = 0.67), suggesting that, similar to calprotectin, serum sST2 levels might have a better sensitivity than endoscopic procedure to estimate the activity of UC patients. Furthermore, we demonstrated that serum sST2 levels behave similarly to other serum inflammation marker, such as TNF-α, in relation to endoscopic and histopathologic activity indexes. However, sST2 is potentially a better biomarker as is more stable than the previously reported cytokine (Dieplinger et al., 2010). Finally, we also showed that total levels of ST2 in colonic mucosa of UC patients positively correlated with endoscopic (r = 0.62) and histopathologic (r = 0.60) UC activity indexes similar to what was described for serum levels. The clear association between intestinal and serum ST2 levels illustrate a valid activity biomarker, unbiased and distinctive of inflammatory process taking place in the intestinal mucosa of UC patients. Thus, ST2 detection might help physicians in the decision making on whether to periodically send patients to colonoscopy, an invasive and expensive test, or use alternative assessment techniques.

3. Conclusion

Current methodology, especially those related to genomics and transcriptomes, will soon allow the improvement in differential diagnosis in patients who show great clinical heterogeneity, with less invasive procedures than colonoscopy and biopsies. Measurement of serum ST2 levels is a reliable, quick and low cost technique for differential diagnosis in IBD and other gastrointestinal diseases, and might allow the assessment of disease activity. Furthermore, in certain subgroups of patients with well-known diagnosis, sST2 has been assigned to have a predictive value to define the course of the disease, ever since genetic analysis of *st2* gene might relate to higher surgery rates, as has been previously shown for NOD2/CARD15 in CD. Here lies the biggest advantage of new biomarkers based on intestinal specific inflammation mechanisms. The future development of molecular classification of IBD, according to molecular biomarkers, may allow a better accuracy in diagnosis, clinical course and response to a determined therapy to induce and sustain remission in IBD.

4. References

Abraham C., Cho J.H. (2009) Inflammatory bowel disease. N Engl J Med 361:2066-78.

Akhabir L., Sandford A. (2010) Genetics of interleukin 1 receptor-like 1 in immune and inflammatory diseases. Curr Genomics 11:591-606.

Ali M., Zhang G., Thomas W.R., McLean C.J., Bizzintino J.A., Laing I.A., Martin A.C., Goldblatt J., Le Souef P.N., Hayden C.M. (2009) Investigations into the role of ST2 in acute asthma in children. Tissue Antigens 73:206-12.

Alvarez-Lobos M., Arostegui J.I., Sans M., Tassies D., Plaza S., Delgado S., Lacy A.M., Pique J.M., Yague J., Panes J. (2005) Crohn's disease patients carrying Nod2/CARD15 gene variants have an increased and early need for first surgery due to stricturing disease and higher rate of surgical recurrence. Ann Surg 242:693-700. Allakhverdi

Z., Smith D.E., Comeau M.R., Delespesse G. (2007) Cutting edge: The ST2 ligand IL-33 potently activates and drives maturation of human mast cells. J Immunol 179:2051-4.

Annese V., Lombardi G., Perri F., D'Inca R., Ardizzone S., Riegler G., Giaccari S., Vecchi M., Castiglione F., Gionchetti P., Cocchiara E., Vigneri S., Latiano A., Palmieri O., Andriulli A. (2005) Variants of CARD15 are associated with an aggressive clinical course of Crohn's disease--an IG-IBD study. Am J Gastroenterol 100:84-92.

Baekkevold E.S., Roussigne M., Yamanaka T., Johansen F.E., Jahnsen F.L., Amalric F., Brandtzaeg P., Erard M., Haraldsen G., Girard J.P. (2003) Molecular characterization of NF-HEV, a nuclear factor preferentially expressed in human high endothelial venules. Am J Pathol 163:69-79.

Barrett J.C., Hansoul S., Nicolae D.L., Cho J.H., Duerr R.H., Rioux J.D., Brant S.R., Silverberg M.S., Taylor K.D., Barmada M.M., Bitton A., Dassopoulos T., Datta L.W., Green T., Griffiths A.M., Kistner E.O., Murtha M.T., Regueiro M.D., Rotter J.I., Schumm L.P., Steinhart A.H., Targan S.R., Xavier R.J., Libioulle C., Sandor C., Lathrop M., Belaiche J., Dewit O., Gut I., Heath S., Laukens D., Mni M., Rutgeerts P., Van Gossum A., Zelenika D., Franchimont D., Hugot J.P., de Vos M., Vermeire S., Louis E., Cardon L.R., Anderson C.A., Drummond H., Nimmo E., Ahmad T., Prescott N.J., Onnie C.M., Fisher S.A., Marchini J., Ghori J., Bumpstead S., Gwilliam R., Tremelling M., Deloukas P., Mansfield J., Jewell D., Satsangi J., Mathew C.G., Parkes M., Georges M., Daly M.J. (2008) Genome-wide association defines more than 30 distinct susceptibility loci for Crohn's disease. Nat Genet 40:955-62.

Baumgart D.C., Carding S.R. (2007) Inflammatory bowel disease: cause and immunobiology. Lancet 369:1627-40.

Beltran C.J., Candia E., Erranz B., Figueroa C., Gonzalez M.J., Quera R., Hermoso M.A. (2009) Peripheral cytokine profile in Chilean patients with Crohn's disease and ulcerative colitis. Eur Cytokine Netw 20:33-8.

Beltran C.J., Nunez L.E., Diaz-Jimenez D., Farfan N., Candia E., Heine C., Lopez F., Gonzalez M.J., Quera R., Hermoso M.A. (2010) Characterization of the novel ST2/IL-33 system in patients with inflammatory bowel disease. Inflamm Bowel Dis 16:1097-107.

Bergers G., Reikerstorfer A., Braselmann S., Graninger P., Busslinger M. (1994) Alternative promoter usage of the Fos-responsive gene Fit-1 generates mRNA isoforms coding for either secreted or membrane-bound proteins related to the IL-1 receptor. EMBO J 13:1176-88.

Bernstein C.N., Wajda A., Blanchard J.F. (2005) The clustering of other chronic inflammatory diseases in inflammatory bowel disease: a population-based study. Gastroenterology 129:827-36.

Bischoff S.C., Wedemeyer J., Herrmann A., Meier P.N., Trautwein C., Cetin Y., Maschek H., Stolte M., Gebel M., Manns M.P. (1996) Quantitative assessment of intestinal eosinophils and mast cells in inflammatory bowel disease. Histopathology 28:1-13.

Bouma G., Strober W. (2003) The immunological and genetic basis of inflammatory bowel disease. Nat Rev Immunol 3:521-33.

Bristol I.J., Farmer M.A., Cong Y., Zheng X.X., Strom T.B., Elson C.O., Sundberg J.P., Leiter E.H. (2000) Heritable susceptibility for colitis in mice induced by IL-10 deficiency. Inflamm Bowel Dis 6:290-302.

Brunner M., Krenn C., Roth G., Moser B., Dworschak M., Jensen-Jarolim E., Spittler A., Sautner T., Bonaros N., Wolner E., Boltz-Nitulescu G., Ankersmit H.J. (2004) Increased levels of soluble ST2 protein and IgG1 production in patients with sepsis and trauma. Intensive Care Med 30:1468-73.
Bulek K., Swaidani S., Aronica M., Li X. (2010) Epithelium: the interplay between innate and Th2 immunity. Immunol Cell Biol 88:257-68.
Burns K., Janssens S., Brissoni B., Olivos N., Beyaert R., Tschopp J. (2003) Inhibition of interleukin 1 receptor/Toll-like receptor signaling through the alternatively spliced, short form of MyD88 is due to its failure to recruit IRAK-4. J Exp Med 197:263-8.
Canto E., Ricart E., Monfort D., Gonzalez-Juan D., Balanzo J., Rodriguez-Sanchez J.L., Vidal S. (2006) TNF alpha production to TLR2 ligands in active IBD patients. Clin Immunol 119:156-65.
Cario E. (2010) Toll-like receptors in inflammatory bowel diseases: a decade later. Inflamm Bowel Dis 16:1583-97.
Cario E., Rosenberg I.M., Brandwein S.L., Beck P.L., Reinecker H.C., Podolsky D.K. (2000) Lipopolysaccharide activates distinct signaling pathways in intestinal epithelial cell lines expressing Toll-like receptors. J Immunol 164:966-72.
Carriere V., Roussel L., Ortega N., Lacorre D.A., Americh L., Aguilar L., Bouche G., Girard J.P. (2007) IL-33, the IL-1-like cytokine ligand for ST2 receptor, is a chromatin-associated nuclear factor in vivo. Proc Natl Acad Sci U S A 104:282-7.
Carter M.J., di Giovine F.S., Jones S., Mee J., Camp N.J., Lobo A.J., Duff G.W. (2001) Association of the interleukin 1 receptor antagonist gene with ulcerative colitis in Northern European Caucasians. Gut 48:461-7.
Cayrol C., Girard J.P. (2009) The IL-1-like cytokine IL-33 is inactivated after maturation by caspase-1. Proc Natl Acad Sci U S A 106:9021-6.
D'Haens G., Sandborn W.J., Feagan B.G., Geboes K., Hanauer S.B., Irvine E.J., Lemann M., Marteau P., Rutgeerts P., Scholmerich J., Sutherland L.R. (2007) A review of activity indices and efficacy end points for clinical trials of medical therapy in adults with ulcerative colitis. Gastroenterology 132:763-86.
Diaz-Jimenez D., Nunez L.E., Beltran C.J., Candia E., Suazo C., Alvarez-Lobos M., Gonzalez M.J., Hermoso M.A., Quera R. (2011) Soluble ST2: A new and promising activity marker in ulcerative colitis. World J Gastroenterol 17:2181-90.
Dieplinger B., Gegenhuber A., Kaar G., Poelz W., Haltmayer M., Mueller T. (2010) Prognostic value of established and novel biomarkers in patients with shortness of breath attending an emergency department. Clin Biochem 43:714-9.
Diez J. (2008) Serum soluble ST2 as a biochemical marker of acute heart failure: future areas of research. J Am Coll Cardiol 52:1466-7.
Enoksson M., Lyberg K., Moller-Westerberg C., Fallon P.G., Nilsson G., Lunderius-Andersson C. (2011) Mast cells as sensors of cell injury through IL-33 recognition. J Immunol 186:2523-8.
Fefferman D.S., Farrell R.J. (2005) Endoscopy in inflammatory bowel disease: indications, surveillance, and use in clinical practice. Clin Gastroenterol Hepatol 3:11-24.
Gachter T., Werenskiold A.K., Klemenz R. (1996) Transcription of the interleukin-1 receptor-related T1 gene is initiated at different promoters in mast cells and fibroblasts. J Biol Chem 271:124-9.

Gisbert J.P., Gomollon F. (2007) [Common errors in the management of the seriously ill patient with inflammatory bowel disease]. Gastroenterol Hepatol 30:294-314.

Gisbert J.P., McNicholl A.G. (2009) Questions and answers on the role of faecal calprotectin as a biological marker in inflammatory bowel disease. Dig Liver Dis 41:56-66.

Gisbert J.P., Gonzalez-Lama Y., Mate J. (2007) [Role of biological markers in inflammatory bowel disease]. Gastroenterol Hepatol 30:117-29.

Gomes P., du Boulay C., Smith C.L., Holdstock G. (1986) Relationship between disease activity indices and colonoscopic findings in patients with colonic inflammatory bowel disease. Gut 27:92-5.

Gudbjartsson D.F., Bjornsdottir U.S., Halapi E., Helgadottir A., Sulem P., Jonsdottir G.M., Thorleifsson G., Helgadottir H., Steinthorsdottir V., Stefansson H., Williams C., Hui J., Beilby J., Warrington N.M., James A., Palmer L.J., Koppelman G.H., Heinzmann A., Krueger M., Boezen H.M., Wheatley A., Altmuller J., Shin H.D., Uh S.T., Cheong H.S., Jonsdottir B., Gislason D., Park C.S., Rasmussen L.M., Porsbjerg C., Hansen J.W., Backer V., Werge T., Janson C., Jonsson U.B., Ng M.C., Chan J., So W.Y., Ma R., Shah S.H., Granger C.B., Quyyumi A.A., Levey A.I., Vaccarino V., Reilly M.P., Rader D.J., Williams M.J., van Rij A.M., Jones G.T., Trabetti E., Malerba G., Pignatti P.F., Boner A., Pescollderungg L., Girelli D., Olivieri O., Martinelli N., Ludviksson B.R., Ludviksdottir D., Eyjolfsson G.I., Arnar D., Thorgeirsson G., Deichmann K., Thompson P.J., Wjst M., Hall I.P., Postma D.S., Gislason T., Gulcher J., Kong A., Jonsdottir I., Thorsteinsdottir U., Stefansson K. (2009) Sequence variants affecting eosinophil numbers associate with asthma and myocardial infarction. Nat Genet 41:342-7.

Hampe J., Franke A., Rosenstiel P., Till A., Teuber M., Huse K., Albrecht M., Mayr G., De La Vega F.M., Briggs J., Gunther S., Prescott N.J., Onnie C.M., Hasler R., Sipos B., Folsch U.R., Lengauer T., Platzer M., Mathew C.G., Krawczak M., Schreiber S. (2007) A genome-wide association scan of nonsynonymous SNPs identifies a susceptibility variant for Crohn disease in ATG16L1. Nat Genet 39:207-11.

Haraldsen G., Balogh J., Pollheimer J., Sponheim J., Kuchler A.M. (2009) Interleukin-33 - cytokine of dual function or novel alarmin? Trends Immunol 30:227-33.

Hardy J., Singleton A. (2009) Genomewide association studies and human disease. N Engl J Med 360:1759-68.

Hayakawa H., Hayakawa M., Kume A., Tominaga S. (2007) Soluble ST2 blocks interleukin-33 signaling in allergic airway inflammation. J Biol Chem 282:26369-80.

Heller F., Florian P., Bojarski C., Richter J., Christ M., Hillenbrand B., Mankertz J., Gitter A.H., Burgel N., Fromm M., Zeitz M., Fuss I., Strober W., Schulzke J.D. (2005) Interleukin-13 is the key effector Th2 cytokine in ulcerative colitis that affects epithelial tight junctions, apoptosis, and cell restitution. Gastroenterology 129:550-64.

Henckaerts L., Pierik M., Joossens M., Ferrante M., Rutgeerts P., Vermeire S. (2007) Mutations in pattern recognition receptor genes modulate seroreactivity to microbial antigens in patients with inflammatory bowel disease. Gut 56:1536-42.

Ho L.H., Ohno T., Oboki K., Kajiwara N., Suto H., Iikura M., Okayama Y., Akira S., Saito H., Galli S.J., Nakae S. (2007) IL-33 induces IL-13 production by mouse mast cells independently of IgE-FcepsilonRI signals. J Leukoc Biol 82:1481-90.

Hunt K.A., Zhernakova A., Turner G., Heap G.A., Franke L., Bruinenberg M., Romanos J., Dinesen L.C., Ryan A.W., Panesar D., Gwilliam R., Takeuchi F., McLaren W.M., Holmes G.K., Howdle P.D., Walters J.R., Sanders D.S., Playford R.J., Trynka G., Mulder C.J., Mearin M.L., Verbeek W.H., Trimble V., Stevens F.M., O'Morain C., Kennedy N.P., Kelleher D., Pennington D.J., Strachan D.P., McArdle W.L., Mein C.A., Wapenaar M.C., Deloukas P., McGinnis R., McManus R., Wijmenga C., van Heel D.A. (2008) Newly identified genetic risk variants for celiac disease related to the immune response. Nat Genet 40:395-402.

Iikura M., Suto H., Kajiwara N., Oboki K., Ohno T., Okayama Y., Saito H., Galli S.J., Nakae S. (2007) IL-33 can promote survival, adhesion and cytokine production in human mast cells. Lab Invest 87:971-8.

Iizuka M., Konno S. (2011) Wound healing of intestinal epithelial cells. World J Gastroenterol 17:2161-71.

Iwahana H., Yanagisawa K., Ito-Kosaka A., Kuroiwa K., Tago K., Komatsu N., Katashima R., Itakura M., Tominaga S. (1999) Different promoter usage and multiple transcription initiation sites of the interleukin-1 receptor-related human ST2 gene in UT-7 and TM12 cells. Eur J Biochem 264:397-406.

Kamada N., Hisamatsu T., Okamoto S., Chinen H., Kobayashi T., Sato T., Sakuraba A., Kitazume M.T., Sugita A., Koganei K., Akagawa K.S., Hibi T. (2008) Unique CD14 intestinal macrophages contribute to the pathogenesis of Crohn disease via IL-23/IFN-gamma axis. J Clin Invest 118:2269-80.

Karoui S., Ouerdiane S., Serghini M., Jomni T., Kallel L., Fekih M., Boubaker J., Filali A. (2007) Correlation between levels of C-reactive protein and clinical activity in Crohn's disease. Dig Liver Dis 39:1006-10.

Kaser A., Zeissig S., Blumberg R.S. (2010) Inflammatory bowel disease. Annu Rev Immunol 28:573-621.

Kawai T., Akira S. (2010) The role of pattern-recognition receptors in innate immunity: update on Toll-like receptors. Nat Immunol 11:373-84.

Kobori A., Yagi Y., Imaeda H., Ban H., Bamba S., Tsujikawa T., Saito Y., Fujiyama Y., Andoh A. (2010) Interleukin-33 expression is specifically enhanced in inflamed mucosa of ulcerative colitis. J Gastroenterol 45:999-1007.

Komai-Koma M., Xu D., Li Y., McKenzie A.N., McInnes I.B., Liew F.Y. (2007) IL-33 is a chemoattractant for human Th2 cells. Eur J Immunol 37:2779-86.

Kristjansson G., Venge P., Wanders A., Loof L., Hallgren R. (2004) Clinical and subclinical intestinal inflammation assessed by the mucosal patch technique: studies of mucosal neutrophil and eosinophil activation in inflammatory bowel diseases and irritable bowel syndrome. Gut 53:1806-12.

Kuhn R., Lohler J., Rennick D., Rajewsky K., Muller W. (1993) Interleukin-10-deficient mice develop chronic enterocolitis. Cell 75:263-74.

Kumagai Y., Akira S. (2010) Identification and functions of pattern-recognition receptors. J Allergy Clin Immunol 125:985-92.

Kuroiwa K., Arai T., Okazaki H., Minota S., Tominaga S. (2001) Identification of human ST2 protein in the sera of patients with autoimmune diseases. Biochem Biophys Res Commun 284:1104-8.

Lamkanfi M., Dixit V.M. (2009) IL-33 raises alarm. Immunity 31:5-7.

Langhorst J., Elsenbruch S., Koelzer J., Rueffer A., Michalsen A., Dobos G.J. (2008) Noninvasive markers in the assessment of intestinal inflammation in inflammatory bowel diseases: performance of fecal lactoferrin, calprotectin, and PMN-elastase, CRP, and clinical indices. Am J Gastroenterol 103:162-9.

LeBouder E., Rey-Nores J.E., Rushmere N.K., Grigorov M., Lawn S.D., Affolter M., Griffin G.E., Ferrara P., Schiffrin E.J., Morgan B.P., Labeta M.O. (2003) Soluble forms of Toll-like receptor (TLR)2 capable of modulating TLR2 signaling are present in human plasma and breast milk. J Immunol 171:6680-9.

Lee D.M., Friend D.S., Gurish M.F., Benoist C., Mathis D., Brenner M.B. (2002) Mast cells: a cellular link between autoantibodies and inflammatory arthritis. Science 297:1689-92.

Leung B.P., Xu D., Culshaw S., McInnes I.B., Liew F.Y. (2004) A novel therapy of murine collagen-induced arthritis with soluble T1/ST2. J Immunol 173:145-50.

Li M.C., He S.H. (2004) IL-10 and its related cytokines for treatment of inflammatory bowel disease. World J Gastroenterol 10:620-5.

Li X., Conklin L., Alex P. (2008) New serological biomarkers of inflammatory bowel disease. World J Gastroenterol 14:5115-24.

Lichtenstein G.R., Rutgeerts P. (2010) Importance of mucosal healing in ulcerative colitis. Inflamm Bowel Dis 16:338-46.

Luthi A.U., Cullen S.P., McNeela E.A., Duriez P.J., Afonina I.S., Sheridan C., Brumatti G., Taylor R.C., Kersse K., Vandenabeele P., Lavelle E.C., Martin S.J. (2009) Suppression of interleukin-33 bioactivity through proteolysis by apoptotic caspases. Immunity 31:84-98.

Manolio T.A. (2010) Genomewide association studies and assessment of the risk of disease. N Engl J Med 363:166-76.

McGovern D.P., Gardet A., Torkvist L., Goyette P., Essers J., Taylor K.D., Neale B.M., Ong R.T., Lagace C., Li C., Green T., Stevens C.R., Beauchamp C., Fleshner P.R., Carlson M., D'Amato M., Halfvarson J., Hibberd M.L., Lordal M., Padyukov L., Andriulli A., Colombo E., Latiano A., Palmieri O., Bernard E.J., Deslandres C., Hommes D.W., de Jong D.J., Stokkers P.C., Weersma R.K., Sharma Y., Silverberg M.S., Cho J.H., Wu J., Roeder K., Brant S.R., Schumm L.P., Duerr R.H., Dubinsky M.C., Glazer N.L., Haritunians T., Ippoliti A., Melmed G.Y., Siscovick D.S., Vasiliauskas E.A., Targan S.R., Annese V., Wijmenga C., Pettersson S., Rotter J.I., Xavier R.J., Daly M.J., Rioux J.D., Seielstad M. (2010) Genome-wide association identifies multiple ulcerative colitis susceptibility loci. Nat Genet 42:332-7.

Medzhitov R. (2001) Toll-like receptors and innate immunity. Nat Rev Immunol 1:135-45.

Medzhitov R. (2010) Inflammation 2010: new adventures of an old flame. Cell 140:771-6.

Mok M.Y., Huang F.P., Ip W.K., Lo Y., Wong F.Y., Chan E.Y., Lam K.F., Xu D. (2010) Serum levels of IL-33 and soluble ST2 and their association with disease activity in systemic lupus erythematosus. Rheumatology (Oxford) 49:520-7.

Moritz D.R., Rodewald H.R., Gheyselinck J., Klemenz R. (1998) The IL-1 receptor-related T1 antigen is expressed on immature and mature mast cells and on fetal blood mast cell progenitors. J Immunol 161:4866-74.

Mosser D.M., Zhang X. (2008) Interleukin-10: new perspectives on an old cytokine. Immunol Rev 226:205-18.

Nishida Y., Murase K., Isomoto H., Furusu H., Mizuta Y., Riddell R.H., Kohno S. (2002) Different distribution of mast cells and macrophages in colonic mucosa of patients with collagenous colitis and inflammatory bowel disease. Hepatogastroenterology 49:678-82.

Oboki K., Nakae S., Matsumoto K., Saito H. (2011) IL-33 and Airway Inflammation. Allergy Asthma Immunol Res 3:81-8.

Osada T., Ohkusa T., Yokoyama T., Shibuya T., Sakamoto N., Beppu K., Nagahara A., Otaka M., Ogihara T., Watanabe S. (2010) Comparison of several activity indices for the evaluation of endoscopic activity in UC: inter- and intraobserver consistency. Inflamm Bowel Dis 16:192-7.

Oshikawa K., Kuroiwa K., Tokunaga T., Kato T., Hagihara S.I., Tominaga S.I., Sugiyama Y. (2001a) Acute eosinophilic pneumonia with increased soluble ST2 in serum and bronchoalveolar lavage fluid. Respir Med 95:532-3.

Oshikawa K., Kuroiwa K., Tago K., Iwahana H., Yanagisawa K., Ohno S., Tominaga S.I., Sugiyama Y. (2001b) Elevated soluble ST2 protein levels in sera of patients with asthma with an acute exacerbation. Am J Respir Crit Care Med 164:277-81.

Palmer G., Gabay C. (2011) Interleukin-33 biology with potential insights into human diseases. Nat Rev Rheumatol 7:321-9.

Palmer G., Lipsky B.P., Smithgall M.D., Meininger D., Siu S., Talabot-Ayer D., Gabay C., Smith D.E. (2008) The IL-1 receptor accessory protein (AcP) is required for IL-33 signaling and soluble AcP enhances the ability of soluble ST2 to inhibit IL-33. Cytokine 42:358-64.

Papp M., Norman G.L., Altorjay I., Lakatos P.L. (2007) Utility of serological markers in inflammatory bowel diseases: gadget or magic? World J Gastroenterol 13:2028-36.

Pastorelli L., Garg R.R., Hoang S.B., Spina L., Mattioli B., Scarpa M., Fiocchi C., Vecchi M., Pizarro T.T. (2010) Epithelial-derived IL-33 and its receptor ST2 are dysregulated in ulcerative colitis and in experimental Th1/Th2 driven enteritis. Proc Natl Acad Sci U S A 107:8017-22.

Pecaric-Petkovic T., Didichenko S.A., Kaempfer S., Spiegl N., Dahinden C.A. (2009) Human basophils and eosinophils are the direct target leukocytes of the novel IL-1 family member IL-33. Blood 113:1526-34.

Pezzilli R., Barassi A., Morselli Labate A.M., Finazzi S., Fantini L., Gizzi G., Lotzniker M., Villani V., Melzi d'Eril G., Corinaldesi R. (2008) Fecal calprotectin levels in patients with colonic polyposis. Dig Dis Sci 53:47-51.

Pierik M., Joossens S., Van Steen K., Van Schuerbeek N., Vlietinck R., Rutgeerts P., Vermeire S. (2006) Toll-like receptor-1, -2, and -6 polymorphisms influence disease extension in inflammatory bowel diseases. Inflamm Bowel Dis 12:1-8.

Pineton de Chambrun G., Peyrin-Biroulet L., Lemann M., Colombel J.F. (2010) Clinical implications of mucosal healing for the management of IBD. Nat Rev Gastroenterol Hepatol 7:15-29.

Podolsky D.K. (2002) Inflammatory bowel disease. N Engl J Med 347:417-29.

Poullis A., Foster R., Northfield T.C., Mendall M.A. (2002) Review article: faecal markers in the assessment of activity in inflammatory bowel disease. Aliment Pharmacol Ther 16:675-81.

Rakoff-Nahoum S., Paglino J., Eslami-Varzaneh F., Edberg S., Medzhitov R. (2004) Recognition of commensal microflora by toll-like receptors is required for intestinal homeostasis. Cell 118:229-41.
Rank M.A., Kobayashi T., Kozaki H., Bartemes K.R., Squillace D.L., Kita H. (2009) IL-33-activated dendritic cells induce an atypical TH2-type response. J Allergy Clin Immunol 123:1047-54.
Regueiro M., Rodemann J., Kip K.E., Saul M., Swoger J., Baidoo L., Schwartz M., Barrie A., Binion D. (2011) Physician assessment of ulcerative colitis activity correlates poorly with endoscopic disease activity. Inflamm Bowel Dis 17:1008-14.
Rehman S.U., Mueller T., Januzzi J.L., Jr. (2008) Characteristics of the novel interleukin family biomarker ST2 in patients with acute heart failure. J Am Coll Cardiol 52:1458-65.
Rennick D.M., Fort M.M., Davidson N.J. (1997) Studies with IL-10-/- mice: an overview. J Leukoc Biol 61:389-96.
Rioux J.D., Xavier R.J., Taylor K.D., Silverberg M.S., Goyette P., Huett A., Green T., Kuballa P., Barmada M.M., Datta L.W., Shugart Y.Y., Griffiths A.M., Targan S.R., Ippoliti A.F., Bernard E.J., Mei L., Nicolae D.L., Regueiro M., Schumm L.P., Steinhart A.H., Rotter J.I., Duerr R.H., Cho J.H., Daly M.J., Brant S.R. (2007) Genome-wide association study identifies new susceptibility loci for Crohn disease and implicates autophagy in disease pathogenesis. Nat Genet 39:596-604.
Risch N., Merikangas K. (1996) The future of genetic studies of complex human diseases. Science 273:1516-7.
Rodgers A.D., Cummins A.G. (2007) CRP correlates with clinical score in ulcerative colitis but not in Crohn's disease. Dig Dis Sci 52:2063-8.
Roseth A.G., Kristinsson J., Fagerhol M.K., Schjonsby H., Aadland E., Nygaard K., Roald B. (1993) Faecal calprotectin: a novel test for the diagnosis of colorectal cancer? Scand J Gastroenterol 28:1073-6.
Roussel L., Erard M., Cayrol C., Girard J.P. (2008) Molecular mimicry between IL-33 and KSHV for attachment to chromatin through the H2A-H2B acidic pocket. EMBO Rep 9:1006-12.
Rutgeerts P., Vermeire S., Van Assche G. (2007) Mucosal healing in inflammatory bowel disease: impossible ideal or therapeutic target? Gut 56:453-5.
Sanada S., Hakuno D., Higgins L.J., Schreiter E.R., McKenzie A.N., Lee R.T. (2007) IL-33 and ST2 comprise a critical biomechanically induced and cardioprotective signaling system. J Clin Invest 117:1538-49.
Schleimer R.P., Kato A., Kern R., Kuperman D., Avila P.C. (2007) Epithelium: at the interface of innate and adaptive immune responses. J Allergy Clin Immunol 120:1279-84.
Schmitz J., Owyang A., Oldham E., Song Y., Murphy E., McClanahan T.K., Zurawski G., Moshrefi M., Qin J., Li X., Gorman D.M., Bazan J.F., Kastelein R.A. (2005) IL-33, an interleukin-1-like cytokine that signals via the IL-1 receptor-related protein ST2 and induces T helper type 2-associated cytokines. Immunity 23:479-90.
Schoepfer A.M., Beglinger C., Straumann A., Trummler M., Vavricka S.R., Bruegger L.E., Seibold F. (2010) Fecal calprotectin correlates more closely with the Simple Endoscopic Score for Crohn's disease (SES-CD) than CRP, blood leukocytes, and the CDAI. Am J Gastroenterol 105:162-9.

Seidelin J.B., Bjerrum J.T., Coskun M., Widjaya B., Vainer B., Nielsen O.H. (2010) IL-33 is upregulated in colonocytes of ulcerative colitis. Immunol Lett 128:80-5.

Seiderer J., Brand S., Herrmann K.A., Schnitzler F., Hatz R., Crispin A., Pfennig S., Schoenberg S.O., Goke B., Lohse P., Ochsenkuhn T. (2006) Predictive value of the CARD15 variant 1007fs for the diagnosis of intestinal stenoses and the need for surgery in Crohn's disease in clinical practice: results of a prospective study. Inflamm Bowel Dis 12:1114-21.

Shih D.Q., Targan S.R. (2008) Immunopathogenesis of inflammatory bowel disease. World J Gastroenterol 14:390-400.

Shimizu M., Matsuda A., Yanagisawa K., Hirota T., Akahoshi M., Inomata N., Ebe K., Tanaka K., Sugiura H., Nakashima K., Tamari M., Takahashi N., Obara K., Enomoto T., Okayama Y., Gao P.S., Huang S.K., Tominaga S., Ikezawa Z., Shirakawa T. (2005) Functional SNPs in the distal promoter of the ST2 gene are associated with atopic dermatitis. Hum Mol Genet 14:2919-27.

Silverberg M.S., Satsangi J., Ahmad T., Arnott I.D., Bernstein C.N., Brant S.R., Caprilli R., Colombel J.F., Gasche C., Geboes K., Jewell D.P., Karban A., Loftus Jr E.V., Pena A.S., Riddell R.H., Sachar D.B., Schreiber S., Steinhart A.H., Targan S.R., Vermeire S., Warren B.F. (2005) Toward an integrated clinical, molecular and serological classification of inflammatory bowel disease: Report of a Working Party of the 2005 Montreal World Congress of Gastroenterology. Can J Gastroenterol 19 Suppl A:5-36.

Sipponen T., Savilahti E., Kolho K.L., Nuutinen H., Turunen U., Farkkila M. (2008) Crohn's disease activity assessed by fecal calprotectin and lactoferrin: correlation with Crohn's disease activity index and endoscopic findings. Inflamm Bowel Dis 14:40-6.

Solem C.A., Loftus E.V., Jr., Tremaine W.J., Harmsen W.S., Zinsmeister A.R., Sandborn W.J. (2005) Correlation of C-reactive protein with clinical, endoscopic, histologic, and radiographic activity in inflammatory bowel disease. Inflamm Bowel Dis 11:707-12.

Stolarski B., Kurowska-Stolarska M., Kewin P., Xu D., Liew F.Y. (2010) IL-33 exacerbates eosinophil-mediated airway inflammation. J Immunol 185:3472-80.

Summerton C.B., Longlands M.G., Wiener K., Shreeve D.R. (2002) Faecal calprotectin: a marker of inflammation throughout the intestinal tract. Eur J Gastroenterol Hepatol 14:841-5.

Suzukawa M., Iikura M., Koketsu R., Nagase H., Tamura C., Komiya A., Nakae S., Matsushima K., Ohta K., Yamamoto K., Yamaguchi M. (2008a) An IL-1 cytokine member, IL-33, induces human basophil activation via its ST2 receptor. J Immunol 181:5981-9.

Suzukawa M., Koketsu R., Iikura M., Nakae S., Matsumoto K., Nagase H., Saito H., Matsushima K., Ohta K., Yamamoto K., Yamaguchi M. (2008b) Interleukin-33 enhances adhesion, CD11b expression and survival in human eosinophils. Lab Invest 88:1245-53.

Takezako N., Hayakawa M., Hayakawa H., Aoki S., Yanagisawa K., Endo H., Tominaga S. (2006) ST2 suppresses IL-6 production via the inhibition of IkappaB degradation induced by the LPS signal in THP-1 cells. Biochem Biophys Res Commun 341:425-32.

Talabot-Ayer D., Lamacchia C., Gabay C., Palmer G. (2009) Interleukin-33 is biologically active independently of caspase-1 cleavage. J Biol Chem 284:19420-6.

Thompson A.I., Lees C.W. (2011) Genetics of ulcerative colitis. Inflamm Bowel Dis 17:831-48. DOI: 10.1002/ibd.21375.

Tibble J., Sigthorsson G., Foster R., Sherwood R., Fagerhol M., Bjarnason I. (2001) Faecal calprotectin and faecal occult blood tests in the diagnosis of colorectal carcinoma and adenoma. Gut 49:402-8.

Tibble J.A., Bjarnason I. (2001) Non-invasive investigation of inflammatory bowel disease. World J Gastroenterol 7:460-5.

Tibble J.A., Sigthorsson G., Foster R., Forgacs I., Bjarnason I. (2002) Use of surrogate markers of inflammation and Rome criteria to distinguish organic from nonorganic intestinal disease. Gastroenterology 123:450-60.

Tominaga S., Jenkins N.A., Gilbert D.J., Copeland N.G., Tetsuka T. (1991) Molecular cloning of the murine ST2 gene. Characterization and chromosomal mapping. Biochim Biophys Acta 1090:1-8.

Vermeire S., Van Assche G., Rutgeerts P. (2004) C-reactive protein as a marker for inflammatory bowel disease. Inflamm Bowel Dis 10:661-5.

Vermeire S., Van Assche G., Rutgeerts P. (2006) Laboratory markers in IBD: useful, magic, or unnecessary toys? Gut 55:426-31.

Vermeire S., Van Assche G., Rutgeerts P. (2010) Role of genetics in prediction of disease course and response to therapy. World J Gastroenterol 16:2609-15.

Verri W.A., Jr., Souto F.O., Vieira S.M., Almeida S.C., Fukada S.Y., Xu D., Alves-Filho J.C., Cunha T.M., Guerrero A.T., Mattos-Guimaraes R.B., Oliveira F.R., Teixeira M.M., Silva J.S., McInnes I.B., Ferreira S.H., Louzada-Junior P., Liew F.Y., Cunha F.Q. (2010) IL-33 induces neutrophil migration in rheumatoid arthritis and is a target of anti-TNF therapy. Ann Rheum Dis 69:1697-703.

Wang F., Tahara T., Arisawa T., Shibata T., Nakamura M., Fujita H., Iwata M., Kamiya Y., Nagasaka M., Takahama K., Watanabe M., Hirata I., Nakano H. (2007) Genetic polymorphisms of CD14 and Toll-like receptor-2 (TLR2) in patients with ulcerative colitis. J Gastroenterol Hepatol 22:925-9.

Wang T., Lafuse W.P., Zwilling B.S. (2001) NFkappaB and Sp1 elements are necessary for maximal transcription of toll-like receptor 2 induced by Mycobacterium avium. J Immunol 167:6924-32.

Weinberg E.O. (2009) ST2 protein in heart disease: from discovery to mechanisms and prognostic value. Biomark Med 3:495-511.

Weinberg E.O., Shimpo M., Hurwitz S., Tominaga S., Rouleau J.L., Lee R.T. (2003) Identification of serum soluble ST2 receptor as a novel heart failure biomarker. Circulation 107:721-6.

Xavier R.J., Podolsky D.K. (2007) Unravelling the pathogenesis of inflammatory bowel disease. Nature 448:427-34.

Zhao W., Hu Z. (2010) The enigmatic processing and secretion of interleukin-33. Cell Mol Immunol 7:260-2.

Zhernakova A., Festen E.M., Franke L., Trynka G., van Diemen C.C., Monsuur A.J., Bevova M., Nijmeijer R.M., van 't Slot R., Heijmans R., Boezen H.M., van Heel D.A., van Bodegraven A.A., Stokkers P.C., Wijmenga C., Crusius J.B., Weersma R.K. (2008) Genetic analysis of innate immunity in Crohn's disease and ulcerative colitis identifies two susceptibility loci harboring CARD9 and IL18RAP. Am J Hum Genet 82:1202-10.

3

Ulcerative Colitis and Microorganisms

José Miguel Sahuquillo Arce and Agustín Iranzo Tatay
Hospital Universitari i Politècnic La Fe
Spain

1. Introduction

The gut, due to its anatomical and functional characteristics, forms the largest area of contact with the outside world. Unlike skin that acts as a defensive barrier, digestive and absorptive processes in the intestine require a certain amount of permeability. This facilitates and creates an optimal niche for the development of a large community of microorganisms that maintains, ideally, a commensal relationship with the host. This ecosystem, known as microbiota, is essential for the digestion of certain carbohydrates, the production and metabolism of nutrients necessary for life and for proper development and maturation of the immune system.

The aim of this chapter is to offer a thorough review of recent publications and scholarly work in order to explain, and somehow clarify, the always complex interaction between humans and microorganisms, as well as the implications that the later have in Ulcerative Colitis.

1.1 The human microbiota

Should we consider the number of microorganisms that live in the mucous linings of human beings, we should be considered merely as the base that supports and nourishes a large microbial ecosystem. Indeed, the total amount of bacteria that colonize our gut reaches about 100 trillion, while the number of cells in our body is no more than 10 trillion. The physiological and environmental differences of each part of the body determine the existence of many different niches, each with its unique microflora adapted to the nutritional resources, pH and presence of antibacterial substances. The capabilities inherent to the colonizing organisms such as the presence of pili or fimbriae which facilitate adherence to epithelial cells, the specific metabolic pathways that each genus is able to develop or the cell wall components that confer increased resistance to the environment are also vital.

The large intestine is by far the location with the greatest number of microorganisms which establish a symbiotic relationship that is broadly beneficial to the host. Over 98% of the microbiota that is found past the ileocaecal valve consists of strict anaerobes, outnumbering aerobic bacteria in a ratio of 1/1,000- 1/10,000. Numerous studies performed hitherto describe microbiota as having between 200 and 1,000 different species of bacteria in healthy subjects any given time, with horizontal transmission of genetic material between species. This means that there is great diversity among the microbiota of different people, and that there is no common core related to all humans, since no particular species is more than 1%

of the total. Only about 50-100 bacteria were found in most individuals regardless of their number. On the other hand, it has been observed that the changes that occur over the lifetime of a healthy person are minimal, the most dramatic being at the beginning of life, since initial colonization after birth until weaning, when the microbiota begins to transform and becomes gradually very similar to that of an adult. These changes are determined by the geographic location with their characteristic eating habits, by the type of birth (caesarean versus vaginal delivery), and the type of feeding after birth (breast vs. bottle). Eventually, the microbiota is composed mostly (> 90%) by bacteria of the genera *Bacteroides* and *Bifidobacterium*, and the rest by *Eubacterium*, *Lactobacillus*, coliforms, *Streptococcus*, *Clostridium*, and a variable number of yeasts.

As an indirect consequence of the large number and variety of microorganisms, the balance achieved between the components of the microbiota and the competition for nutritional resources exert a protective effect on the host by preventing colonization and proliferation of potential pathogens.

This huge set of microorganisms contains approximately three million of unique genes, i.e. 150 times more genes than our own genome. This metagenome or microbiome is essential for proper homeostasis and good health, as it provides metabolic pathways that allow implementations that we would be unable to perform without the assistance of the intestinal microbiota, like digestion of some sugars, production of vitamins or removal of hydrogen in the distal intestine. Recent studies have demonstrated a common set of around 500,000 unique genes shared by the microbiota of different subjects, in other words, a common metagenome. For all this, it has been suggested that the microbiota serves as an organ for human beings (Zhu et al., 2010).

In addition to these functions, the intestinal epithelium requires intestinal flora and the substances excreted by it in order to develop properly, given that these metabolic by-products promote growth and epithelial differentiation.

1.2 Microbiota and immune system

The intestinal lumen is comparable to a battlefield; there is a continuous struggle even when the host does not show any type of pathology. Indeed, the intestinal epithelium is extensively infiltrated by lymphocytes with defensive functions. More profoundly, in the lamina propria, dendritic cells are responsible for monitoring the presence of pathogenic antigens and activate surrounding lymphocytes if necessary. It has been established that there is a continuous exchange of information and regulation between epithelial and immune cells present in the intestinal mucosa, mainly through Toll-like receptors on the cell membrane and the Nucleotide-binding oligomerization domains in the cell cytosol, but also, by other substances that need further investigation so their functioning is utterly understood. The end result of this cross-talk is the development and maturation of lymphocytes Th 1, Th 2, Th 17 (a type of lymphocyte abundant in the intestine but scarce elsewhere in the body), regulatory T cells, IgA-secreting plasma cells and the release into the intestinal lumen of bactericidal substance like the defensins (Tanoue et al., 2010; Sansonetti , 2010). All this leads to the subsequent inflammatory response or tolerance reaction; but also to systemic immune defence maturation, as neutrophils, in the absence of intestinal flora, lack the necessary priming to be effective (Takeshi et al., 2010).

Several studies have shown that a plural and abundant microbiota is essential to maintain a balance between defensive immune responses and tolerance towards commensal bacteria

(Salzman, 2010; Tanoue et al., 2010; Lidar et al., 2009). But some bacteria seem to have a more significant role than others:

- Segmented Filamentous Bacteria, a Gram-positive bacteria related to *Clostridium*, also known as *Candidatus arthromitus*, is capable by itself of stimulating the differentiation of Th 17 cells, which by producing IL-17 attracts neutrophils and macrophages to the gut mucosa. But on the other hand, these bacteria also stimulate the IgA-producing plasma cells, an antibody that blocks bacterial antigens in the intestinal lumen and prevents the possible infiltration and local inflammation while regulating the ecological balance of the commensal flora. This bacterium is not found in the mucus above the epithelial layer, instead, it attaches intimately to the epithelial cells (Takeshi et al., 2010).
- A Gram-negative bacterium, *Bacteroides thetaiotaomicron*, whose presence down-regulates inflammation by activation of the nuclear export of RelA, subunit of Nuclear Factor kappa B, a substance with inflammatory properties that enhances gene transcription when located inside the nucleus (Takeshi et al., 2010). This protein complex is related to the receptor responsible for the anti-inflammatory properties of 5-aminosalicylic acid.
- Two species of Gram-positive rods, *Lactobacillus* spp. and *Bifidobacterium* spp., and a Gram-negative rod, *Bacteroides fragilis*, induce the maturation of regulatory T cells in the lamina propria, stimulating the production of IL-10, an immunosuppressive interleukin (Danase, 2011; Takeshi et al., 2010).

1.3 Microorganisms as causative agents in ulcerative colitis

Since the description of inflammatory bowel disease as an independent clinical entity, attempts have been made to associate it with a particular microorganism as an aetiological agent, as happened with *Helycobacter pylori* and gastric ulcer. Several studies have shown some involvement of a number of pathogens in the onset of Ulcerative Colitis flares, but to date, no study has concluded a positive relation between a microorganism and this disease:

- *Cytomegalovirus* and *Clostridium difficile* are able to develop a condition similar to Ulcerative Colitis, precipitate a relapse or worsen the course (Lawlor et al., 2010; Sonnenberg, 2010). In addition, it has been found a linear geographical relationship between Ulcerative Colitis cases and colitis due to *C. difficile.*
- *Escherichia coli, Campylobacter jejuni, Salomonella enterica* and *Shigella* spp. have been associated with this disease because of their ability to disrupt the intestinal epithelium, promote a displacement of commensal flora and trigger an excessive inflammatory response (Gasull et al., 2007; Phalipon & Sansonetti, 2003; Siegel et al.,2005).
- *Mycobacterium avium paratuberculosis* has been associated with Crohn's disease, but some studies suggest it may have some relevance in patients with impaired intracellular bacteria destruction by a continuous augmented state of inflammation.

The most recent lines of research point to the dysbiosis as the cause of up-regulated inflammation. Several studies have discovered that the microbiota of Ulcerative Colitis patients is significantly different from that of healthy controls (Danase, 2011; Scarpa et al., 2011). Although, a causal relationship was not establish because these changes in the microbiota could be either the cause or the consequence of the alterations observed in the intestinal epithelium. Thus far, this hypothesis is to some extent supported by some other studies that point toward the transplant of healthy microbiota as a solution to the disease, with very promising results (Do et al., 2010; Kahn et al., 2011; Ng et al., 2010).

The main theories that try to explain Ulcerative Colitis aetiopathogenesis by means of an infectious agent can be summarized as follows:

- Dysbiosis hypothesis which implies that an imbalance between beneficial versus detrimental resident intestinal bacterial species may incite chronic inflammatory responses (Friswell et al. 2010).
- Persistent infection hypothesis which proposes that Ulcerative Colitis may arise as a result of persistent infection with enteric pathogens (Khan et al., 2011).
- Luminal antigen translocation hypothesis which indicates that defects in the intestinal barrier function or impaired mucosal clearance facilitate increased translocation of luminal antigens, including intestinal commensal bacteria, across the intestinal barrier where they may prime mucosal immune responses that lead to loss of immunological tolerance toward the luminal antigens (Fava & Danes, 2011).
- Hygiene hypothesis which postulates that helminthic colonization of the gut shifts immune response towards Th 2 and Th 3, i.e., humoural and regulatory pathways. Thus, prevention of parasitic helminths by means of improved hygiene, may be one factor leading to Ulcerative Colitis through a excessive Th 1 immune response (Weinstock & Elliot, 2008).

In summary, the relationship between the microbiota and its host is very complex and studies to date suggest that the aetiology of Ulcerative Colitis is equally complex. Beyond the characteristics of the patient, a myriad of microorganisms capable of modulating the inflammatory response come into play. To find a single responsible among them challenges conventional models of infectious disease, and small variations in the concentration or location of commensal microorganisms may be the key.

2. Immunosuppressive therapy in ulcerative colitis

Immunosuppressive drugs are used increasingly and earlier for the treatment of Ulcerative Colitis. This implies an important risk factor for these patients since they become partially defenceless against possible microbiological pathogens. Moreover, the degree of immunosuppression may be exacerbated by factors such as older age (Cottone et al., 2010), severity of symptoms and comorbidities, recent surgery or malnutrition. In addition, more severe conditions or those that do not respond to treatment involve a greater degree of immunosuppression due to the fact that the combination of two or more drugs is required (Koutroubakis, 2010). Table 1 summarizes immunosupression impairments and the most common microorganisms associated.

2.1 Corticosteroids

Corticosteroids suppress the Th 1 response by inhibiting the transcription of genes encoding pro-inflammatory interleukins, chiefly IL-2; thereby reducing the proliferation and activation of T cells. However, the Th 2 response is also altered, given that B lymphocytes express fewer IL-2 receptors and consequently, there is a reduction in the production of antibodies (Elenkov, 2004).

This reduction in pro-inflammatory cytokines tampers the chemotactic migration of neutrophils to the inflammatory focus, diminishing also its ability to adhere and its phagocytic function.

Phagocytosis of opsonised microorganisms is also disturbed as the expression of FC receptors in macrophages is down-regulated too (Franchimont, 2004).

Immune response impairment	Microorganisms
Neutropenia	*Staphylococcus aureus*, Gram-negative rods, *Aspergillus*, *Candida*
Phagocytic function	*Streptococcus pneumoniae*, *Haemophilus influenzae*
Chemotaxis	*Sataphylococcus aureus*, *Mucor*
T lymphocytes (Th 1 response)	*Mycobacterium*, *Nocardia*, *Legionella*, *Aspergillus*, *Candida*, *Cryptococcus neoformans*, *Pneumocystis jiroveci*, Cytomegalovirus, *Herpes simplex virus*, *Varicella-Zoster virus*, respiratory viruses, *Strongyloides*, *Toxoplasma*, *Leishmania*
B lymphocytes (Th 2 response)	*Staphylococcus aureus* , *Streptococcus pneumoniae*, *Haemophilus influenzae*, *Pneumocystis jiroveci*, *Enterobacteriaceae*

Table 1. Immune System impairment and most common associated microorganisms

2.2 Purine analogues: Azathioprine and 6-mercaptopurine

Azathioprine is a pro-drug that is converted into 6-mercaptopurine by human metabolism. 6-thioguanine nucleotides, the resulting metabolites, accumulate in tissues where they exert their cytotoxic effects by inhibiting purine synthesis and consequently, DNA and RNA. Therefore, a decrease in the production of T and B lymphocytes is achieved; they also promote apoptosis of activated T lymphocytes. Thus, both the Th 1 and Th 2 immune responses are impaired (Sahasranaman et al., 2008; Tiede et al. 2003).

The therapeutic effects of these drugs are achieved within 2-3 months from administration, and duration of treatment depends on adverse effects and patient's tolerance, so that the time period of immunosuppression that the patient will face can be considerable (Maltzman & Koretzky, 2003).

2.3 Calcineurin inhibitors: Tacrolimus and cyclosporine

Calcineurin inhibitors decrease the cellular immune response by inhibiting T-dependent antibody production and several cytokines, chiefly IL-2 but also IL-3, IL-4, IL-5, Tumour Necrosis Factor alpha and beta. A reduction in the number of activated T lymphocytes is achieved with a significant decrease in the Th 1 response. Numerous studies have shown that calcineurin inhibitors can be effective for short-term clinical improvement in patients with refractory disease, but also could be used in situations that require an early and powerful response as in fulminant Ulcerative Colitis. The use of these drugs requires careful assessment of risks and benefits, and close surveillance of adverse effects.

2.4 Biological therapies

Biological drugs block the action of Tumour Necrosis Factor alpha, a pro-inflammatory cytokine, and promote apoptosis of activated T cells, inhibiting Th 1 immune response and local inflammation. Monoclonal antibodies anti-Tumour Necrosis Factor alpha mechanism of action includes the neutralization of both soluble and transmembrane portion of this molecule; also neutralizes Tumour Necrosis Factor alpha-producing (Sandborn, 2010; Smolen, 2011). Monoclonal antibodies anti-Tumour Necrosis Factor alpha were first used in the treatment of Crohn's disease but have been used successfully in severe, unresponsive to treatment Ulcerative Colitis or as rescue therapy (Hoentjen & van Bodegraven, 2009; Lees et al. 2007).

3. Ulcerative colitis and infection

Patients suffering from Ulcerative Colitis may develop infections just like any healthy person. However, there are a number of situations and conditions that make these infections critical; hence they must be addressed as soon as possible in order to avoid unwanted or unexpected complications.

On the one hand, these patients present an altered immunity, which predisposes them to face a number of opportunistic microorganisms that seldom cause disease in healthy people. Second, they are challenged with infections from typical and common pathogens, but in their state of immunosuppression this microorganisms may have a more aggressive course and a worse prognosis (Harbaum et al., 2010; Nagasaki et al., 2010). Local disorders in the digestive tract result in another source for potential complications, allowing the displacement of bacteria from the normal microbiota which are harmless otherwise (Sahuquillo-Arce et al., 2008). Finally, these patients may need surgical treatment, aggravating local immunosuppression as well as increasing susceptibility to infection (Scarpa et al. 2011).

Although large studies of patients with Ulcerative Colitis show a low prevalence of opportunistic infections, there are numerous articles about specific cases reports or short series of such infections, which confirm the severity that these infections can acquired in Ulcerative Colitis patients (Aoyagi et al., 1999; Chuang et al., 2010; Escher et al., 2010; Kudo et al., 2010; Rodríguez-Peláez et al., 2010).

An early suspicion of these complications is essential to enhance prognosis in this group of patients, so physicians must improve their knowledge and be aware about these infections. The management of immunocompromised patient is difficult; therefore, an early diagnosis and a prompt establishment of an adequate therapeutic regimen remain the two fundamental pillars that will determine the course and outcome of infection.

3.1 Management of the patient before infection

The infectious and immunological history of the patient should be defined when Ulcerative Colitis is first diagnosed, and whenever possible, before starting immunosuppressive therapy (Viguet et al., 2008). This will require a thorough knowledge about the patient and a systematic record of every detail (Rahier et al., 2009) in order to assess:

- The history of past infections and travels to areas with endemic infections, even if those travels are distant in time.
- A methodical review of systems, including regular dental and gynaecological evaluation.
- A serological screening to evaluate the immune status against the following viruses: rubella, measles, mumps, *Varicella-Zoster*, *Cytomegalovirus*, *Epstein-Barr*, hepatitis B, hepatitis C, HIV, poliovirus; and against tetanus, diphtheria and *Toxoplasma gondii*.

- Any contact with *Mycobacterium tuberculosis* by means of a chest X-ray and tuberculin skin test (with a booster if negative) or interferon-gamma release assays (Schoepfer et al. 2009), in patients who have not suffered from tuberculosis in the past. These tests should always be performed, but they are mandatory before initiating therapy with anti-Tumour Necrosis Factor alpha drugs.

The use of vaccines is another important step in managing these patients. Besides the recommended vaccinations for the general population, the following should also be considered (Aberra & Lichtenstein, 2005):

- *Varicella-Zoster* in seronegative patients, preferably before starting immunosuppressive therapy since this vaccine contains attenuated viruses. Passive immunization should be considered in seronegative high risk immunosupressed patients after exposure to the virus.
- Pneumococcal vaccination with booster after 3-5 years.
- Hepatitis B, which may require a booster due to immunosuppressive therapy.
- *Influenzavirus* annually.
- *Papillomavirus* in young women, according to national guidelines.
- Travel vaccines; the practitioner must bear in mind that vaccines which contain live viruses should be avoided.

3.2 Management of patients with suspicion of infection

The diagnosis of infection begins with a thorough anamnesis, which should reflect the degree and time length of immunosuppression of the patient, concomitant diseases, use of antineoplastic or antimicrobial treatments, presence of catheters, previous infections and any possible exposure to nosocomial, occupational or unusual pathogens, such as travels to endemic areas of histoplasmosis, coccidioidomycosis, etc. These factors will be crucial in establishing an empirical treatment (Gómez Gómez & Gobernado, 2011).

A systematic physical examination will be the next step. Given that very often the symptoms that immunosuppressed patients present are scarce or absent, and that fever can be the only one, the physician's attitude should be aggressive in order to locate the source of infection. To describe all the necessary tests for the diagnosis of these patients is beyond the scope of this chapter, but there are a number of important considerations that must be taken into account:

- A CT yields better performance than X-ray in pulmonary infections (Sahuquillo-Arce & Menéndez-Villanueva, 2010).
- Infections of the digestive tract can be misleading and may be interpreted as an Ulcerative Colitis relapse. It may require tissue biopsy for microbiological and histopathological studies, as well as all the usual non-invasive tests such as stool culture, study of parasites or detection of *C. difficile* toxins.
- Central nervous system infections may require a MRI or even a biopsy, especially if space-occupying lesions are observed.

3.3 Opportunistic microorganisms and common infectious agents

The following is a brief description of the most frequent opportunistic microorganisms found in immunosuppressed patients; but we will also discuss about typical pathogens that may have a ominous prognosis chiefly due to the poor immune system of the host (Murray et al., 2003; Rahier et al., 2009).

3.3.1 Bacteria

These microorganisms constitute the commonest group of infectious agents in both gastrointestinal and other systems infections. Three different groups can be distinguished:

- Nosocomial infections by pathogens that may present antimicrobial multi-resistance such as *Pseudomonas aeruginosa.*
- Community-acquired microorganisms which, in these patients, may be more devastating and with greater tendency to spread, such as *Streptococcus pneumoniae.*
- Endogenous microorganisms which were under control before immunosuppression (Qu et al., 2009).

The following are the most relevant of bacterial pathogens, both common and opportunistic. Recommended treatments for opportunistic and common bacterial pathogens are shown in table 2.

- *Pseudomonas aeruginosa* is a Gram-negative rod found in nature, which colonizes the hospital setting. Among the many virulence factors it has, adhesion to the epithelium, toxin production, biofilm formation and quorum sensing are essential for its great adaptation and survivability. This bacterium is associated with nosocomial infections, mechanical ventilation infection, wound infections and community-acquired pneumonia, chiefly in immunosuppressed patients who have been in contact with the hospital environment. The most challenging infection is pneumonia, as it is rapidly progressive and radiographically indistinguishable from other pyogenic infections. Patients present with productive cough, fever, dyspnoea, micro-abscesses and focal haemorrhage. Mortality is very high among immunosuppressed patients because of its rapid course, it reaches up to 40%, and this ratio increases if there is bacteraemia. Antimicrobial treatment is problematic because of its intrinsic resistance to many broad-spectrum antibiotics, especially considering that hospital-acquired strains present a greater number of resistances due to selection in a hostile antimicrobial environment.
- *Staphylococcus aureus* is a Gram-positive coccus that colonizes the skin and is a major nosocomial pathogen. Between 10-40% of people are nasal carriers. It has several virulence factors, including toxin production and antibiotic resistance. Methicillin resistant strains (MRSA) vary in proportion between countries (2% in the Netherlands, 28% in Spain, 54% in Portugal). It is more frequent in hospitals and health-care associated settings. This pathogen is very versatile and can produce different clinical syndromes ranging from conditions like skin or surgical wound infection to bacteraemia, meningitis, or a highly aggressive type of pneumonia that occurs after an Influenzavirus infection.
- *Streptococcus pneumoniae* is a Gram-positive coccus that can be found in the nasopharynx of healthy carriers. It is an important agent of community-acquired pneumonia, but it can also emerge as sinusitis, otitis, bacteraemia or meningitis.
- *Nocardia* spp. is a Gram-positive partially acid-fast branched rod. Ubiquitous in the environment, it is acquired primarily by inhalation. Pulmonary nocardiosis supposes over 40% of all forms, and *Nocardia asteroides complex* is responsible for up to 90%. It can follow an acute course, but chronic forms are more likely, presenting as a recurrent suppurative process with or without abscess formation, cavitation, or fistula. Other types include surgical wound infection or disseminated forms that can affect the central nervous system. The prognosis depends on the patient's immunosuppression level and bacterial dissemination.

Microorganism	Treatment	Alternative treatment
Empirical treatment	Amikacin + piperacillin-tazobactam, imipenem or meropenem	Empirical treatment should be adapted to more likely microoganisms, local antimicrobial resistance patterns and prior infections.
Pseudomonas aeruginosa	Ceftazidime; cefepime; aztreonam; Piperacillin-tazobactam or carbapenem Associate aminoglycoside + ciprofloxacin or colistin in severe systemic infection.	
Staphylococcus aureus	Methicilin susceptible *S. aureus*: Cloxacillin + gentamicin. Methicilin resistant *S. aureus*: glycopeptide. If vancomycin MIC is > 1 mg/l then linezolid or daptomycin.	MSSA: amoxicillin-clavulanate; ampicillin-sulbactam; 1st-2nd generation cephalosporins; clindamycin; levofloxacin or moxifloxacin. MRSA: Linezolid; tigecycline or minocycline
Listeria monocytogenes	Ampicillin alone or associated with gentamicin	Cotrimoxazole alone or associated with ampicillin or rifampicin. Clarithromycin, doxycycline, rifampicin, moxifloxacin, levofloxacin, meropenem, linezolid and vancomycin are also active
Nocardia spp.	Cotrimoxazole + amikacin, cefotaxime, ceftriaxone or imipenem.	Linezolid; levofloxacin; moxifloxacin, tigecycline; doxycycline; minocycline or amoxicillin-clavulanate
Stenotrophomonas maltophilia	Cotrimoxazole + minocycline, tigecycline, moxifloxacin, levofloxacin, aztreonam, ceftazidime, rifampicin or colistin.	Tigecycline; fluorquinolone or ceftazidime
Acinetobacter baumannii	Imipenem + sulbactam or amikacin	Associate two or more of the following according to antibiogram: Tigecycline, colistin, doripenem, ceftazidime, doxycycline, minocycline piperacillin-tazobactam, tobramycin, rifampicin and levofloxacin

Microorganism	Treatment	Alternative treatment
Enterobacter spp.	Carbapenem or fluoroquinolone	Cefepime; Piperacillin-tazobactam; aminoglycosides; tigecycline; cotrimoxazole or colistin.
M. tuberculosis	Isoniazid+rifampicin+pyrazinamide for two months, then 4 months on isoniazid + rifampicin. Add ethambutol the first two months if high suspicion of Multi-drug resistance.	Ethambutol or streptomycin instead of pyrazinamide. Ethambutol + levofloxacin or moxifloxacin instead of isoniazid. isoniazida + pyrazinamide + ethambutol for 12 months if rifampicin is not possible. Levofloxacin o moxifloxacin can be added the first two months.
M. kansasii	Isoniazid + rifampicin + ethambutol	Amikacin; clarithromycin; streptomycin; fluoroquinolone or ethambutol if rifampicin resistance. Sulfamethoxazole; linezolid or cycloserine can be used instead of ethambutol
M. avium complex	Macrolides (azithromycin or clarithromycin) + ethambutol + rifampicin or rifabutin three times a week, or dialy if cavitation or dissemination	Streptomycin or amikacin + ethambutol + rifampicin or ribabutin if macrolide resistance. Consider addition of moxifloxacin. Consider surgical excision in antimicrobial therapy failure.
M. xenopi	Isoniazid + rifampicin + ethambutol and/or streptomycin	

Table 2. Recommended treatments for bacterial pathogens in immunocompromised patients (Mensa et al., 2011)

- *Listeria monocytogenes* is a Gram-positive rod widely distributed in the environment, circumstance that facilitates its incorporation into food production and processing. Moreover, it can grow at 4°C and become a food-borne disease. Typically, it causes meningitis, encephalitis and sepsis in cell-mediated immunocompromised patients. It has also been linked to intestinal lesions in Ulcerative Colitis patients.
- *Legionella pneumophila* is an intracellular Gram-negative rod widely distributed in aquatic environments. Pneumonia by this pathogen in immunocompromised patients can be severe and life threatening. Corticosteroid treatment is a major risk factor.
- Nonfermentative Gram-negative bacilli and *Enterobacteriaceae* such as *Acinetobacter baumannii, Stenotrophomonas maltophilia* or *Enterobacter* spp. are increasingly becoming relevant as nosocomial pathogens which endanger the lives of patients during the

immediate postoperative period. Furthermore, these bacteria have multiple acquired and intrinsic antimicrobial resistances that complicate treatment.

Microorganism	**Treatment**	**Alternative treatment**
Escherichia coli	Aminopenicillin + betalactamase inhibitor; 2nd- 3rd generation cephalosporin or aztreonam. Fosfomycin or nitrofurantoin can be used in urinary tract infections. Enteritis: fluoroquinolone or cotrimoxazole (Patients with enterohaemorrhagic *E. coli* who are treated can develop HUS)	Carbapemen; tygecycline or colistina if Extended-Spectrum Betalactamase *E.coli*.
Shigella spp.	Ciprofloxacin	Cotrimoxazole, ceftriaxone, cefixime or azithromycin
Salmonella enterica	Typhoid fever: ceftriaxone; cefixime or azithromycin. Enteritis: fluoroquinolone. Bacteraemia: 3rd generation cephalosporin; aztreonam or ciprofloxacin for a month.	Typhoid fever: ciprofloxacin; aminopenicillin; chloramphenicol or cotrimoxazole. Bacteraemia: Aminopenicillin.
Yersinia spp. (other than *Y. pestis*)	Ciprofloxacin 3rd generation cephalosporin + gentamicin for systemic infection	Doxycycline or Cotrimoxazole
Campilobacter jejuni	Erithromycin or azithromycin	Imipenem or aminopenicillin + betalactamase inhibitor
Clostridium difficile	Mild course: metronidazole p.o. More aggressive forms: vancomycin Consider association with metronidazole i.v. or gammaglobulin in severe forms	Teicoplanin; fusidic acid; nitazoxanide; rifampicin p.o. or tygecycline i.v.

Table 3. Recommended treatments for enteric bacterial pathogens in immunocompromised patients (Mensa et al., 2011)

- *Mycobacterium tuberculosis* presents a low incidence around 2%, despite the fact that the risk of active tuberculosis in immunosuppressed patients is 30-50 times higher than in the general population. The main risk factor is reactivation of latent infection, thus screening for tuberculosis before initiating therapy is required, in particular in those who will receive anti-Tumour Necrosis Factor alpha antibodies. In immunocompromised patients, *M. tuberculosis* is often more rapidly progressive and disseminates more frequently. Multi-drug resistant isolates are a worldwide concern that jeopardizes the final outcome.

- Other mycobacteria such as *M. kansasii, M. avium complex* or *M. xenopi,* can appear as opportunistic pathogens primarily affecting the lung. They all have, in immunocompromised patients, an incidence similar to that of *M. tuberculosis.* Diagnosis is difficult because it requires the presence of symptoms, isolation of the microorganism in at least three respiratory samples and radiological signs or response to antimicrobial treatment.

Recommended treatments for enteric bacterial pathogens are shown in table 3.

- *Campylobacter jejuni* is a Gram-negative curve-shaped rod and the most common cause of community-acquired acute bacterial diarrhoea. It is normally accompanied by fever and abdominal pain. Campylobacter diarrhoea may contain blood or mucous. The majority of patients with Campylobacter diarrhoea have some component of segmental colitis, usually beginning in the small bowel and progressing distally to the caecum and colon.
- *Shigella* spp. is a Gram-negative rod belonging to the *Enterobacteriaceae* family. It causes bacillary dysentery in humans, an acute recto-colitis that reflects the capacity of the microorganism to invade, and cause the inflammatory destruction of the intestinal epithelium barrier, which will disrupt the homeostatic balance that protects the gut against inflammation in the presence of its commensal microbiota. The activation of pro-inflammatory molecules can initiate an Ulcerative Colitis-like process or trigger a relapse (Sansonetti, 2006).
- Adherent and invasive *Escherichia coli, Salmonella enterica* and *Yersinia* spp. all have the same potential as Shigella spp. to cause disease, although some serotypes of the *Escherichia* genus seem to have a healing capacity in Ulcerative Colitis patients, similar to that of 5-ASA drugs, by restoring mucosal homeostasis (Sartor & Muelhbauer, 2007). All three can cause life-threatening disease, but *E. coli* is much more frequent and versatile.
- *Clostridium difficile* is a Gram-positive anaerobic rod that produces two toxins -named A and B- with cytopathic effects. It has been associated with Ulcerative Colitis onset and can also worsen its clinical manifestations or mimic an acute flare. Unlike healthy persons, colitis in immunocompromised patients is mostly community-acquired.

3.3.2 Fungi

This group represents a constellation of opportunistic pathogens associated with high mortality. One of the main reasons is that they are often overlooked due to its difficult and intricate diagnosis. Recommended treatments for fungi are shown in table 4.

- *Aspergillus* spp. is a filamentous fungus present in the environment and generates high concentrations of spores in the air. It is not a common pathogen in healthy people since the inhaled spores are eliminated by the mucociliary apparatus of the respiratory tract, alveolar macrophages or neutrophils. But, it poses a serious challenge to neutropenic patients. Neutropenia and impaired cellular immunity are predisposing factors for colonization and development of invasive pulmonary aspergillosis. The most frequently isolated species in humans are *A. fumigatus* (73%) and *A. flavus* (15%), followed to a lesser extent by A. niger, *A. terreus*, and so on. The incidence of this disease in immunosuppressed patients varies between 1-15%, and although there are limited data in patients with Ulcerative Colitis, case reports do exist that reflect its severity. The classic symptoms of invasive pulmonary aspergillosis are dyspnoea, chest pain and haemoptysis, even though 25% of patients may be asymptomatic at the time of diagnosis. A chest radiograph may be normal in up to 10% of cases, so CT is essential for diagnosis. Initially, one or more nodules with or without cavitation are detected. The presence of halo sign indicates vascular invasion by the microorganism, but other fungi such as *Fusarium* or diseases such as carcinomatous metastases can produce similar patterns. The aetiological diagnosis is based on direct examination and culture of non-invasive or invasive respiratory specimens such as sputum, bronchial aspirate or bronchoalveolar lavage, and the detection in blood or bronchoalveolar lavage of DNA or galactomannan, an antigen from the cell-wall of *Aspergillus*. Treatment is based on the administration of antifungals, the reconstitution of the immune status and surgery if it presents with severe haemoptysis, persistence of the organism despite treatment, or committed major vascular structures.

- *Pneumocystis jiroveci* is a non-filamentous fungus that colonizes the respiratory epithelium of humans and is transmitted by air from person to person. Recent studies suggest that the reservoir comprises young children and immunocompromised patients. In all cases, over 90% of patients have received continued treatment with corticosteroids. The typical presentation is the emergence of non-productive cough, fever, dyspnoea and tachypnoea in a one-week period time. X-ray shows a bilateral interstitial pattern, but may be normal in up to 20% of cases, CT being more sensitive. The most informative samples for diagnosis are the bronchoalveolar lavage and transbronchial biopsy, but induced sputum, nasopharyngeal washings or biopsies are also useful. Prophylaxis is not as clear as in HIV-positive patients, but is recommended in subjects who have received prolonged treatment with corticosteroids, or who have received anti-T cell therapy, those suffering from a prolonged neutropenia or have a CMV lung infection, and those with prior P. jiroveci or other opportunistic pathogens pneumonia.
- *Cryptococcus neoformans* is a yeast widely distributed in nature which is acquired by inhaling small dried forms of the microorganism. In immunosuppressed patients, it is capable of a rapidly progressive pulmonary infection with spread to other organs, with great predilection for central nervous system. The most common symptoms are fever, pleurisy, dyspnoea, chronic cough, haemoptysis and weight loss. Neurological manifestations such as sub-acute meningitis with possible development of hydrocephalus may precede pulmonary symptoms. Chest X-rays shows calcified nodules, bilateral infiltrates and hilar or mediastinal lymphadenopathy, cavitation and pleural effusion may also be observed. The aetiological diagnosis is done through the vision of encapsulated yeasts in respiratory samples or cerebrospinal fluid, cultivation and identification by biochemical tests. Detection and titration of capsular antigen in cerebrospinal fluid, blood or respiratory specimens facilitate an early diagnosis, but it is also useful to acknowledge the disease prognosis and progression.

Prophylaxis with fluconazole is not recommended because of the low incidence of this disease.

- *Candida* spp. is a yeast that frequently colonizes the respiratory and gastrointestinal tracts of immunosuppressed patients or of those who have received broad spectrum antibiotics. It seldom causes disease but it may arise as oral mucositis, colonization of catheters and surgical wounds, and even as haematogenous dissemination. Diagnosis may be difficult in some cases because it is necessary to distinguish between colonization and infection. Prophylaxis with fluconazole in different immunocompromised patients has led to increasing numbers of antifungal resistant strains of Candida other than *C. albicans*, such as *C. glabrata* or *C. krusei*.
- *Histoplasma capsulatum* is endemic along the Ohio, Mississippi and St. Lawrence rivers, but it can be found throughout the world. Histoplasmosis can reactivate years after primary infection and may mimic tuberculosis or neoplastic disease chiefly in the nervous central system and mucocutaneous surfaces.

Microorganism	**Treatment**	**Alternative treatment**
Empirical	Caspofungin or voriconazole	Amphotericin B lipid formulation
Aspergillus spp.	Voriconazole Combination with equinocandine is recommended Withholding immunosuppressive treatment and surgical excision should be considered	Caspofungin; amphotericin B lipid formulation or the combination of both.
Pneumocystis jiroveci	Cotrimoxazole	Pentamidin; clindamycin + primaquine; dapsone + trimethoprim; atovaquone 750 mg/8 h.
Cryptococcus neoformans	Amphotericin B + flucytosine	Fluconazole + flucytosine
Candida spp.	Equinocandine (except for *C. parapsilosis* and *C. guilliermondii*); fluconazole (except for *C. krusei* or *C. glabrata*)	Voriconazole or amphotericin

Table 4. Recommended treatments for fungal pathogens in immunocompromised patients (Mensa et al., 2011)

3.3.3 Viruses

Viruses are a group of pathogens whose incidence is increasing and may have a high morbidity and mortality. Disease in these patients may be community-acquired, but reactivation of latent viruses such as Herpesviridae is more characteristic and challenging. Recommended treatments for common viruses are shown in table 5.

- *Cytomegalovirus* is a herpes virus that remains in a latent form after primary infection. The disease is acquired by infection from another person or by reactivation after immunosuppressive therapy. CMV colitis can imitate an Ulcerative Colitis flare. Symptoms range from fever and abdominal pain to haemorrhagic diarrhoea or fulminant colitis. Moreover, it has been associated with steroid-resistant Ulcerative Colitis (Ayre et al., 2009). Pneumonitis is also a major complication; radiologically, it shows interstitial or bilateral reticulonodular infiltrates. CT shows bronchial wall thickening and ground-glass opacification. In addition to infectious conditions, CMV produces local immunosuppression that promotes super-infection with other opportunistic pathogens. The presence of CMV in the lung is a risk factor for infection with *Aspergillus* or *Pneumocystis jiroveci*. The etiological diagnosis is complicated by the presence of co-infection and similarity with other pathogens. Interestingly, the histopathological detection of CMV means infection, but not necessarily disease. The most predictive diagnosis is achieved with the detection of CMV in blood either by cell cultures (shell vial + immunofluorescence staining), detection of pp65 antigen in peripheral blood leukocytes, or detection of viral load with molecular biology techniques (PCR, real-time PCR).

Microorganism	**Treatment**	**Alternative treatment**
Citomegalovirus	Ganciclovir	Foscarnet or cidofovir
Varicella-Zoster virus	Valaciclovir; acyclovir or famciclovir	Foscarnet
Herpes simplex virus	Acyclovir	Foscarnet or cidofovir
Herpes 8 virus	Unknown	Foscarnet; cidofovir; adefovir; valaciclovir or ganciclovir
Epstein-Barr virus	Acyclovir or ganciclovir	
Respiratory sincitial virus	Inhaled ribavirin Consider association with palivizumab	
Influenzavirus	Oseltamivir or zanamivir	Amantadine or ribavirin (in severe pneumonia by B or C serotypes)

Table 5. Recommended treatments for viral pathogens in immunocompromised patients (Mensa et al., 2011)

- *Respiratory syncytial virus* is a seasonal pathogen that affects mostly in winter and spring. It may cause pneumonitis on its own or alonside other opportunistic microorganisms with similar clinical and radiological findings (CMV, *P. jiroveci*). Thus, suspicion is essential for diagnosis. Prevention is the best therapeutic tool because, although there are treatments with ribavirin or monoclonal antibodies, the results are yet inconclusive.

- *Herpes simplex virus*, immunosuppressed patients frequently develop symptomatic HSV disease which can be life-threatening. Undoubtedly, disseminated HSV with pulmonary, hepatic, colonic or brain involvement have a very high mortality rate. Early treatment reduces mortality and morbidity.
- *Varicella-Zoster virus* primary infection in immunocompromised patients can develop pneumonia or encephalic complications. Reactivation of the virus presents the risk of disseminated zoster, with mortality rates similar to those for varicella.
- *Epstein-Barr virus* can reactivate in patients on immunosuppressive therapy and, although the clinical relevance has not yet been established, its capability to produce lymphomas demands careful attention. Cessation of immunosuppressive agents often leads to lymphoma spontaneous regression.
- *Herpes* 8 is not a very common pathogen, although colonic Kaposi's sarcoma that required total colectomy has been described in an Ulcerative Colitis patient under immunosuppressive therapy.
- There is little evidence about **Hepatitis C virus** and Ulcerative Colitis, but immunotherapy does not seem to have any adverse effect on its course. Nevertheless, liver function and viraemia must be monitored as well as patient's immunosuppression level in order to make a decision on treatment.
- Corticosteroids and anti-Tumour Necrosis Factor alpha appear to have a deleterious effect on **Hepatitis B virus**-positive patients. Consequently, prophylactic antiviral treatment should be started prior to immunosuppressive therapy.
- **HIV**-positive patients on immunosuppressive therapy should be closely observed due to their underlaying condition. Although the interactions between these diseases fall beyond the scope of this chapter, doctors should be very cautious and suspend immunosuppressive therapy if concomitant opportunistic infections arise or there is no response to Highly Active Anti Retroviral Therapy.
- Other respiratory viruses such as *Influenza, Parainfluenza, Metapneumovirus* and *Adenovirus*, are a growing cause of morbidity and mortality in immunocompromised patients, reaching 10-20% of all pulmonary infections in some studies. The course of infection may also be aggravated by *Haemophilus influenzae, Streptococcus pneumoniae* or *Staphylococcus aureus* bacterial pneumonia (Sahuquillo-Arce & Menéndez-Villanueva, 2010).

3.4 Parasites

They are a group of rare lung infections, but physicians must be observant due to its remarkable clinical relevance. Recommended treatments for common parasites are shown in table 6.

- *Strongyloides stercoralis* is an intestinal nematode of tropical and subtropical climates. The larvae penetrate the skin and migrate via the blood to the lungs, from where they will reach the intestine. In immunosuppressed patients, it can produce Ulcerative Colitis-like colitis but also hyperinfestation which implies very poor prognosis since diffuse bronchopneumonia and alveolar bleeding can be present. The diagnosis is done by observing larvae in faecal extensions, but also in the sputum or bronchoalveolar lavage from hyperinfestation cases.
- *Toxoplasma gondii* is a parasite of cats. It rarely causes disease in healthy patients, but it remains dormant and can reactivate in immunosuppressed patients. Toxoplasmosis is

usually due to reactivation, and commonly causes central nervous system disease which is uniformly fatal if untreated, but also interstitial pneumonia, haemorrhagic pneumonia, lung consolidation, myocarditis or chorioretinitis. The high mortality observed is related to diagnosis delay. The diagnosis of choice is the direct view of the parasite by histological staining or isolation in cell cultures.

- *Leishmania* spp. are obligate intracellular protozoa transmitted to humans from infected sandflies. In visceral leishmaniasis, the parasite migrates to the internal organs such as liver, spleen and bone marrow. Signs and symptoms include fever, weight loss, malaise, anaemia, substantial swelling of the liver and spleen, and frequently, diarrhoea. Visceral leishmaniasis is a zoonosis rare in Western Europe, but life-threatening in immunocompromised patients. The course of infection depends on the type of the patient's immune reaction; patients with Th 1 response often present an asymptomatic or oligo-symptomatic disease, and after recovery they are immune to re-infection (Badaró et al., 1986; Hagenah et al., 2007). The disease can relapse after treatment in immunocompromised patients.

Microorganism	Recommended treatment	Alternative treatment
Toxoplasma gondii	sulfadiazine + pyrimethamine + folinic acid Pregnant woman: spiramycin until delivery	Cotrimoxazole; clindamycine + pyrimethamine + folinic; pyrimethamine + folinic acid + dapsone, atovacuona or clarithromycin; sulfadiazine + atovaquone, dapsone or clarithromycin.
Strongyloides stercoralis	Ivermectin for 5-7 days Consider addition of albendazole in hyperinfestation	Albendazole (once every month during 3 months after therapeutic success) Thiabendazole or mebendazole
Leishmania spp.	Amphotericin B liposomal on days 1, 5, 10, 17, 24, 31 and 38	Pentamidine; meglumine antimoniate; amphotericin B deoxycholate or paramomicin

Table 6. Parasitic infections treatment in immunocompromised patients (Mensa et al., 2011)

4. Conclusions

The relationship between the microbiota and its host is based on a very delicate equilibrium. Recent research has enlarged our knowledge about the interactions between humans and microbiota to an extent that admiration is the only possible reply at the sight of all the associations and its connotations. Trillions of microorganisms live and interact inside our bodies, and they are not only useful, but valuable for us.

Immune responses are modulated in such a fine way as to differentiate beneficial microorganisms from pathogens, and this happens at every moment without even noticing. As we have seen, in normal circumstances different bacteria play different roles; some have pro-inflammatory faculties, others protect from inflammation and at least one, *Candidatus arthromitus*, can have both. In the end, the microbiota and the immune system achieve a balance that preserves intestinal homeostasis. But, when the barrier between the two worlds

fails, this cross-talk between bacteria and immune cells is disturbed and inflammation reactions take place.
The involvement of bacteria in Ulcerative Colitis is not yet utterly understood, but unquestionably, microorganisms found in gut microbiota have the potential to induce and maintain inflammatory processes. Needless is to say that more research is needed, but the picture drawn so far brings to light that, interestingly, the human microbiota could be both the cause and the solution to this disease.
While a total comprehension of the aetiopatholgy is found so an accurate cure may be developed, Ulcerative Colitis patients are treated with immunosuppressive drugs. This fact involves that their immune response against challenging microorganisms are impaired. Thus they are exposed to infectious diseases with a worst course and prognosis, but also to opportunistic pathogens. A better knowledge and awareness about this scenario is necessary by both doctors and patients for a correct and early management of infection. On the other hand, specialist in gastroenterology, internal medicine, microbiology and infectious diseases need to collaborate for a successful management of these patients.
In conclusion, Ulcerative Colitis, due to the intrinsic characteristics of the patient and immunosuppressive therapies, features a multifaceted relationship with microorganisms which we are just beginning to unveil.

5. Acknowledgment

The authors are indebted to Dr. Guillermo Bastida for his assistance in finding recent evidence-based bibliography.

6. References

Aberra, FN & Lichtenstein, GR. (2005). Methods to avoid infections in patients with inflammatory bowel disease. *Inflammatory Bowel Diseases*. Vol. 11, No. 7 (July 2005), pp. 685-95, ISSN 1536-4844

Álvarez-Sala, Walter, JL; Casan Clarà, P; Rodríguez de Castro, P; Rodríguez Hermosa, JL & Villena Garrido, V. (Eds.). 2010. *Neumología Clínica*, Elsevier España S.L., ISBN 978-84-8086-298-1, Barcelona, Spain.

Aoyagi, H; Chikamori, F; Takase, Y & Shibuya, S. (1999). [Infectious complications in patients with ulcerative colitis]. *Nippon Rinsho*. Vol. 57, No. 11 (November 1999), pp. 2580-2583, ISSN: 0047-1852

Ayre, K; Warren, BF; Jeffery, K & Travis, SP. (2009). The role of CMV in steroid-resistant ulcerative colitis: A systematic review. *Journal of Crohn's & colitis*. Vol. 3, No, 3 (September 2009), pp. 141-148, ISSN:1873-9946

Badaró, R; Carvalho, EM; Rocha, H; Queiroz, AC & Jones, TC. (1986). Leishmania donovani: an opportunistic microbe associated with progressive disease in three immunocompromised patients. *Lancet*. Vol 1, No. 8482 (March 1986), pp. 647-649, ISSN 0140-6736

Chuang, MH; Singh, J; Ashouri, N; Katz, MH & Arrieta, AC. (2010). Listeria meningitis after infliximab treatment of ulcerative colitis. *Journal of Pediatric Gastroenterology and Nutrition*. Vol. 50, No. 3 (March 2010), pp. 337-339, ISSN 0277-2116

Cottone, M; Kohn, A; Daperno, M; Armuzzi, A; Guidi, L; D'Inca, R; Bossa, F; Angelucci, E; Biancone, L; Gionchetti, P; Ardizzone, S; Papi, C; Fries, W; Danese, S; Riegler, G;

Cappello, M; Castiglione, F; Annese, V & Orlando, A. (2010). Advanced age is an independent risk factor for severe infections and mortality in patients given anti-tumor necrosis factor therapy for inflammatory bowel disease. *Clinical Gastroenterology and Hepatology*. Vol 9, No. 1 (January 2011), pp. 30-35, ISSN 1542-3565

Do, VT; Baird, BG & Kockler, DR. (2010). Probiotics for maintaining remission of ulcerative colitis in adults. *The Annals of Pharmacotherapy*. Vol. 44, No. 3 (March 2010), pp. 565-571, ISSN 1060-0280

Elenkov, IJ. (2004). Glucocorticoids and the Th1/Th2 balance. *Annals of the New York Academy of Sciences*. Vol. 1024 (June 2004), pp. 138-146, ISSN 0077-8923

Escher M; Stange EF & Herrlinger KR. (2010). Two cases of fatal Pneumocystis jirovecii pneumonia as a complication of tacrolimus therapy in ulcerative colitis--a need for prophylaxis. *Journal of Crohn's & colitis*. Vol. 4. No. 5 (November 2010), pp., 606-609, ISSN 1873-9946

Fava, F & Danese, S. (2011). Intestinal microbiota in inflammatory bowel disease: friend of foe? *World Journal of Gastroenterology*. Vol. 17, No. 5 (February 2011), pp. 557-566, ISSN 1007-9327

Franchimont, D. (2004). Overview of the actions of glucocorticoids on the immune response: a good model to characterize new pathways of immunosuppression for new treatment strategies. *Annals of the New York Academy of Sciences*. Vol. 1024 (June 2004), pp.124-137, ISSN 0077-8923

Friswell, M; Campbell, B and Rhodes, J. (2010). The role of bacteria in the pathogenesis of inflammatory bowel disease. *Gut and Liver*. Vol. 4, No. 3 (September 2010), pp. 295-306, ISSN 2005-1212

Gassull, MA; Gomollón, F; Hinojosa, J & Obrador, A. (Eds.). 2007. Enfermedad Inflamatoria Intestinal, *Arán ediciones* S.L., ISBN 978- 84-86725-98-3, Madrid, Spain.

Gómez Gómez, J & Gobernado, M. (Eds.). 2011. Síndromes Infecciosos, Ergon, ISBN 978-84-8473-934-0, Madrid

Hagenah, GC; Wündisch, T; Eckstein, E; Zimmermann, S; Holst, F; Grimm, W; Neubauer, A & Lohoff, M. (2007). Sepsisähnliches Krankheitsbild bei Immunsuppression nach früherem Mallorcaurlaub. *Der Internist*. Vol. 48, No. 7 (July 2007), pp. 727-730, ISSN 1432-1289

Harbaum, L; Siebert, F & Langner, C. (2010). Opportunistic streptococcal gastritis in a patient with ulcerative colitis mimicking gastric involvement by inflammatory bowel disease. *Inflammatory Bowel Diseases*. Vol. 16, No. 12 (December 2010), pp. 2008-2009, ISSN 1536-4844

Hoentjen, F & van Bodegraven, AA. (2009). Safety of anti-tumor necrosis factor therapy in inflammatory bowel disease. *World Journal of Gastroenterology* . Vol 15, No. 17 (May 2009), pp. 2067-2073. , ISSN 1007-9327

Kahn, SA; Gorawara-Bhat, R & Rubin, DT. (2011). Fecal bacteriotherapy for ulcerative colitis: Patients are ready, are we? *Inflammatory Bowel Diseases*. (May 2011), ISSN 1536-4844

Khan, KJ; Ullman, TA; Ford, AC; Abreu, MT; Abadir, A; Marshall, JK; Talley, NJ & Moayyedi, P. (2011). Antibiotic therapy in inflammatory bowel disease: a systematic review and meta-analysis. *The American Journal of Gastroenterology*. Vol 106, No. 4 (April 2011), pp. 661-673, ISSN 1572-0241

Koutroubakis, IE. (2010). Recent advances in the management of distal ulcerative colitis. *World Journal of Gastrointestinal Pharmacology and Therapeutics* . Vol 1, No. 2 (April 2010), pp. 43-50, ISSN 2150-5349

Kudo, T; Aoyagi, Y; Fujii, T; Ohtsuka, Y; Nagata, S & Shimizu T. (2010). Development of Candida albicans colitis in a child undergoing steroid therapy for ulcerative colitis. *Journal of Pediatric Gastroenterology and Nutrition*. Vol. 51, No. 1 (July 2010), pp. 96-99, ISSN 0277-2116

Lawlor G; Moss AC. (2010). Cytomegalovirus in inflammatory bowel disease: pathogen or innocent bystander? *Inflammatory Bowel Diseases*. Vol. 16, No. 9 (September 2010), pp.1620-1627, ISSN 1536-4844

Lees, CW; Heys, D; Ho, GT; Noble, CL; Shand, AG; Mowat, C; Boulton-Jones, R; Williams, A; Church, N; Satsangi, J; Arnott, ID & Scottish Society of Gastroenterology Infliximab Group. (2007). A retrospective analysis of the efficacy and safety of infliximab as rescue therapy in acute severe ulcerative colitis. *Alimentary Pharmacology & Therapeutics*. Vol. 26, No. 3 (August 2007), pp. 411-419, ISSN 1365-2036

Lidar, M; Langevitz, P & Shoenfeld, Y. (2009). The role of infection in inflammatory bowel disease: initiation, exacerbation and protection. *Israel Medical Association Journal*. Vol. 11, No. 9 (September 2009), pp. 558-563, ISSN 1565-1088

Maltzman, JS & Koretzky, GA. (2003). Azathioprine: old drug, new actions. *The Journal of clinical investigation*. Vol. 111, No. 8 (April 2003), pp. 1122-1124, ISSN 0021-9738

Mensa, J; Gatell, JM; García-Sánchez, JE; Letang, E; López Suñé, E and Marco, F. (Eds.). 2011. *Guía de terapia antimicrobiana*, Antares, ISBN 978-84-88825-07-0, Barcelona, Spain.

Murray, P; Baron, EJ; Jorgensen, JH; Pfaller, MA & Yolken, RH. (Eds.). 2003. Manual of Clinical Microbiology, ASM Press, ISBN 1-55581-255-4, Washington, USA.

Nagasaki, A; Takahashi, H; Iinuma, M; Uchiyama, T; Watanabe, S; Koide, T; Tokoro, C; Inamori, M; Abe, Y & Nakajima, A. (2010). Ulcerative colitis with multidrug-resistant Pseudomonas aeruginosa infection successfully treated with bifidobacterium. *Digestion*. Vol. 81, No. 3 (January 2010), pp. 204-205, ISSN 0012-2823

Ng, SC; Plamondon, S; Kamm, MA; Hart, AL; Al-Hassi, HO; Guenther, T; Stagg, AJ & Knight, SC. (2010) Immunosuppressive effects via human intestinal dendritic cells of probiotic bacteria and steroids in the treatment of acute ulcerative colitis. *Inflammatory Bowel Diseases*. Vol. 16, No. 8 (August 2010), pp. 1286-1298, ISSN 1536-4844

Phalipon, A & Sansonetti, PJ. (2003). Shigellosis: innate mechanisms of inflammatory destruction of the intestinal epithelium, adaptive immune response, and vaccine development. *Critical Reviews in Immunology*. Vol. 23, No. 5-6 (2003) pp. 371-401, ISSN 1040-8401

Qu, Z; Kundu, UR; Abadeer, RA & Wanger, A. (2009). Strongyloides colitis is a lethal mimic of ulcerative colitis: the key morphologic differential diagnosis. *Human Patholology*. Vol. 40, No. 4 (April 2009), pp. 572-577, ISSN 0046-8177

Rahier, JF; Yazdanpanah, Y; Colombel, JF & Travis, S. (2009). The European (ECCO) Consensus on infection in IBD: what does it change for the clinician? *Journal of Crohn's and Colitis*. Vol. 3 (February 2009), pp. 47–91, ISSN 1873-9946

Rodríguez-Peláez, M; Fernández-García, MS; Gutiérrez-Corral, N; de Francisco, R; Riestra, S; García-Pravia, C; Rodríguez, JI & Rodrigo, L. (2010). Kaposi's sarcoma: an opportunistic infection by human herpesvirus-8 in ulcerative colitis. *Journal of Crohn's & colitis*. Vol 4, No. 5 (November 2010), pp. 586-590, ISSN 1873-9946

Sahasranaman, S; Howard, D & Roy, S. (2008). Clinical pharmacology and pharmacogenetics of thiopurines. Eur J Clin Pharmacol. Vol. 64, No, 8(August 2008), pp. 753-767, ISSN 0031-6970

Sahuquillo-Arce, JM & Menéndez-Villanueva, R. (2010). Infecciones pulmonares en otras inmunodepresiones, In: *Neumología Clínica*, Álvarez-Sala Walter, JL; Casan Clarà, P; Rodríguez de Castro, P; Rodríguez Hermosa, JL; Villena Garrido, V, pp. 383-392, Elsevier España SL, ISBN 978-84-8086-298-1, Barcelona, Spain.

Sahuquillo-Arce, JM; Ramirez-Galleymore, P; Garcia J; Marti, V & Arizo, D. (2007). Mobiluncus curtisii bacteremia. *Anaerobe*. Vol. 14, No. 2 (April 2008), pp. 123-124, ISSN 1075-9964

Salzman, NH. (2010). Microbiota-immune system interaction: an uneasy alliance. *Current opinion in microbiology*. Vol. 14, No. 1 (February 2011), pp. 99-105, ISSN 1369-5274

Sandborn, WJ. (2010). State-of-the-art: Immunosuppression and biologic therapy. *Digestive Diseases*. Vol. 28, No. 3 (September 2010), pp. 536-542, ISSN 0257-2753

Sansonetti PJ. (2010). To be or not to be a pathogen: that is the mucosally relevant question. *Mucosal Immunology*. Vol. 4, No. 1 (January 2011), pp. 8-14, ISSN 1933-0219

Sansonetti, PJ. (2006). The bacterial weaponry: lessons from Shigella. *Annals of the New York Academy of Sciences*. Vol. 1072 (August 2006), pp. 307-312, ISSN 0077-8923

Sartor, RB & Muehlbauer, M. (2007). Microbial host interactions in IBD: implications for pathogenesis and therapy. *Current Gastroenterology Reports*. Vol. 9, No. 6 (December 2007), pp. 497-507, ISSN 1522-8037

Scarpa, M; Grillo, A; Faggian, D; Ruffolo, C; Bonello, E; D'Incà, R; Scarpa, M; Castagliuolo, I & Angriman, I. (2011). Relationship between mucosa-associated microbiota and inflammatory parameters in the ileal pouch after restorative proctocolectomy for ulcerative colitis. *Surgery*. Vol. 150, No. 1 (July 2011), pp. 56-67, ISSN 0039-6060

Schoepfer, AM; Flogerzi, B; Fallegger, S; Schaffer, T; Mueller, S; Nicod, L & Seibold, F. (2008). Comparison of interferon-gamma release assay versus tuberculin skin test for tuberculosis screening in inflammatory bowel disease. *The American Journal of Gastroenterology*. Vol. 103, No. 11 (November 2008), pp. 2799-2806, ISSN 1572-0241

Siegal, D; Syed, F; Hamid, N & Cunha, BA. (2005). Campylobacter jejuni pancolitis mimicking idiopathic ulcerative colitis. *Heart & lung: the journal of critical care*. Vol. 34, No. 4 (July 2005), pp. 288-290, ISSN 0147-9563

Smolen, JS & Emery, P. (2011). Infliximab: 12 years of experience. *Arthritis research & therapy*. Vol.13, No. 1:S2 (May 2011), ISSN 1478-6354

Sonnenberg, A. (2010). Similar geographic variations of mortality and hospitalization associated with IBD and Clostridium difficile colitis. *Inflammatory Bowel Diseases*. Vol 16, No. 3 (March 2010), pp. 487-493, ISSN 1536-4844

Tanoue, T; Umesaki, Y & Honda, K. (2010). Immune responses to gut microbiota-commensals and pathogens. *Gut Microbes*. Vol. 1, No. 4 (July 2010), pp.224-233, ISSN 1949-0976

Tiede, I; Fritz, G; Strand, S; Poppe, D; Dvorsky, R; Strand, D; Lehr, HA; Wirtz, S; Becker, C; Atreya, R; Mudter, J; Hildner, K; Bartsch, B; Holtmann, M; Blumberg, R; Walczak,

H; Iven, H; Galle, PR; Ahmadian, MR & Neurath, MF. (2003). CD28-dependent Rac1 activation is the molecular target of azathioprine in primary human CD4+ T lymphocytes. *The Journal of clinical investigation*. Vol. 111, No. 8 (April 2003), pp. 1133-1145, ISSN 0021-9738

Viget, N; Vernier-Massouille, G; Salmon-Ceron, D; Yazdanpanah, Y & Colombel, JF. (2008). Opportunistic infections in patients with inflammatory bowel disease: prevention and diagnosis. *Gut*. Vol. 57, No. 4 (April 2008), pp. 549-558, ISSN 1468-3288

Weinstock JV, Elliott DE. (2009). Helminths and the IBD hygiene hypothesis. *Inflammatory Bowel Diseases*. Vol. 15, No. 1 (January 2009), pp. 128-133, ISSN 1536-4844

Weisser, M; Khanlari, B; Terracciano, L; Arber, C; Gratwohl, A; Bassetti, S; Hatz, C; Battegay, M & Flückiger, U. (2007). Visceral leishmaniasis: a threat to immunocompromised patients in non-endemic areas? *Clinical microbiology and infection: the official publication of the European Society of Clinical Microbiology and Infectious Diseases*. Vol. 13, No. 8 (August 2007), pp. 751-713, ISSN 1469-0691

Zhu, B; Wang, X & Li, L. (2010). Human gut microbiome: the second genome of human body. *Protein Cell*. Vol. 1, No. 8 (August 2010), pp. 718-725, ISSN 1674-800X

4

Primary Sclerosing Cholangitis and Ulcerative Colitis

Sophia Jagroop and Ramona Rajapakse
Division of Gastroenterology, Stonybrook University Medical Center, Stony Brook, New York USA

1. Introduction

Primary Sclerosing Cholangitis (PSC) is a chronic hepatobiliary disease characterized by progressive inflammation and fibrosis of the intra and extra biliary tree. This phenomenon leads to diffuse stricturing of the biliary tree and, if left untreated, can result in cirrhosis, portal hypertension and end stage liver disease. There are treatments aimed at delaying the progression of disease and reducing symptoms. However, the definitive treatment at the end stage of this disease is liver transplant.

The etiology and pathogenesis of the disease is largely unknown although some researchers have speculated that immunologic and genetic factors may be involved. Ulcerative colitis (UC) is also a chronic inflammatory disorder of the colon of unknown etiology with possible genetic and environmental triggers. The correlation between both these diseases would suggest that the etiology could be immune mediated.

2. Immune system involvement

Current theories postulate that an autoimmune process leading to lymphocytic infiltrate causes biliary destruction (Aron 2009). Some studies have found an increased number of serum autoantibodies being expressed in patients with PSC. For example, antineutrophil cytoplasmic, antinuclear, and anticardiolipin antibodies are seen with increased frequency in PSC (Angulo 2000). A study of 73 patients with definite PSC found that 81% were positive for the above listed antibodies (Angulo 2000). Also, a study of 25 PSC patients showed that 75% tested positive for pANCA (Gur 1995). These serum markers lack specificity for PSC. Nonetheless, the involvement of the immune system remains apparent.

In addition, some other autoimmune disorders are associated with the occurrence of PSC. A few case reports found males under the age of 25 that were diagnosed with PSC, to have UC and Type 1 Diabetes Mellitus (Gluch 1999 and Kay 1993). Chronic liver diseases, such as Primary Biliary Cirrhosis and Autoimmune Hepatitis have also been noted to have some overlapping features. More importantly, there is evidence that PSC has significant overlap features with autoimmune hepatitis. Three patients with elevated liver function tests, positive Antinuclear Antibody and/or Anti-smooth muscle antibodies were found to have histological and cholangiographic evidence of PSC (Gohike 1996). This supports the overall theory that the immune system is significantly involved with the development of PSC.

Undoubtedly an association between UC and PSC exists, however the mechanism by which they are related remains largely unknown. Some have suggested that a shared autoantibody between biliary and colon epithelium exists. An epitope that was common to the colon and biliary epithelial cells was discovered. Using this finding, a study was conducted to determine if a cross-reactive antibody exists that is common to PSC and UC (Mandal 1994). This study found that sera from patients with PSC contained autoantibodies against a cross-reactive peptide shared by colon and biliary epithelial cells. Therefore, this antibody could suggest a molecular association between PSC and UC.

Based on the premise that PSC and UC are strongly related, some theorist have postulated that infectious agents may be involved in the development of PSC. That is, when the colonic mucosa is significantly inflamed, toxic agents can invade the blood circulation and thereby cause PSC. 26 patients with AIDS-related cholangiopathy were found to have CMV and Cryptosporidium infection (Benhamou 1993). The most common infectious agents isolated from patients with AIDS-related cholangiopathy include microsporidium and cryptosporidium. Non-infectious agents have been linked to the development of PSC. For example, patients receiving hepatic artery infusion of chemotherapeutic agents were reported to have cholangiographic evidence of PSC (Barnett 2001). However, UC disease activity does not correlate with the appearance of PSC.

3. Genetics

The understanding of certain genetic associations between US and PSC has gained increased importance. For example, one study illustrated that several members of three families had PSC and UC (Quigley 1983). It has been suggested that specific human leukocyte antigen (HLA) haplotypes may be more likely to occur in the setting of well-defined PSC. Several specific HLA haplotypes have been found to strongly correlate with the development of PSC. In one study, HLA-DRw52a was present in 100% of 29 patients studied with PSC (Prochazka 1990). Also, of these patients 15 shared a common haplotype 12 of who had previously diagnosed UC (Prochazka 1990). The most common haplotypes associated with PSC include the following: HLA-B8, DR3, Dr2 and DR6 (Prochazka 1990). Also, in patients with both PSC and UC an increased presence of MICA and MICB alleles were demonstrated (Wiencke 2001). These alleles are primarily expressed in the gastrointestinal epithelium (Wiencke 2001). Some authors have suggested that this may represent a link between colonic and biliary disease. However, whether one specific gene is involved with the occurrence of PSC remains controversial.

The use of certain HLA haplotypes to determine disease progression is also under investigation. One study found that the HLA-DR3, DQ2 heterozygote genotype was associated with rapid progression of PSC and that the DR4, DQ8 haplotype was related to the development of cholangiocarcinoma (Boberg 2001). This finding could have an impact on determining disease progression. However, this genetic association requires further investigation before it can take center stage in determining prognosis and therapy.

4. Epidemiology

PSC is most often seen in Northern European populations. In some Nordic countries it is considered the primary indication for liver transplant (16). According to the NIH, PSC affects less than 200,000 people in the United States Population. This disease is most commonly seen between the ages of 20-30 years and is most common in men. PSC occurs in

5 % of patients with UC, and, conversely, UC occurs in 60-75 % of patients with PSC. The mean survival is 10- 12 years after diagnosis, with an increased risk for cholangiocarcinoma. Despite the known association with UC, there is a small subset of patients with retroperitoneal fibrosis who have been diagnosed with PSC (Bartholomew 1963). There are varying reports of the actual incidence and prevalence of PSC, which is likely due to the inconsistency in its presentation and lack of sufficient data. A population-based study in the United States demonstrated that the incidence of PSC was approximately 0.54 to 1.3 per 100,000, and the prevalence is 6.3 to 20.9 per 100,000 (Bambha 2009). Most of the patients described in this study had underlying UC.

5. Clinical presentation and diagnosis

Most patients are initially asymptomatic and therefore present with abnormal liver function tests or hepatomegaly on physical exam. The most common lab abnormalities include, an elevated serum alkaline phosphatase level, usually twice the upper limit of normal, and an

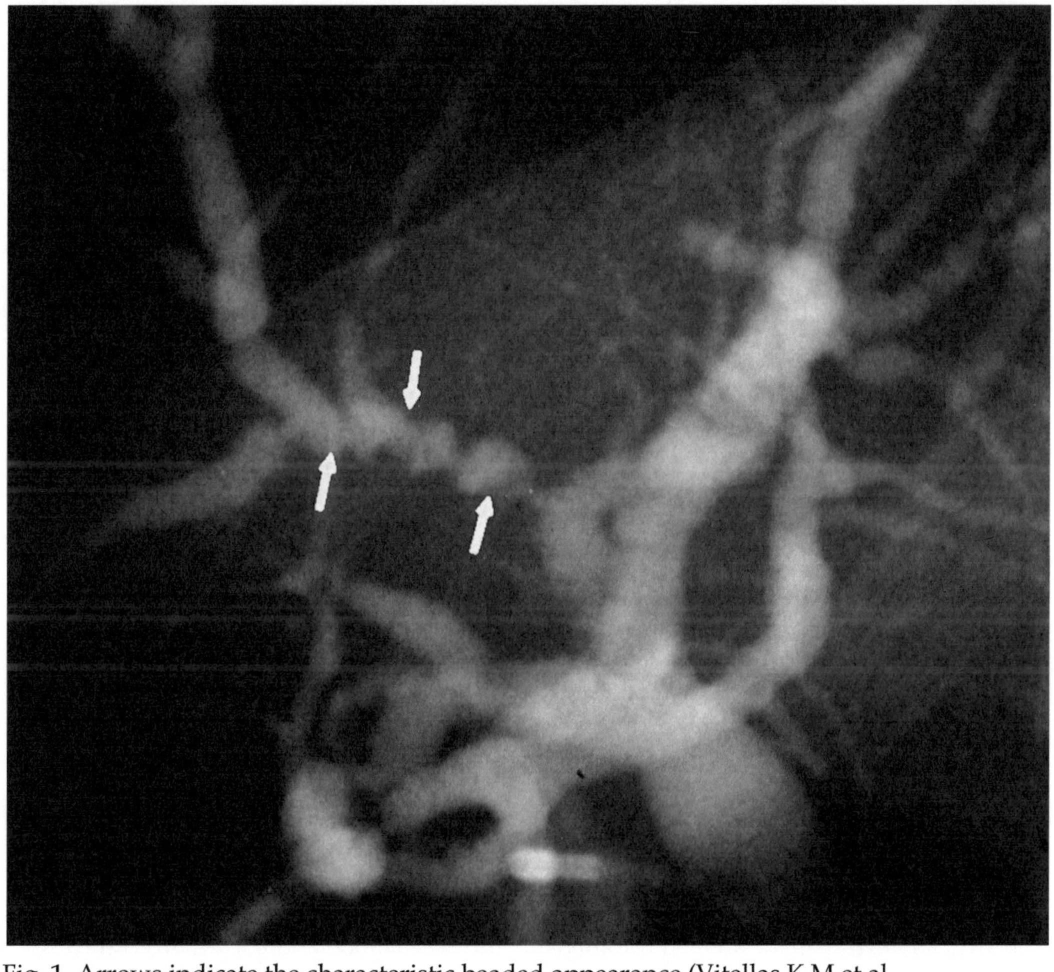

Fig. 1. Arrows indicate the characteristic beaded appearance (Vitellas K M et al. Radiographics 2000;20:959-975)

elevated Gamma glutamyltransferase. Also, the serum bilirubin and transaminases will demonstrate a cholestatic pattern. PSC develops insidiously and symptoms are often non-specific in their initial presentation. However, as the disease progresses, the most notable symptoms include, jaundice, right upper quadrant pain, pruritis, fever, weight loss and fatigue. Waxing and waning symptoms are typical of PSC.

The diagnosis of PSC can be confirmed by liver biopsy or characteristic changes on cholangiogram. Endoscopic Retrograde Cholangio Pancreatography (ERCP) has been considered the gold standard in diagnosing PSC. However, ERCP is more invasive in

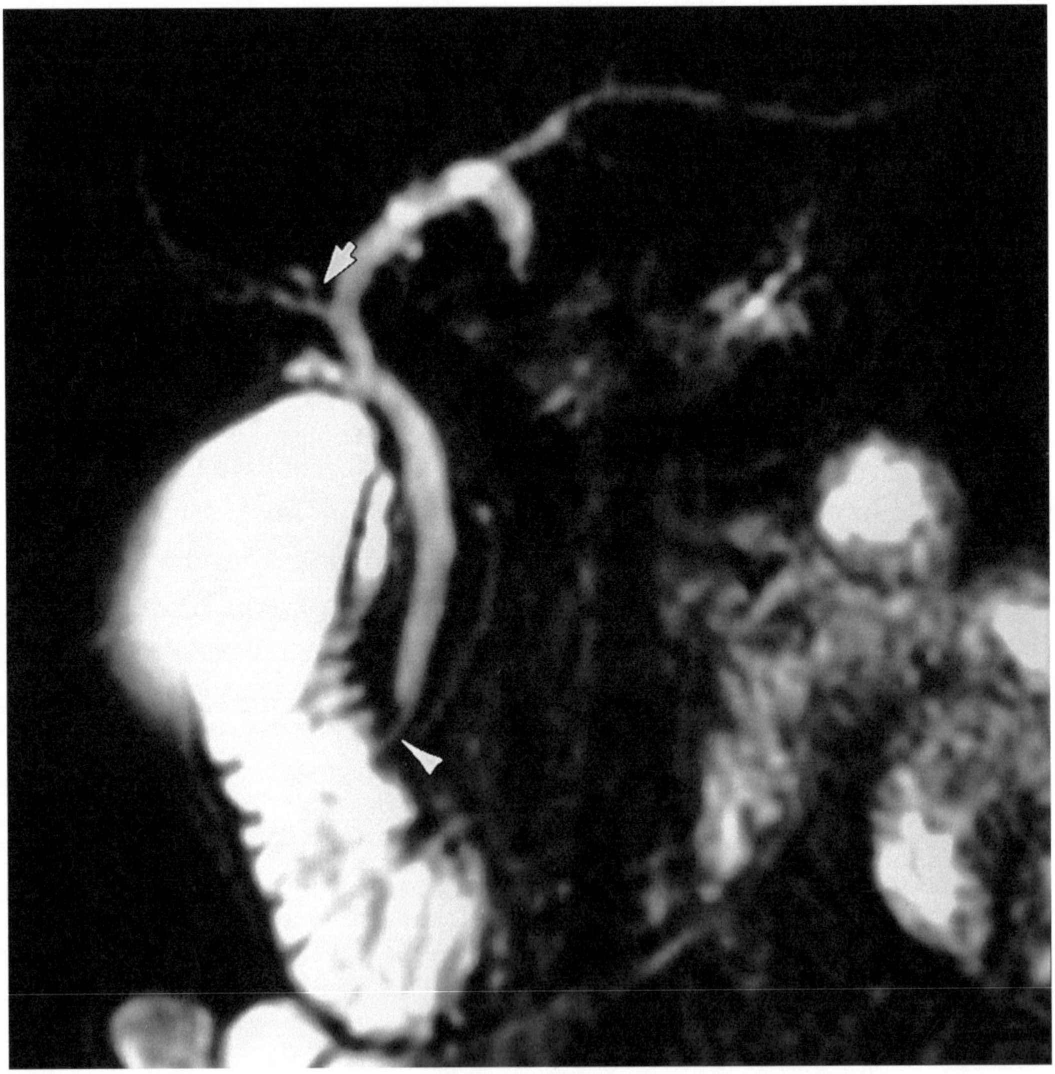

Fig. 2. Early PSC in a 45-year-old man with ulcerative colitis and elevated results of liver function tests. Coronal MRCP image shows a stricture at the distal common bile duct (arrowhead), extrahepatic and left intrahepatic ductal dilatation and irregularity, and a subtle stricture at the bifurcation of the posterior right hepatic duct (arrow). (Vitellas K M et al. Radiographics 2000;20:959-975)

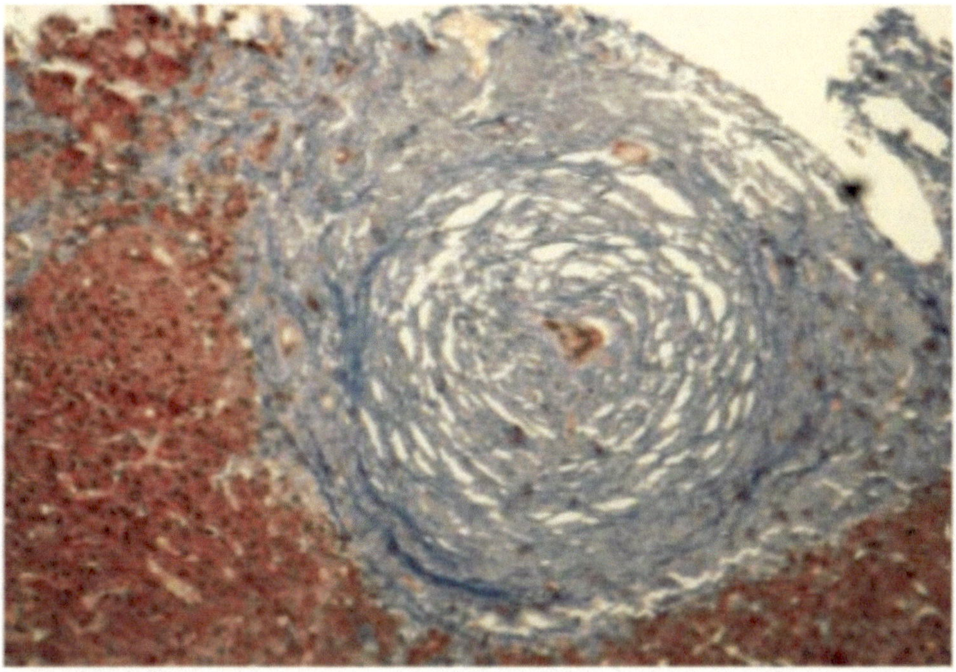

Fig. 3. Stage 2 lesion (Lee, Young-Mee, Kaplan M. Primary sclerosing cholangitis. NEJM 1995)

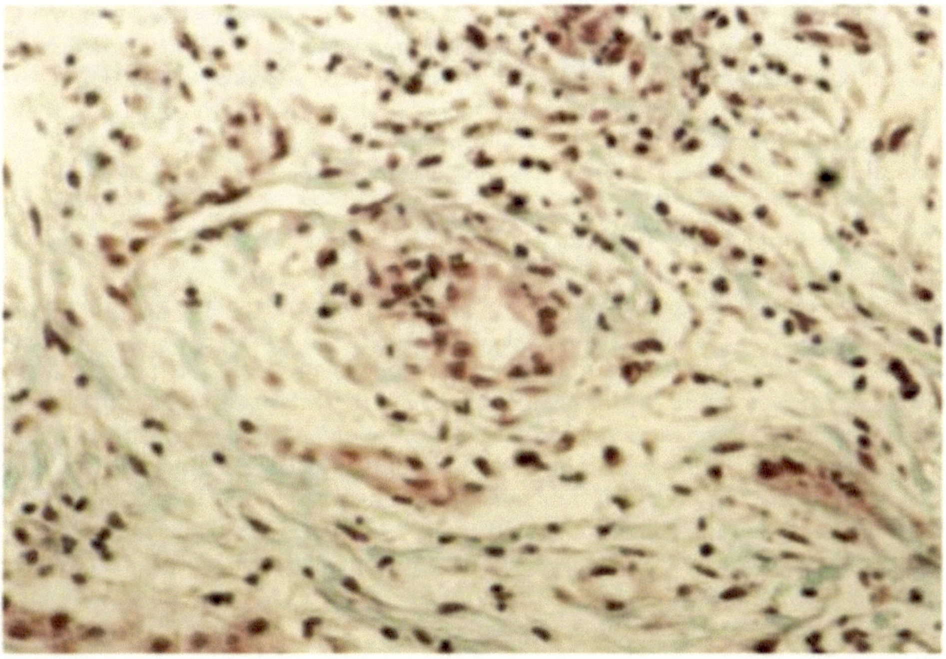

Fig. 4. Early stage 1 disease (Lee, Young-Mee, Kaplan M. Primary sclerosing cholangitis. NEJM 1995)

comparison to Magnetic Resonance CholangioPancreatography (MRCP), which has comparable accuracy. In cases with a high pretest probability of PSC with a negative MRCP, an ERCP would be indicated to visualize small ductal disease. The characteristic findings on imaging include, multiple segmental strictures with intervening segments that appear normal, otherwise known as a "beaded appearance"(figure 1). Figure 2 is an image of a patient with UC and abnormal LFTS that was found to have a stricture in the common bile duct and the bifurcation of the hepatic duct, with luminal irregularities.
Liver biopsy is not indicated for diagnosis in cases with a positive finding on cholangiogram. However, liver histology can be useful in staging the disease. The characteristic histological feature of PSC is the "onion skin appearance", which occurs due to periductal fibrosis (figure 3). However, this finding is rarely found on biopsy specimens. Stage 1 is defined as the portal triad of edema, scarring and mono/polynuclear cell infiltrate (figure 4). Stage 1 remains confined to the portal triad. Stage 2 refers to expansion of the portal triads with fibrosis into parenchyma (fig 3). Stage 3 and 4 are defined by bridging fibrosis and eventual cirrhosis.

6. PSC & UC association

There is a high prevalence of UC in patients with PSC while a minority of patients with UC have PSC as an extra intestinal manifestation. The current data approximates that 50-75% of all patients with PSC have IBD, and in contrast the incidence of patients with UC developing PSC is 2.5-7.5 % (Raj 1999). This association is an important one for many reasons. A study of 1500 cases of UC established that 3.7 % had PSC and within this subset the prevalence of substantial colitis was 5.5%, in contrast to 0.5 % with distal colitis (Olsson1991). This suggests that cases with more severe and extensive UC are more likely to develop PSC. However, a few case reports have demonstrated a milder course of colonic disease in patients that developed PSC (Schrumpf 2001 ad Moayyeri 2005). Therefore, regardless of the strong association between these two diseases, for the most part they seem to progress autonomously.
The definitive treatment for UC when patients remain refractory to medical management is surgery. Proctocolectomy with ileal reservoir is the most widely accepted surgical procedure. A common issue with this ileal reservoir, referred to as the pouch, includes the development of pouchitis. This diagnosis is characterized by diarrhea that is occasionally bloody and abdominal discomfort. In the subset of UC patients that develop PSC, pouchitis after ileal pouch-anal anastomosis (IPAA) is being diagnosed with increasing frequency.
A study was performed to determine the frequency of pouchitis in patients with and without PSC who had an IPAA for UC (Penna 1995). Patients with indeterminate colitis or other constructions of reservoirs were excluded in this study. The results showed that one or more episodes of pouchitis occurred in 63% of patients with PSC (Penna 1995). In addition, of these patients the overall risk for pouchitis increased at 1, 2, 5, and 10 years after IPAA.
Interestingly Aitola et al also demonstrated that patients with PSC had more chronic, but not acute inflammation in the pouch mucosa than patients without cholangitis (Aitola 1998). In comparison to patients receiving IPAA for other diseases such as Familial Adenomatous Polyposis, the frequency of pouchitis was higher in the PSC-UC patient. Therefore, based on this data it is unlikely that the cause of pouchitis is surgery and more likely a consequence of PSC-UC. A matched case control study was performed to describe the clinical features and outcomes in patients with PSC and IBD. This study found that a significant number of

patients in the PSC-IBD group developed back wash ileitis and had an increased incidence of colorectal neoplasia (Loftus 2005).
Some speculate that the significant bowel inflammation is due to a possible change in bile acid fecal output. This phenomenon is thought to lead to the development of pouchitis, but, this is purely speculation. Nonetheless, an underlying immunologic association exists between UC-PSC patients and the later development of pouchitis.

7. Malignancy

In comparison to the general population, patients with PSC are at higher risk for developing Cholangicarcinoma. This malignancy is defined as an adenocarcinoma of the biliary ducts that is rapidly progressive, with an average life expectancy of 5 months at the time of diagnosis. It is considered a rare disease within the general population, with a lifetime risk of less than 1 %. In contrast, PSC patients have an estimated lifetime risk of 10-15% for developing cholangiocarcinoma (Berqquist 2002). This disease is the second leading cause of death in PSC patient. Cholangiocarcinomas are most commonly found in the common hepatic duct or common bile duct, but can also be detected at the cystic duct. The sites at which this disease originates allows rapid dissemination to the liver, gallbladder, pancreas and duodenum. Also, intra-peritoneal seeding is not an uncommon consequence of this disease. Therefore, cholangiocarcinoma is most frequently diagnosed when it's metastatic.
The pathogenesis of PSC is believed to be due to chronic inflammation and obstruction of the bile ducts. This ongoing insult to the biliary epithelium is believed to result in malignant conversion of the biliary epithelium. In support of this theory, south Asian patients with Clonorchis sinesis were at increased risk for developing cholangiocarcinoma (Schwartz 1986). The precise molecular mechanism by which chronic inflammation leads to cholangiocarcinoma still remains unclear.
Early diagnosis of cholangiocarcinoma is important, especially in PSC patients because it is considered a contraindication to liver transplantation. The diagnosis of Cholangiocarcinoma in PSC patients is significantly difficult. The use of tumor markers to detect early disease has been studied. The CA 19-9 and carcinoembryonic antigen (CEA) has been noted to be significantly elevated in patients with cholangiocarcinoma. However, whether they are useful as markers of early cholangiocarcinoma is debatable. A study was conducted to investigate the utility of measuring CA 19-9 and CEA in patients with PSC for early diagnosis of cholangiocarcinoma (Bjournsson 1999). This study found that the levels of CA 19-9 could rise along with elevations in alkaline phosphatase, which indicates a relapse of PSC. However, the sensitivity of the combination of CA 19-9 and CEA was low, but the specificity was high (88%). Bile levels of these tumor markers were evaluated in this study and didn't reveal any clinically useful differences. Therefore, the use of these tumor markers for detection of cholangiocarcinoma remains controversial.
The use of conventional radiologic imaging such as Magnetic resonance or CT scans are of low sensitivity in diagnosing cholangiocarcinoma. Patients with PSC often have cholangiographic evidence of biliary strictures, which make malignant strictures indistinguishable. Hence, obtaining tissue is essential for diagnosis. The use of advanced endoscopic techniques, such as, Endoscopic Ultrasound (EUS) with fine needle aspiration (FNA) is increasingly important for obtaining cytology.
The combination of brush cytology and FNA increases sensitivity for diagnosis of Cholangiocarcinoma (Eloubeidi 2004). The reported sensitivity of EUS with FNA is 89 %

(Eloubeidi 2004). Figure 5 is an image of EUS diagnosing cholangiocarcinoma. Other endoscopic techniques, such as Intraductal Ultrasound (IDUS) and Choledoscopy have increased sensitivity in cases of negative brush cytology or tissue biopsy using EUS. IDUS uses a smaller caliber probe that can be passed through an endoscope into the biliary and pancreatic duct. This procedure increases the sensitivity of the ultrasound to detect lesions in the pancreatic or biliary ducts. In PSC patients, this technique can assist in distinguishing between benign and malignant strictures (Tischendorf 2007). Cholangioscopy is also useful because it allows for direct visualization of the biliary stricture (Figure 6). The use of these endoscopic procedures increases the overall sensitivity for detection of cholangiocarcinoma especially in patients with PSC.

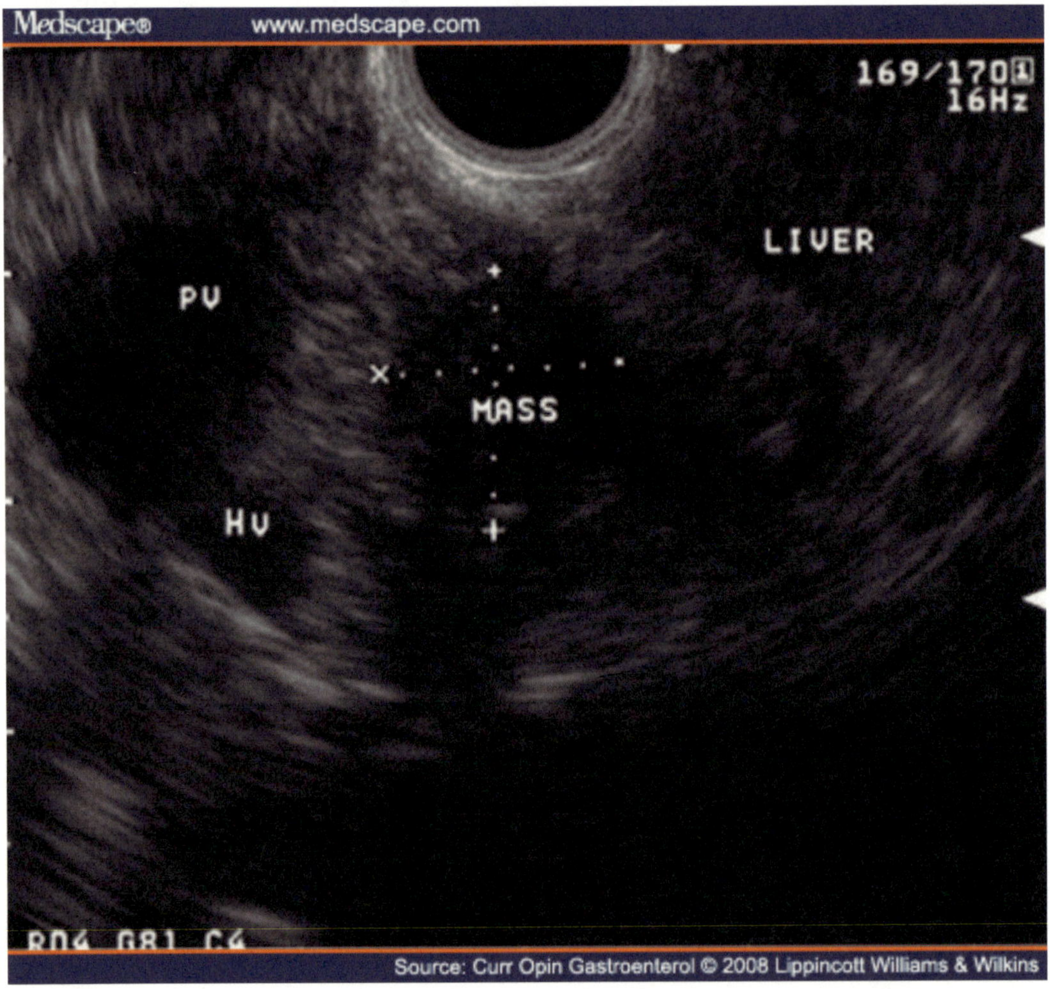

Fig. 5.

UC has a well-known association with the development of colorectal neoplasia. The risk in these patients increases with the duration and extent of disease. A study published in the New England Journal of Medicine found that the relative risk of colorectal cancer (CRC) was 14.8 for patients with pan colitis, 2.8 for those with left-sided colitis, and 1.7 for those with

Proctitis (Ekbom 1990). It has been suggested that patients with both PSC and UC are at even higher risk for CRC. A cohort study was performed comparing patients with UC and PSC, and random samples of UC controls without PSC (Shetty 1999). These patients were analyzed from diagnosis of the disease until an outcome. They found that thirty-three (25%) of 132 UC patients with PSC developed CRC or dysplasia compared with 11 (5.6%) of 196 controls (adjusted relative risk 3.15, 95% confidence interval 1.37-7.27) (Shetty 1999). They also found that patients with PSC and CRC were more likely to have more proximal and advanced CRC. This finding has a significant impact on disease surveillance and management.

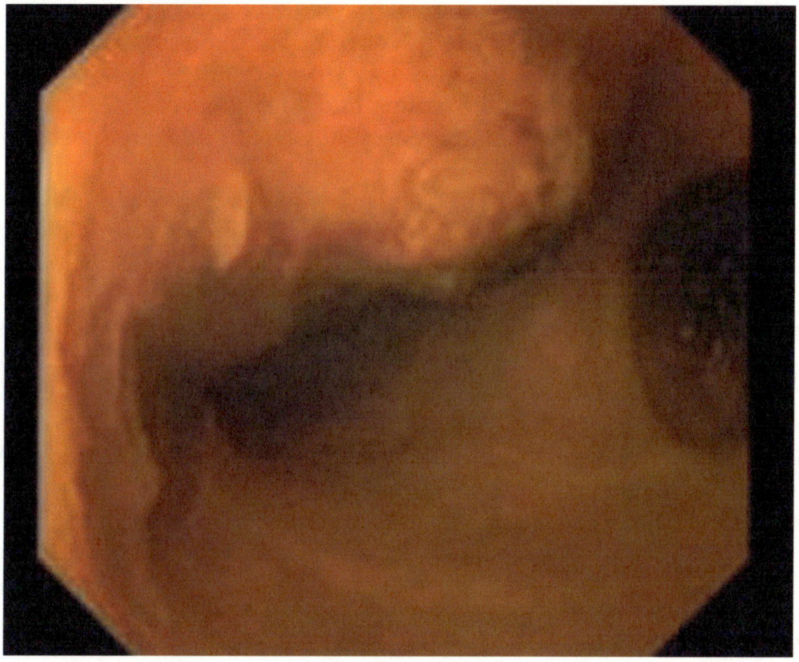

Fig. 6. Bile duct tumor on direct video cholongioscopy (www.cpmc.org/liver)

There are several theories regarding the pathogenesis of CRC in patients with PSC and UC. Some suggest that the increased bile acids in the colon may contribute to the development of dysplasia. Based on this notion, a study was conducted to evaluate the effect of ursodeoxycholic acid in preventing the occurrence of colonic dysplasia. This was a cross-sectional study that evaluated patients with UC and PSC that were undergoing routine endoscopic colonic surveillance. This study found that ursodiol use was associated with a statistically significant decrease in prevalence of colonic dysplasia (Tung 2001). However, this medication has not been evaluated in prospective study, therefore its utility remains controversial.

The risk of CRC has been noted to increase with the length of UC exposure. PSC patient are a t even higher risk for CRC and therefore require yearly surveillance colonoscopies (Eaden 2002). It has been suggested that the cumulative risk of CRC in PSC patients is estimated to be 9 % after 10 yrs, 31% after 20 yrs and 50 % after 25 yrs of disease (Broome 1995). A study of PSC patients undergoing Liver transplants with hx of UC and pancolitis were found to be at increased risk of CRC (Silva 2004). Therefore, in post-transplant patients yearly colonoscopies are still recommended.

8. Medical treatment for PSC

Various medications have been studied to evaluate whether they would have a curative role in PSC. Immunosuppressive medications have been extensively studied because of their role in suppressing inflammatory cytokines. These medications include, glucocorticoids, azathioprine, methotrexate, and pentoxifylline. It has been postulated that the upregulation of inflammatory cells leads to biliary ductal destruction. Bharucha et al gave 20 patients with PSC sustained release pentoxifylline for approximately one year. The serum bilirubin, transaminases and alkaline phosphatase were followed every three months. The overall study showed no significant improvements in the liver biochemistry and the disease (Bharucha 2000). Also, a prospective study using pulse dosing of methotrexate was conducted on patients with clinical and histologic evidence of PSC (Knox 1994). This study also showed no significant benefit in preventing the progression of PSC. Therefore, the data overwhelmingly shows that these immunosuppressive agents are unable to halt the progression of the disease.

The use of ursodeoxycholic acid (UDCA) may have a role in reducing the levels of the liver biochemistries. UDCA assists in the regulation of cholesterol by reducing the rate at which the intestine absorbs cholesterol. Some studies have suggested that it acts as an immunosuppressant. In PSC patients, UDCA is thought to be protective to the cholangiocytes by reducing bile exposure. Some studies have shown a mild improvement in serum liver chemistry, however the evidence on liver histology remains unchanged. A study was done to evaluate the use of high dose UDCA to determine whether the change in the bile acid pool would affect the outcome of PSC patients (Cullen 2008). Thirty-one patients were randomized to 10 mg/kg, 20 mg/kg or 30 mg/kg of UDCA daily for 2 years. They found that the higher doses of UDCA were well tolerated and the mayo survival risk score improved over 1-4 year period. However, some other studies have found contradicting results. A study also aimed at evaluating high dose UDCA and its effects on survival, symptoms, and quality of life was conducted. This study was a randomized placebo-controlled trial that included 219 patients followed for a 5-year period (Olsson 2005). The endpoints included quality of life assessments, changes in liver biochemistry, death and liver transplantation. They found that the serum alkaline phosphatase and alanine aminotransferase decreased within the first 6 months. However, there were no significant differences in overall symptoms, survival and quality of life. Despite the findings of an initial decrease in liver biochemistry, the use of UDCA as an aid in symptomatic management still remains controversial.

Managing the complications associated with PSC with use of medications and supplements is still useful. These complications include the development of bacterial cholangitis, deficiency in fat-soluble vitamins and pruritis. In PSC, recurrent episodes of bacterial cholangitis is not uncommon and if not managed appropriately can become life threatening. Antibiotic prophylaxis can be used and is helpful in these recurrent cases. Any procedure that involves manipulation of the biliary always requires antibiotic prophylaxis. The antibiotics commonly used are cephalosporins, fluroquinolones and beta lactamase inhibitors. Ultimately, these patients will require liver transplantation given the severity of the disease.

9. Prognostic models

In an effort to appropriately counsel patients regarding prognosis, models have been created to predict survival and indication for liver transplant. The most popular models include, Mayo clinic, Kings College, Multicenter, and Revised Mayo (Table 1).

MAYO CLINIC MODEL	REVISED MAYO MODEL	MULTICENTER MODEL	KINGS COLLEGE MODEL
Age	Age	Age	Age
Bilirubin	Bilirubin	Bilirubin	Hepatomegaly
Histologic Stage	Albumin	Splenomegaly	Splenomegaly
Hemoglobin	AST	Histologic Stage	Histologic Stage
IBD	Variceal Bleed		Alkaline Phosphatase

Table 1. Predictors of Survival

The Mayo clinic model was able to predict blood usage, length of stay in ICU and occurrence of significant complications in patients undergoing liver transplant (Dickson 1992 and Kim 1999).

The revised Mayo Model predicts survival based upon age, liver biochemistry and history of variceal bleed (Kim 2000). The estimated probability of survival is based on a scale over 1-4 yr period. The Multicenter Model was based upon a survival analysis that identified significant variables, which predicted survival in approximately four hundred patients with PSC (Dickson 1992). The Kings College Model was based upon a multivariate analysis that found hepatomegaly, splenomegaly, serum alkaline phosphatase and histologic stage to be independent prognostic factors (Farrant 1991). All of these models utilize mathematic formulas to determine the management of PSC. The models can be used to assess the appropriate time to consider liver transplant. Also, it helps to determine survival post liver transplant. The Child-Pugh classification can also be used to determine overall survival. These models however, are unable to predict the development of associated malignancies or harmful effects of PSC.

Determining the rate of recurrence of PSC post-transplant has also been evaluated. A large cohort study was conducted, which followed patients for 55 months after liver transplant (Graziadei 1999). This study found that 20 % of PSC patients developed histologic features of PSC and biliary strictures. Also, the average time to diagnosis of PSC was 360 and 1350 days respectively. However, this study was unable to delineate the factors that lead to the recurrence of PSC. In the current literature, there is limited information on what clinical variables may influence recurrence. A retrospective analysis was performed, which focused on the risk factors leading to allograft failure in PSC patients (Alexander 2008). The three most important factors that lead to failure included; acute cellular rejection, steroid-resistant acute cellular rejection and HLA-DRB1 association. These findings suggest that a strong immunologic association exist. What implications this may have on future liver transplant decision-making remains controversial.

10. Conclusion

Primary Sclerosing Cholangitis is a well known but uncommon extraintestinal manifestation of Ulcerative Colitis. This disease association can have a significant impact on the overall management and prognosis of both diseases. The focus of this literature review and chapter was to present the most current understanding of the pathophysiology, diagnosis and management of PSC as an extra intestinal manifestation of UC and to enumerate the special circumstances pertaining to patients having both diseases. Overall, the reader should have gained an understanding of the many ways in which PSC can manifest and how the association with UC can alter their overall management and prognosis.

11. References

Aitola, Matikainen et al: Chronic Inflammatory Changes in the Pouch Mucosa Are associated with Cholangitis Found on Peroperative Liver Biopsy Specimens at Restorative Protocolectomy for Ulcerative Colitis. Scandinavian Journal of Gastroenterology 1998, Vol 33, No. 3, Pgs 289-293

Alexander J et al: Risk factors for recurrence of primary sclerosing cholangitis after liver transplantation. Liver Transpl. 2008 Feb;14(2):245-51

Angulo P, PeterJB, Gershwin ME, DeSotel CK, Shoenfeld Y, Ahmed AE, Lindor KD. Serum autoantibodies in patients with primary sclerosing cholangitis. J Hepatol 2000 Feb;32(2):182-7.

Aron JH, Bowlus CL. The immunobiology of primary sclerosing cholangitis. Semin Immunopathol. 2009 Sep;31(3):383-97.

Bambha K, Kim WR, Talwalkar J, Torgerson H, et al. Incidence, clinical spectrum, and outcomes of primary scerosing cholangitis in a United States community. Gastroenterology. 2009 Nov;125 (5):1364-9.

Barnett KT, Malafa MP: Complications of hepatic artery infusion: A review of 4580 reported cases. Int J Gastrointest Cancer 2001; 30:147-60.

Bartholomew Lg et al. Sclerosing Cholangitis: Its possible association with riedels stauma and fibrous retroperitonitis- report of 2 cases. N Engl J Med 1963;269;8-12.

Benhamou Y, Caumes E, Gerosa Y, et al: AIDS-related cholangiopathy. Critical analysis of a prospective series of 26 patients. Dig Dis Sci 1993; 38:1113-18

Bergquist A, Ekbom A, Olsson R, Kornfeldt D, Lööf L, Danielsson A, Hultcrantz R, Lindgren S, Prytz H, Sandberg-Gertzén H, Almer S, Granath F, Broomé U (2002). Hepatic and extrahepatic malignancies in primary sclerosing cholangitis. J Hepatol 36 (3): 321–7.

Bharucha AE, Jorgensen R, Lichtman SN, et al: A pilot study of pentoxifylline for the treatment of primary sclerosing cholangitis. Am J Gastroenterol 2000; 95:2338-42

Bjornsson E, Kilander A, Olsson R: CA 19-9 and CEA are unreliable markers for cholangiocarcinoma in patients with primary sclerosing cholangitis. Liver 1999; 19:501-8.

Boberg KM, Spurkland A, Rocca G, Egeland T, Saarinen S et al. The HLA-DR3, DQ 2 heterozygous genotype is associated with an accelerated progression of primary sclerosing cholangitis. Scand J Gastroenterol. 2001 Aug;36(8): 886-90.

Broome U, Lofberg R, Veress B, et al. Primary sclerosing cholangitis and ulcerative colitis. Evidence for increased neoplastic potential. Hepatology1995;22:1404–8.

Cullen SN, Rust C, Fleming K, et al: High dose ursodeoxycholic aid for the treatment of primary sclerosing cholangitis is safe and effective. J Hepatol 2008; 48:792.

Dickson ER, Murtaugh PA, Wiesner RH, et al: Primary sclerosing cholangitis: Refinement and validation of survival models. Gastroenterology 1992; 103:1893-901

Eaden et al. Guidelines for screening and surveillance of asymptomatic colorectal cancer in patients with inflammatory bowel disease Gut 2002; 51:v10-v12 doi:10.1136/gut.51.suppl_5.v10

Ekbom A et al: Ulcerative colitis and colorectal cancer. A population based study. N Engl J Med 1990 Nov 1;323 (18):1228-33

Eloubeidi MA, Chen VK, Jhala NC, et al: Endoscopic ultrasound-guided fine needle aspiration biopsy of suspected cholangiocarcinoma. Clin Gastroenterol Hepatology 2004; 2:209-13

Farrant JM, Hayllar KM, Wilkinson ML, et al: Natural history and prognostic variables in primary sclerosing cholangitis. Gastroenterology 1991; 100:1710-17

Gluch J, Glaser J. Primary sclerosing cholangits, Ulcerative colitis and Type 1 diabetes mellitus. Z Gastroenterology. 1999 Aug; 37(8):735-8.

Gohike F, Lohse AW, Dienes HP, Lohr H et al. evidence for an overlap syndomeof autoimmune hepatitis and primary sclerosing cholangitis. J hepatol. 1996 Jun; 24(6)699-705.

Graziadei IW et al: Recurrence of primary sclerosing cholangitis following liver transplantation. Hepatology. 1999 Apr;29(4):1050-6

Gur H, Shen G, Sutjita M, Terrberry J, Alosachie I, Barka N, Lin HC, Peter JB, Meroni PL, Kaplan M et al. Autoantibody profile of primary sclerosing cholangitis. Pathobiology. 1995;63(2):76-82.

JJW Tischendorf, PN Meier et al. Transpapillary intraductal ultrasound in the evaluation of dominant bile duct stenosis in patients with primary sclerosing cholangitis. Scandinavian 2007

Kay M, Wyllie R, Michener W, Caufield M, Steffen R. Associated ulcerative colitis, sclerosing cholangits, and insulin-dependent diabetes mellitus. Cleve Clin J Med. 1993 Nov-dec;60(6):473-8.

Kaya M, Petersen BT, Angulo P, et al: Balloon dilation compared to stenting of dominant strictures in primary sclerosing cholangitis. Am J Gastroenterol 2001; 96:1059-66.

Kim WR, Therneau TM, Wiesner RH, et al: A revised natural history model for primary sclerosing cholangitis. Mayo Clinic 2000

Knox TA, Kaplan MM: A double-blind controlled trial of oral-pulse methotrexate therapy in the treatment of primary sclerosing cholangitis. Gastroenterology 1994; 106:494-9.

Loftus, Harewood et al: PSC-IBD: a unique form of inflammatory bowel disease associated with primary sclerosing cholangitis. Gut 2005; 54: 91-96

Mandal A, Dasgupta A, Jeffers L, Squillante L, Hyder S, Reddy R, Schiff, Das KM. Autoantibodies in sclerosing cholangitis against a shared peptide in biliary and colon epithelium. Gastroenterlogy. 1994 Jan;106(1):185-92.

Moayyeri, Ebrahimi et al: Clinical course of ulcerative colitis in patients with and without primary sclerosing cholangitis. Journal of Gastroenterology and Hepatology, Vol 20, Issue 3, pgs 3366-370, March 2005

Olsson R, Danielsson A, Jarnerot G, Lindstrom E et al: Prevalence of primary sclerosing cholangitis in patients with ulcerative colitis. Gastroenterology. 1991 May;100 (5 pt 1):1319-23.

Olsson R, Boberg KM, de Muckadell OS, et al: High dose ursodeoxycholic acid for the treatment of primary sclerosing cholangitis: A 5-year multicenter, randomized, controlled study. Gastroenterology 2005; 129:1464-72

Penna, Dozois et al: Pouchitis after ileal pouch-anal anastomosis for ulcerative colitis occurs with increased frequency in patients with associated primary sclerosing cholangitis. Gut 1995

Prochazka EJ, Terasaki PI, Park MS, Goldstein LI, Busuttil RW. Association of primary sclerosing cholangitis with HLA-DRw52a. N Engl J Med. 1990 Jun 28;322(26):1842-4

Quigley EM, Larusso NF, Ludwig J, MacSween RN, Birnie GG, Watkinson G. Familial occurrence of primary sclerosing cholangitis and ulcerative colitis. Gastroenterology 1983 Nov;85 (5): 1160-5.

Raj V, Lichtenstein DR. Hepatobilliary manifestations of inflammatory bowel disease. Gastroenterol Clin North Am. 1999;28(2):491-51

Schrumpf Erik MD et al: Epidemiology of primary sclerosing cholangitis. Best Practice and Research Clinical Gastroenterology. Vol 15; Issue 4, August 2001, Pgs 553-562.

Schwartz DA: Cholangiocarcinoma associated with liver fluke infection: A preventable source of morbidity in Southeast Asian immigrants. Am J Gastroenterol 1986; 81:76-9

Shetty K, Rybicki L, Brzezinski A, et al: The risk for cancer or dysplasia in ulcerative colitis patients with primary sclerosing cholangitis. Am J Gastroenterol 1999; 94:1643-9

Silva et al: Colon Cancer after orthotopic liver transplant. Critical Reviews in Oncology and Hematology;2004: vol 56:147-153

Tung BY, Emond MJ, Haggitt RC, et al: Ursodiol use is associated with lower prevalence of colonic neoplasia in patients with ulcerative colitis and primary sclerosing cholangitis. Ann Intern Med 2001; 134:89-95

W. Ray Kim MD et al.The relative role of the child-pugh classification and the mayo natural history model in the assessment of survival in patients with primary clerosing cholangitis. Hepatology. Vol 29, Issue 6, pages 1643- 1648, June 1999

Wiencke K, Spurkland A, Schrumpf, Boberg KM. Primary sclerosing cholangitis is associated to an extended B8-DR3 haplotype includimg particular MICA and MICB alleles. Hepatology. 2001Oct;34(4 Pt 1):625-30.

5

Colorectal Cancer in Ulcerative Colitis Patients

Joseph D. Feuerstein and Sharmeel K. Wasan
Boston University School of Medicine
USA

1. Introduction

The association between ulcerative colitis (UC) and colorectal cancer (CRC) was first reported in the 1920s (Crohn & Rosenberg, 1925). Since then, numerous studies have confirmed the overall risk of developing colorectal cancer associated with UC, and inflammatory bowel disease (IBD) in general. Many studies incorporate both UC and Crohn's colitis together with regards to their risk of colorectal cancer. While more recent studies have questioned how substantial the increased risk of colorectal cancer truly is in UC, relative to the general population, specific characteristics of UC patients increase their overall risk of developing CRC. In fact, CRC is one of the most serious complications of IBD and accounts for approximately 10-15% of the deaths in IBD patients (Munkholm et al, 2003). To reduce this complication, UC related CRC screening programs should focus on the individuals' risk of developing CRC with the goal of early identification of the cancer and subsequent increased overall survival.

2. Risk factors for developing colorectal cancer

Patients with UC are at an overall increased risk of developing CRC compared to the general population. This risk is additive to the baseline risk of developing sporadic CRC. The average age at diagnosis of UC related CRC ranges from 43.2 to 50.9 years (Eaden et al., 2001a; Lakatos & Lakatos, 2006). In addition to age, significant risk factors include the extent of colonic disease, age of onset and duration of disease, degree of inflammation, and the presence of primary sclerosing cholangitis. All these factors are crucial to prognosticate the patients overall risk and discuss treatment options.

2.1 Overall risk

While the risk of developing CRC in patients with UC is increased, the magnitude is challenging to estimate. Multiple studies with differing methodologies (population based cohorts versus populations from tertiary referral centers) have been performed and have reported varying risk estimates for the development of CRC. This difference may in part be due to the fact that some tertiary care centers opt for earlier colectomy or early therapy with aminosalicylates which may reduce the reported incidence of CRC. In 2001 a meta-analysis by Eaden and Abrams found the cumulative incidence of CRC in UC patients to be 2% at 10 years of disease, 8% after twenty years, and 18% after thirty years of disease. However, even this meta-analysis may overestimate the risk of CRC given the large percentage of patients who were treated only in tertiary care centers. Data from the Olmsted County database in the United States (US) did not find any increased risk of CRC in UC over a fourteen year follow up (Jess et al., 2006). A more recent study in the Netherlands looking at 26,855 patients with IBD (both ulcerative colitis and Crohn's disease) under the age of 65 found an overall incidence of 0.04% colitis related CRC (Baars et al., 2011). Despite these varying estimates, it appears that there is an increased risk of developing CRC, although the exact number is difficult to approximate.

2.2 Anatomic extent of disease

Anatomic extent of disease has been reported as one of the most important predictors of CRC risk in UC. Extent of disease is defined by the most extensivedisease noted histologically or endoscopically at any time (Mathy et al., 2003). Extent of disease is usually classified as pancolitis, left sided colitis, proctosigmoiditis, or proctitis. The definition of left sided colitis, unfortunately, varies in the literature; while most studies report it to be up to the splenic flexure, other studies extend it to the hepatic flexure. Overall, subtotal or pancolitis carried a relativerisk of 14.8 to 19.2, while for left sided disease, the relative risk was 2.8. (Ekbom et al., 1990; Gyde et al., 1988). Isolated proctosigmoiditis or proctitis did not significantly increase the risk of CRC (Jess et al., 2006; Langholz et al., 1992). In more recent studies, presence of backwash ileitis also did not increase the risk of CRC. (Haskell et al., 2005). The increased risk related to extent of disease is most significant in pancolitis patients during the first two decades of disease. By the fourth decade of disease, however, the incidence of CRC among pancolitis and L sided colitis equalizes (Greenstein et al., 1979; Gyde et al., 1988). Thus, these two groups of UC patients are recommended to undergo surveillance colonoscopy with biopsies given their increased risk.

2.3 Age of onset and duration of disease

The younger the age of onset of ulcerative colitis, the higher the patient's risk of cancer. After 35 years of follow-up, patients with extensive colitis diagnosed before the age of 15 had a cumulative risk of CRC of 40%. Patients diagnosed with UC between the ages of 15-39 had a lower, but still substantial, cumulative risk of CRC of 25% (Ekbom et al., 2006). However, this increased risk has not been substantiated in all studies. Greenstein et al estimated that patients aged 10-19 at diagnosis of left sided or pancolitis had an incidence of CRC of 3.6 per 1000 patient years. This incidence was increased to 12.7 per 1000 patient years in patients diagnosed between ages 30-39 (Greenstein et al., 1979). A recent study found a small but statistically significant increased risk of CRC with duration of disease (Baars et al., 2011). However CRC is rarely found when disease duration is less than eight to ten years (Ransohoff, 1988). Even in patients with extensive colitis, no cancers were detected during the first decade of follow up in 1406 patient-years (Lennard-Jones et al., 1990). In cases where CRC was diagnosed, the mean duration of disease from time of diagnosis of UC was seventeen years (Pinczowski et al., 1994). Considerations therefore for CRC screening due to UC are based on disease duration, not patient age. It is important to remember that in addition to UC related risks of CRC, UC patients also develop the same increased risk of age-related sporadic CRC.

2.4 Degree of inflammation

The severity of inflammation noted on colonoscopy is also associated with CRC. A study by Rutter et al reviewed patients with UC and CRC or dysplasia compared to UC patients without CRC or dysplasia. Inflammation was categorized as chronic/quiescent, mild, moderate, or severe by colonoscopic and histologic means. In univarate analysis both colonoscopic and histologic signs of inflammation increased the risk of CRC (odds ratio 2.5 and 5.1 respectively) (Rutter et al., 2004d). The increased risk was more dramatic from histologic scoring (Gupta et al., 2007; Rutter et al., 2004d). A similar study confirmed these results noting the progression from histologic inflammation to dysplasia or CRC (Rubin et al., 2006a). The risk of developing CRC is still present even after areas of severe mucosal inflammation return to normal.

2.5 Risks among males and females

Initial studies found no difference in the risk of developing CRC between men and women. (Ekbom et al., 1990). However, a more recent study of 7,607 patients of whom 4,125 had UC, noted an overall lower risk of CRC amongst women compared to men. Relative to the general population women with UC still had an overall increased risk of CRC. However, compared to their male counterparts, women diagnosed before the age of forty five and with more than ten years of disease had a lower relative risk of CRC (Soderlund et al., 2010).

2.6 Family history

Just like the two to three fold increased risk of CRC in first degree relative of patients in the general population, having a family history of CRC further increases the UC patient's risk of cancer (Askling et al., 2001; Nuako et al., 1998a). This risk was even more substantial when the first degree relative developed CRC prior to the age of fifty (Askling et al., 2001).

2.7 Associated Primary sclerosing cholangitis (PSC)

A small subset of patients with UC (2-5%) who develop PSC are at an even greater increased risk of developing CRC. This risk also increases with duration of disease. The risk of carcinoma or dysplasia in these patients was found to be 9% at ten years, 31% at twenty years, and 50% after twenty five years of disease duration (Broome et al., 1995). While some studies have failed to replicate this finding (Loftus et al., 1996; Nuako et al., 1998b), a meta analysis of studies including patients with UC and PSC found a four fold increased risk of CRC (Soetikno et al., 2002). This risk of CRC was also noted even after orthotopic liver transplant for PSC with an approximate incidence of 1% per person year (Loftus et al., 1998). A study from the United Kingdom noted a much higher cumulative risk post transplantation with risks of 14% at five years and 17% at ten years post-transplantation (Vera et al., 2003). Given the dramatic increase risk of CRC associated with associated PSC, patients having both UC and PSC should initiate annual colonoscopy surveillance at time of PSC diagnosis.

2.8 Miscellaneous risk factors

Additional risk factors that are only noted on colonoscopy include strictures, shortened colon, and pseudopolyps. In a small retrospective study, true strictures were found in 15 of 469 patients with UC. Of these fifteen patients, there were twenty seven strictures noted. Two were cancerous at diagnosis and twenty three showed low or high grade dysplasia. Ultimately, thirteen of the fifteen patients underwent colectomy, and an additional four patients were found to have CRC (Lashner et al., 1990). Another retrospective study of hospitalized patients with UC found the prevalence of strictures to be 5%, with 24% of the strictures being malignant. In all of these cases, the patients had more than twenty years of disease (Gumaste et al., 1992). Similarly, Rutter et al found that both strictures (odds ratio of 4.62) and post-inflammatory polyps (odds ratio of 2.29) conveyed a significantly increased risk of developing CRC (Rutter et al., 2004c). While post-inflammatory polyps do not develop directly into CRC, they are thought to act as a surrogate marker of previous severe inflammation which has been shown to carry significant risk of CRC (Rutter et al., 2004c). The risk of a malignant stricture increased with disease duration, location proximal to the splenic flexure, and presence of a symptomatic large bowel obstruction (Gumaste et al., 1992).

Risk factors for UC related CRC	Relative Risk
Anatomic extent of disease (pancolitis > left sided)	+++
Duration of disease	+++
Co-morbid Primary sclerosing cholangitis	+++
Younger age of onset	++
Inflammation	+
Stricture	+
Pseudopolyps	+
Family history of colorectal cancer	+
Male > female	+
Proctitis/Proctosigmoiditis	-
Backwash ileitis	-
Smoking	-

Table 1. Risk factors for colorectal cancer: + indicates increased risk and – indicates no proven increased risk

3. Genetics of UC related CRC

Similar to most cancers, genetic mutation, loss of function of tumor suppressor genes, oxidative stress, and errors in DNA mismatch repair all play critical roles in the development of UC associated CRC. Some of the genetic changes are similar to sporadic CRC, but key aspects and timing of events differ. Many of these changes occur prior to any detectable mucosal changes. Unlike sporadic CRC which develops in a stepwise process over many years, UC associated CRC can progress rapidly without a classic slow progression.

3.1 Genetics of UC associated CRC

While chronic inflammation is a risk factor for developing cancer, in UC inflammation is only one aspect in the pathophysiology of CRC development. For example, despite the inflammation seen in proctitis and proctosigmoiditis, patients with this extent of disease do not convey an increased risk of cancer. The step-wise process in the development of CRC is similar to the well established "adenoma-carcinoma" sequence in sporadic CRC. Crypt foci or mircoadenoma, progress to large adenoma, to cariconma-in-situ, and then into invasive adenocarcinoma. The most common cause of sporadic CRC arises from chromosomal instability leading to abnormal segregation of chromosomes and aneuploidy. The chromosomal instability leads to loss of heterozygosity and eventually loss of function of tumor suppressor genes. The loss of function of the APC gene is a crucial initiating event in the development of most adenomas. In sporadic colorectal cancer, key underlying features include both chromosomal instability and microsatellite instability. Eventually there is the loss of the p53 tumor suppressor gene which is the transition from adenoma to carcinoma. The remaining 15% of sporadic CRC involve the microsatellite instability pathway involving the loss of function of DNA mismatch repair genes. Two of the genes commonly affected are hMLH1 and hMSH2. (Itzkowitz, 2003; Itzkowitz & Yio, 2004)

Like sporadic CRC, UC related CRC develops from sequential steps of somatic genetic mutation and associated clonal expansion. While the same genetic mutations occur in UC related CRC, the timing and frequency is different. Approximately 80% of the cancers are related to chromosomal instability while 20% are related to microsatellite instability. In UC related CRC the main genetic alteration is in the allelic deletion of p53 in 50-85% of cases (Itzkowitz & Yio, 2004). In review of colectomy specimens, the p53 mutation preceded aneuploidy which in turn preceded p53 loss of heterzygosity (Brentnall et al., 1994). This loss of heterozygosity correlates with malignant progression, and is detected in 63% of low grade dysplasia and 85% of cases involving high grade dysplasia (Burmer et al., 1992). The p53 mutation was also detected at a high frequency (>50%) in patients with UC and inflamed mucosa (Hussain et al., 2000). The APC mutation is extremely rare (0-3%) and only occurs late in high grade dysplasia or cancer (Aust et al., 2002). Similarly, allelic deletion of the APC gene occurs in < 33% of colitis-related neoplasia (Umetani et al., 1999). Also different from sporadic CRC, the k-ras mutation is quite rare in UC related CRC, while BRAF mutation is more common (Lakatos & Lakatos, 2008; Yashiro et al., 2001). Microsatellite instability occurs through the same process as in sporadic CRC, and involves mismatch repair defects of hMLH1, hMSH2, and hMSH6 (Lakatos & Lakatos, 2008). In approximately 25% of cases, microsatellite instability was demonstrated two to twelve years before the diagnosis of CRC (Tahara et al., 2005).

3.2 Oxidative stress

The role of oxidative stress from chronic inflammation seems to play some role in the development of UC related CRC. Oxidative stress has multiple effects including cellular damage, contributing to the pathogenesis of colitis, and contributing to colon cancer carcinogenesis (Ullman & Itzkowitz, 2011). The chronically inflamed tissue release reactive oxygen and nitrogen species (RONS) from cells in the innate immune system. Actively inflamed tissue in UC expresses increased levels of both RONS and nitric oxide synthase (Hussain et al., 2000; Itzkowitz & Yio, 2004; Ullman & Itzkowitz, 2011;). Furthermore, measurements of 8-hydroxydeoxyguanosine, a mutagen formed from hydroxal radicals is found to be increased in UC mucosa and even higher in specimens with dysplasia. . The formulation of free radicals affects metabolic processes that regulate DNA, RNA, proteins, and lipids. Once the genes or proteins affecting colonocyte homeostasis are affected, like p53, dysplasia and carcinoma ensue. Lastly, the oxidative stress has also been found to interfere with DNA mismatch repair enzymes, contributing to microsatellite instability as well (Ullman & Itzkowitz, 2011).

3.3 DNA methylation

DNA methylation also contributes to the development and progression of colitis-related CRC. The resulting methylation of CpG islands in several genes occurs prior to dysplasia and is found diffusely in the UC mucosa (Issa et al., 2001). The hMLH1 hypermethylation is noted in neoplastic mucosa most commonly with high levels of MSI (46%) but is also found with low and no detected MSI (Fleisher et al., 2000; Ullman & Itzkowitz, 2011). Hypermethylation of cell cycle inhibitor $p16^{ink14a}$ is frequently found in neoplastic specimens in colitis-related cancer (Hsieh et al., 1998). While 10% of samples without dysplasia already showed hypermethylation of the p16 promoter, the rates rapidly increased with degree of dysplasia reaching 100% in tumor samples (Ullman, 2011). Similarly, $p14^{ARF}$, which is an indirect regulator of p53, is encoded by the same gene as $p16^{ink14a}$. Loss of expression via hypermethylation is detected in 50% of adenocarcinoma specimens, 33% of dysplasic specimens, and 60% of mucosal samples with no dysplasia (Sato et al. 2002; Ullman & Itzkowitz, 2011).

Chromosomal instability	Microsatellite instability	Hypermethylation	Oxidative stress
Aneuploidy	hMLH1	hMLH1	Free radicals
P53	hMSH2	$p16^{ink14a}$	DNA mismatch repair enzymes
APC	hMSH6	$p14^{ARF}$	
Chromosomal loss of function	DPC4		

Table 2. Summary of genetic changes in colitis related colorectal cancer

4. Pathophysiology of dysplastic lesions in ulcerative colitis

Dysplasia is currently the best indicator of CRC risk in UC (Goldman, 1996). It is defined as neoplastic epithelium confined to the basement membrane that is categorized histologically by a mix of architectural and cytologic features (Guindi & Riddell, 2001; Riddell et al., 1983). 75 to 90% of cancers in UC are noted to have underlying dysplasia with the classic progression from inflammation to dysplasia to carcinoma (Sharan & Schoen, 2002). However, a substantial number of colitis associated cancers arise without any preceding dysplasia, but even these cancers only occur in areas of chronic or active inflammation (Goldman, 1996; Riddell et al., 1983; Woolrich et al., 1992). In studies looking at patients who underwent colectomy for CRC, dysplasia was absent in up to 25% of the specimens (Brackmann et al., 2009; Connell et al., 1994). Consequently, the absence of dysplasia alone does not rule out the possibility of carcinoma.

4.1 Classification of dysplasia

Biopsy specimens are classified based on microscopic morphology as (1) negative for dysplasia, (2) indefinite for dysplasia, or (3) positive for dysplasia (Ridell, 1983). While true dysplasia is classified based on the degree of cytologic and architectural atypia of the crypts and surface epithelium, distinguishing these features can be challenging. Indefinite for dysplasia classifies specimens that possess some cytologic and architectural features of low grade dysplasia but also has active inflammation or ulceration in the area making the neoplastic status unclear. The features include changes that are more extreme than expected in just regenerative changes, nuclear features that seem beyond those considered normal repair, and nuclei in quiescent disease that are larger than expected for that disease state (Guindi & Riddell, 2001). Once a lesion is classified as dysplastic it is further differentiated into (1) low grade dysplasia, (2) high grade dysplasia, and (3) carcinoma (Riddell et al., 1983). Because there is significant inter-observer variability among pathologists, the diagnosis of dysplasia must be confirmed by a second expert IBD pathologist. Histologically, low grade dysplasia is hallmarked by nuclear enlargement, increased nuclear to cytoplasmic ratio, hyperchromasia, pleomorphisms, and increased mitoses. Classically, the nuclei are limited to the basal half of the cell cytoplasm. High grade dysplasia is similar to low grade dysplasia histologically, but more severe. It has prominent nuclear stratification and nuclei that are larger with more open nuclear chromatin patterns compared to low grade dysplasia. Unlike low grade dysplasia, the mitoses are both more frequent and present in the upper levels of the crypts as well as the surface epithelium. Additional general characteristics include: hyperchromatism, crowding, pleomorphism, loss of polarity of nuclei, and architectural aberrations like back to back gland patterns and cribriforming of the crypts (Farraye et al., 2010; Guindi & Riddell, 2001). This category of high grade dysplasia also includes carcinoma in situ, but it is not differentiated in reports (Itzkowitz & Harpaz, 2004). Carcinoma is defined by the presence of cells or glands that penetrate through the lamina propria and or submucosa. In UC-related carcinoma, single cell and small gland infiltration or large dysplastic crypts with irregular jagged contours or a complex cribriform gland pattern are seen. Also commonly seen features include necrosis, hemorrhage, ulceration, and desmoplasia. Ultimately, when determining the degree of dysplasia, pathologists assign the level based on the most severe level of atypical portion found in the biopsy sample (Farraye et al., 2010).

4.2 Dysplasia classification systems

While the United States uses the Ridell based classification of dysplasia (negative, indefinite, low or high grade dysplasia), outside the US, the Vienna system is used. This system was developed to improve standardization of interpretation and terminology of dysplasia. It is slightly different than Ridell's classification and uses a five category system. The five categories are: negative for neoplasia/dysplasia, indefinite for neoplasia/dysplasia,

Vienna	Riddell
1. Negative for neoplasia/dysplasia	1. Negative for dysplasia
2. Indefinite for neoplasia/dysplasia	2. Indefinite for dysplasia
3. Noninvasive low grade neoplasia	3. Low grade dysplasia
4. Noninvasive high grade neoplasia **a. High grade adenoma/dysplasia** **b. Noninvasive carcinoma** **c. Suspicious of invasive carcinoma**	4. High grade dysplasia
5. Invasive neoplasia **a. Intramucosal adenocarcinoma** **b. Submucosal carcinoma or beyond**	

Table 3. Riddell and Vienna classification systems

noninvasive high-grade neoplasia, and invasive neoplasia. The last two categories are further sub-classified histologically (see table 3 for full details) (Schlemper et al., 2000). Clinically though, there are no important differences between the two classification systems.

4.3 Risk of cancer based on degree of dysplasia

Given that the presumed stepwise sequence of developing CRC in UC is inflammation to low grade dysplasia to high grade dysplasia to carcinoma, the risk of progression from levels of dysplasia is important to quantify to help determine surveillance recommendations. Indefinite for dysplasia has classically been considered to be non-cancerous. However, newer studies question if the malignancy risk is underestimated. According to some studies, indefinite for dysplasia should be considered to behave like the subcategory low grade dysplasia (Bernstein et al., 1994). The progression from indefinite dysplasia to CRC ranged from 9% to 28% (Bernstein et al., 1994; Rutter et al., 2006; Ullman et al., 2008). In low grade dysplasia, the overall risk of cancer is reported as a 10% risk of invasive carcinoma (axon, 1994; Bernstein et al., 1994). Unfortunately in high grade dysplasia the risk is even greater, increasing to nearly 40% (Bernstein et al., 1994).

Dysplasia	Risk of CRC
High grade dysplasia	+++
Low grade dysplasia	++
Indefinite for dysplasia	Questionable risk (could be similar to low grade dysplasia)
Negative for dysplasia	No risk

Table 4. Type of dysplasia and risk of CRC

4.4 Dysplastic associated lesions or masses (DALM)

Dysplasia is further sub-classified as flat or elevated lesions (Itzkowitz & Harpaz, 2004). Flat dysplasia is undetectable endoscopically but picked up by random biopsies, while raised is visualized and referred to as "DALM" (dysplastic associated lesion or mass) (Blackstone et al., 1981). DALMs are visible dysplastic lesions with an unacceptably high risk of carcinoma. In a series by Blackstone et al., 58% of these lesions had an underlying carcinoma

Adenoma-like DALMs	Non-adenoma-like DALMs
Sessile/pedunculated polyps	Sessile (broad based)
Well circumscribed	Poorly circumscribed
Smooth	Irregular surface
Clear borders	Indistinct border
	Ulceration/necrosis
	Strictures
	Tethering

Table 5. Features of DALMs

(Blackstone et al., 1981). Others studies, report underlying carcinomas ranging from 34% to 84% (Bernstein et al., 1994; Odze, 1999). DALMs can be further sub-classified into adenoma-like and non-adenoma-like features (Engelsgjerd et al., 1999; Odze et al., 2004; Rubin et al., 1999). Adenoma-like features include well circumscribed, smooth or papillary, non-necrotic, sessile, or pedunculated polyps. Non-adenoma-like polyps include velvety patches, plaques, irregular bumps or nodules, wart-like thickening, stricturing lesions, and broad-based masses (Odze, 2008). The differentiation between adenoma-like and non-adenoma-like is based on gross endoscopic examination. Histologically both types of DALMs are made of tubular, tubulovillous or villous proliferation of adenoma epithelium with dysplastic columnar cells (Torres et al., 1998).

4.5 Treatment of DALMs

One of the challenges related to DALMs is the reliance on the endoscopist to differentiate adenoma-like lesions from a sporadic adenoma. Like the general population, sporadic adenomas increase with age and can be removed via polypectomy. However, some DALMs can develop features similar to a sporadic adenoma making it further difficult to differentiate the two (Guindi & Riddell, 2001; Torres et al., 1998). While there have been studies to differentiate sporadic adenomas from DALMs in UC patients, most did not achieve a level of certainty to confidently differentiate them (Bernstein et al., 1999; Torres et al.. 1998). The only aspect that seems to differentiate the two in UC are that adenoma-like lesions proximal to the start of the UC are likely sporadic adenomas (Torres et al., 1998).

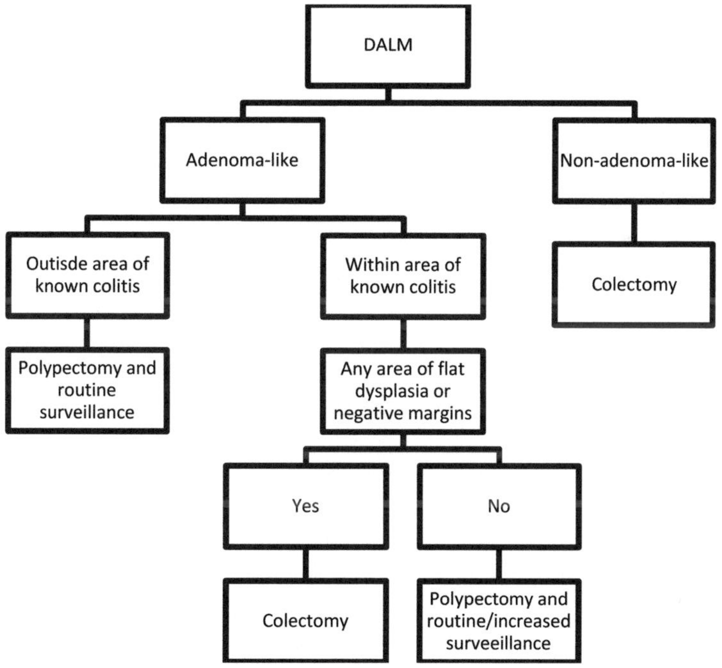

Fig. 1. Treatment algorithm for DALMs

Until recently, treatment differed between sporadic adenomas and adenoma-like DALMs for which colectomy had been recommended. Thirty four patients with adenoma-like DALMs who underwent polypectomy were compared both to UC patients with sporadic adenomas who underwent polypectomy and non-UC patients with sporadic adenomas who underwent polypectomy. The development of recurrent polyps was 62.5% in the adenoma-like DALM group, 50% in UC sporadic adenoma group and 49% in the non-UC sporadic adenoma control group (Engelsgjerd et al., 1999). In another study of eighty seven UC patients who underwent polypectomy, only 4.6% developed dysplasia during a mean follow up of six years (Vieth et al., 2006). Given that polypectomy for adenoma-like DALMs in UC patients affords similar protection against CRC as polypectomy for sporadic adenomas, current consensus recommendations support polypectomy for DALMs. Therefore, if an adenoma-like DALMs is completely resected endoscopically, with negative margins for dysplasia from biopsies around the lesion and no other findings of flat dysplasia in the colon, then routine surveillance following polypectomy is appropriate (Friedman et al., 2003; Odze et al., 2004; Rubin et al., 1999). Similarly, any adenoma-like lesions outside the area of UC can be presumed to be sporadic in nature and treated with polypectomy and routine surveillance alone (Friedman, 2003). For adequate follow up surveillance, tattooing the adjacent mucosa to the resected polyps can aid in future identification and monitoring.

In contrast, non-adenoma-like DALMs carry an unacceptable cancer risk (38% to 83%) even in those lesions considered endoscopically resectable. Therefore, any non-adenoma-like DALMs regardless of their sub-classification as low or high grade dysplasia necessitate colectomy.

4.6 Flat dysplasia

In cases of flat dysplasia, it is important to differentiate between high and low grade dysplasia. In small studies, high grade flat dysplastic lesions had concurrent CRC in 42% to 67% of cases (Bernstein et al., 1999; Connell et al., 1994; Hata et al., 2003). In another study, patients who underwent colectomy for high grade dysplasia, 45% were found to have CRC noted on pathology (Rutter et al., 2006). In patients with high grade dysplasia who chose not to undergo colectomy, 25% to 32% of the cases progressed to CRC (Bernstein et al., 1999; Rutter et al, 2006). Given the high risk for synchronus CRC associated with high grade dysplastic lesions, and the significantly increased risk of progression to CRC, current consensus opinions recommends colectomy.

With regards to low grade flat dysplasia, however, the evidence is more equivocal. Low grade dysplasia can be viewed as an intermediate step in the development of CRC, or it alone may be a marker for synchronous undiagnosed high grade dysplastic lesions or cancer. (Bernstein et al., 1994; Gorfine et al., 2000; Rutter et al., 2006). Studies vary regarding the risks of low grade dysplasia with some equating it to the risk of high grade dysplasia while others find it no more concerning than patients with no dysplasia. Small studies including patients who underwent colectomy for low grade dysplasia found synchronous CRC in 19% to 27% of patients (Bernstein et al., 1994; Farraye et al., 2010; Rutter et al., 2006). A more recent meta-analysis by Thomas et al. included 20 surveillance studies of flat low grade dysplasia or low grade dysplasia DALMs, and found a cancer incidence of 14 per 1000 patient years and 30 per 1000 patient year incidence of advanced lesions (high grade dysplasia or CRC). When low grade dysplasia was detected on colonoscopy it was associated with a nine fold increased risk of developing CRC, and 12 fold risk of developing advanced lesions. For patients who opt to avoid colectomy and prefer continued surveillance of flat dysplasia, according to this meta-analysis the positive predictive value for progression to high grade dysplasia or CRC is approximately 14.6% (Thomas et al., 2007). Other studies list rates of progression to neoplasia ranging from 33% to 54% (Rutter et al., 2006; Ullman et al., 2002). Other studies suggest that the risk of progression from low grade dysplasia to high grade dysplasia or CRC is actually much lower. In a study of patients with long standing extensive UC, the risk of progression to CRC in patients with low grade dysplasia was 10% while patients with extensive UC but no dysplasia progressed to CRC in 4% of the cases. This study concluded that the risk of progression is not much higher than in patients with no dysplasia (0.8 to 3%) and therefore prophylactic colectomy is not appropriate (Lim et al., 2003). Moreover, another study did not find any cases of low grade dysplasia progressing to CRC (Befrits et al., 2002). Since the actual risk of progression is unclear, consensus recommendations favor discussion with the patients and informing them of the risks and benefits of surveillance versus early colectomy. A medical decision analysis of 10,000 patients with UC was performed to assess patient preference when faced with the decision between surveillance and colectomy for unifocal low grade dysplasia. Overall patients preferred immediate colectomy, with slight increase in quality adjusted life years and overall lower costs of treatment (Nguyen et al., 2009).

4.7 Prevalent versus incident dysplasia

Dysplasia is further classified based on when it was found on endoscopic exam. Dysplasia detected on initial colonoscopy is referred to as prevalent dysplasia. Prevalent dysplasia carries a higher rate of progression to CRC. When prevalent low grade dysplasia was found 29% of patients progressed to high grade dysplasia or CRC during follow up (Bernstein et al., 1994). In contrast, dysplasia that was detected on subsequent surveillance colonoscopy is referred to as incident dysplasia. When incident low grade dysplasia was found, only 16% of cases progressed to high grade dysplasia or CRC. In comparison, if no dysplasia was noted on initial colonoscopy, the risk of subsequent CRC ranged from 1.1% to 3.1% (Bernstein et al., 1994; Connell et al., 1994; Lindberg et al., 1996; Nugent et al., 1991).

4.8 Interobserver variability in grading of dysplasia

Unfortunately, there is significant variability in pathologists' agreement in the grading of dysplasia, ranging from 42 to 65% (Melville et al., 1989). This is most prominent in non-gastrointestinal specialized pathologists and between the classification of marked regenerative changes versus low grade dysplasia and between the classification of high grade dysplasia and invasive adenocarcinoma (Riddell et al., 1983). Interobserver studies show only moderate levels of agreement between pathologists' interpretations (Dixon et al., 1988; Eaden et al, 2001b; Melville et al., 1989; Odze et al., 2002). The levels of agreement were lowest in cases of indefinite dysplasia and low grade dysplasia. Unfortunately, even with experienced pathologists, there still remain a significant amount of interobserver variability between indefinite versus low grade (Melville et al., 1989). In contrast, the interobserver validity between negative and high grade dysplasia is quite good (Dixon et al., 1988). Given that treatment decisions are made based on the degree of dysplasia, consensus recommendations recommend that a pathologist specializing in gastroenterology review and confirm any cases of dysplasia (Itzkowitz & Present, 2005).

Levels of dyplasia	Interobserver validity
Indefinite for dysplasia vs. Low grade dysplasia	**Poor**
High grade dysplasia vs. Carcinoma	**Poor**
Negative for dysplasia vs. High grade dysplasia	**Good**

Table 6. Interobserver validity based on level of dysplasia

4.9 Molecular markers

In order to reduce interobserver variability molecular and non-molecular markers have been evaluated to aid in the diagnosis of dysplasia. Majority of the studies on tumor markers are tested from the biopsy samples of dysplasia or no dysplasia which unfortunately does not provide information on the evolution of the dysplasia. Few studies have been designed to study patients longitudinally over time to detect the early expression of tumor markers. The markers that have been evaluated in this format showing increased risk of CRC include aneuploidy, p53, MSI and mucin-associated STn antigen (Farraye et al., 2010). Aneuploidy is an early event in the carcinogenesis pathway often occurring before or coincident with the initial detection of dysplasia (Rubin et al., 1992). Similarly, p53 mutation is also an event that is likely preceding the dysplasia and is an important step in the carcinogenesis progression (Lashner et al., 1999). In some of the patients the p53 mutation was detected eight months to two years prior to dysplastic changes (Ilyas & Talbot, 1995; Lashner et al., 1999). Patients with this mutation had a relative risk of developing dysplasia or cancer of 4.53 (95% CI 2.16-9.48) and was associated with cancer related mortality (Lashner et al., 1999). Likewise, patients who develop microsatellite instability CRC already expressed these changes in non-dysplastic tissue ranging from two to twelve years prior to the diagnosis of CRC (Tahara et al., 2005). The STN antigen expression occurs frequently in dysplastic lesions that often occur earlier than the aneuploidy changes (Karlen et al., 1998b). While these markers seem to portend a poor prognosis like p53, they are not incorporated yet into the overall assessment to choose between colectomy and continued surveillance. The added benefits of these makers are their noted presence in the mucosa long before carcinoma develops. Such an aid could assist pathologists in being more precise in their grading of dysplasia. However, further studies are still needed to determine the niche of molecular profiling in CRC surveillance and risk stratification.

Molecular Markers to assist in determination of dysplasia
AMACR
Aneuploidy
p53
MSI
Mucin-associated STn antigen

Table 7. Potential molecular markers to aid in determination of dysplasia

A potentially promising biomarker is the α-methylacyl-CoA racemase (AMACR). This marker is not found in any non-dysplastic tissue. It is significantly increased in areas of low grade dysplasia (96%), high grade dysplasia (80%) and adenocarcinoma (71%). This marker was only found in 14% of cases of indefinite for dysplasia, but was only focally and weakly positive. In attempting to differentiate high grade dysplasia the specificity is nearly 100% with a sensitivity of 80 to 96% (Dorer & Odze, 2002). While more studies are still needed, this marker does have the potential to significantly assist pathologists in determination of dysplasia versus no dysplasia.

5. Surveillance colonoscopy

While enhanced surveillance colonoscopy in patients with UC is presumed to reduce the risk of developing CRC, it has not been proven through randomized control trials. Only case series suggest a possible benefit (Eaden et al., 2000a; Lofberg et al., 1990; Nugent et al., 1991). A Cochrane database review of these trials in 2004 revealed a reduction in CRC mortality in those patients who underwent at least one screening colonoscopy with a relative risk of 0.28 (95% confidence interval 0.07 to 1.17). This effect was more pronounced in those who had at least two screening colonoscopies (RR 0.22 95% confidence interval 0.03 to 1.74). This effect was less notable for patients who only had one colonoscopy (RR 0.43 95% confidence intervals 0.05 to 3.76). Unfortunately though, all the confidence intervals crossed 1. As a result, the study concluded that there is no clear evidence that surveillance colonoscopy prolongs patient survival. While cancer is detected at an earlier stage in patients with a better prognosis who undergo surveillance screening, there is concern that lead time bias may cause this affect. It seems likely, though, that screening reduces the risk of death and may be cost effective as well. (Mpofu et al., 2004).

5.1 Surveillance colonoscopy recommendations

While classic CRC screening recommends colonoscopy once every ten years given the slow evolution of adenoma to carcinoma, in UC this interval is less clear. Some studies have noted new pathology within one to two years of a reported negative colonoscopy (Connell et al., 1994; Lim et al., 2003). Therefore, surveillance colonoscopy initiation and interval follow up is tailored to the patients underlying risks. All patients with UC should undergo a screening colonoscopy at eight years to ten years after the onset of symptoms with appropriate biopsies to determine the true extent of any microscopic disease (Eaden & Mayberry, 2002).

Extent of disease, which helps determine follow up interval, is based on the most proximal disease noted histologically at any point in the patient's disease. If the patient's disease is isolated proctitis or proctosigmoiditis then UC specific related screening can be terminated. As mentioned earlier, these isolated conditions do not convey a significantly increased risk of UC-related CRC. These patients should follow routine screening CRC prevention guidelines starting at age 50 unless the patient has a concerning family history necessitating earlier screening as per CRC screening guidelines.

If the UC is classified as pancolitis or left sided colitis with negative initial screening, the follow up colonoscopies should be performed every one to two years. In patients who have a negative initial screening colonoscopy, follow up exams should be performed every one to two years until the patient has two negative examinations. After two negative exams, surveillance can be spread to over one to three years until the duration of disease has existed for twenty years. At that time, interval surveillance should be narrowed again to every one to two years.

Patients with associated primary sclerosing cholangitis carry a significantly increased risk of CRC and therefore should begin indefinite screening immediately at the time of diagnosis and every year thereafter. Other high risk patients, like those with a family history of CRC in first degree relatives, ongoing active inflammation (either endoscopic or histologic), foreshortened colon, strictures, or multiple inflammatory pseudopoyps all may benefit from more frequent surveillance exams. However, the exact interval follow up is unclear (Farraye et al., 2010; Itzkowitz & Present, 2005).

Initial screening colonoscopy	Screening recommendations
Ulcerative colitis screening colonoscopy	Initiate 8-10 years after onset of disease
Associated Primary sclerosing cholangitis	Initiate at time of diagnosis
Interval follow up screening after initial negative screening colonoscopy	
UC patient with negative initial screen	Continue surveillance intervals every 1-2 years until 2 negative exams then interval screening is every 1-3 years.
UC patient with 20 years duration of disease	Re-start surveillance intervals every 1-2 years
UC patient with Extensive/Left sided colitis	Continue regular surveillance intervals every 1-2 years
UC patient with PSC	Continue surveillance every year
UC patient with family history of CRC, active inflammation, foreshortened colon, strictures, multiple inflammatory pseduoplyps	May benefit from more frequent surveillance. Exact interval surveillance is unclear.
UC patient with isolated Proctitis/Proctosigmoiditis	Screen per guidelines for age-specific CRC (no increased surveillance)

Table 8. Summary of screening and follow up surveillance recommendations

The British Society of Gastroenterology updated their screening recommendations in 2010. The updates to their guidelines include initiating screening approximately ten years after disease onset. Also, surveillance colonoscopies should only be performed during disease remission, but should not be unduly delayed. Importantly, the risk of cancer is influenced by duration and extent of disease and additional risk factors like primary sclerosing cholangitis and family history of colorectal cancer. Also, both histologic and endoscopic features can also portend an increased risk of CRC. Patients at high risk should have yearly exams, moderate risk every three years, and low risk every five years. Newer modalities of screening are also incorporated in the new guidelines. Pancolonic dye spraying with targeted biopsies of the abnormal area should be performed. If chromoendoscopy is available then it should be used. Otherwise two to four random biopsies of every 10 cm of colon should be obtained. However, in areas of concern, additional biopsy samples should be taken. Finally, if dysplastic lesions can be completely removed it is not necessary to recommend colectomy (Cairns et al., 2010).

5.2 Management of dysplastic lesions

In the event that flat high grade dysplasia is noted anywhere in the colon and confirmed by an expert gastrointestinal pathologist, colectomy is the treatment of choice (Farraye et al., 2010; Thomas et al., 2007). Similarly, multifocal low grade dysplasia is also considered a strong indication for colectomy. Those with pathology termed indefinite for dysplasia should undergo a repeat examination in three to twelve months (Farraye et al., 2010). It is unclear if colectomy or enhanced surveillance should be performed for flat unifocal low grade dysplasia given the potential progression to high grade dysplasia or CRC. If surveillance is chosen, follow up colonoscopy should be done within three to six months. Discussion about risks and benefits of colectomy versus closer surveillance must be discussed with the patient. Similarly, it is unclear if recurrent findings of flat low grade dysplasia on serial colonoscopies increase the risk of synchronous or metachronous CRC compared to the risk associated with the finding of an isolated flat low grade dysplasia. A similar discussion with the patient regarding risks and benefits of screening versus colectomy should be done.

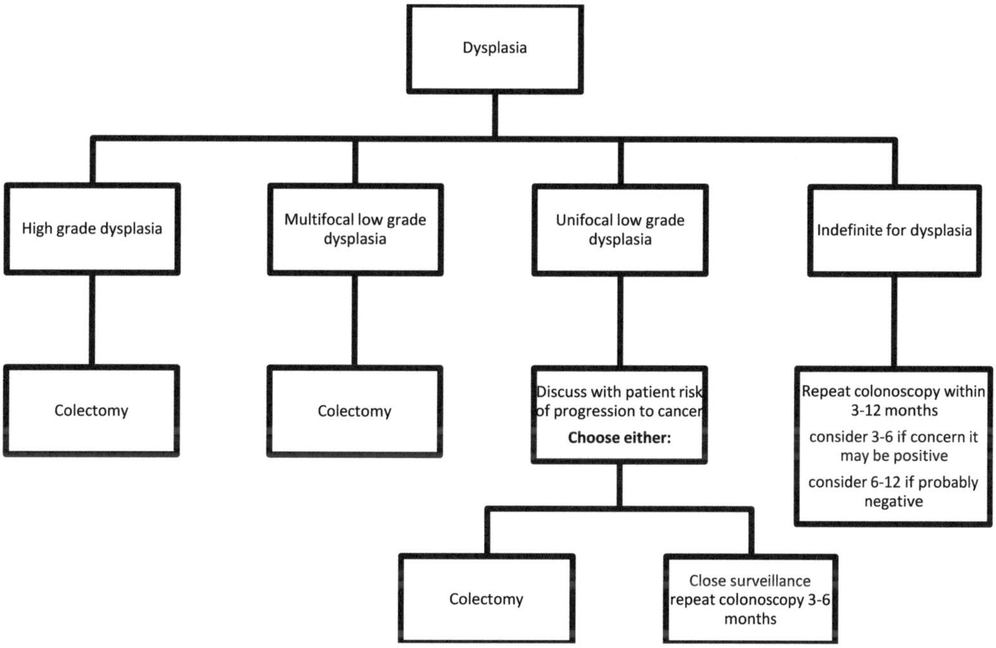

Fig. 2. Management of dysplasia (For DALM management see figure)

5.3 Factors involving successful endoscopy

There are a number of factors that affect the success rate of a screening colonoscopy program. The initial detection of potentially dysplastic lesions relies on endoscopist skill and technique. Unlike sporadic adenomas, some lesions in UC may be flat and difficult to detect. Overall though, up to two thirds of dysplastic lesions are visible on endoscopy (Rutter et al, 2004b). However, a sizable number of potentially dysplastic lesions are missed on routine endoscopic visualization. As a result, a number of newer techniques are being developed to enhance the detection of the remaining dysplastic lesions. Another challenge is the ability to completely resect suspected lesions. While prior studies had recommended colectomy for DALMs, newer studies have demonstrated equal success with complete polypectomy (Engelsgjerd et al., 1999; Vieth et al., 2006). The importance of complete resection is crucial to the success of a surveillance program. Any lesion that cannot be completely resected, should negate continued surveillance and proceed to colectomy. Lastly, the endoscopic must comply with the current consensus recommendations when using their recommended intervals. Overall adherence to consensus guidelines is quite poor (Bernstein et al., 1995; Eaden et al., 2000b).

5.4 Adequate sampling of mucosa

Given that microscopic disease can occur anywhere in the colon, multiple biopsies must be obtained to achieve adequate surveillance. Thirty three samples yielded a 90% probability of detecting any present dysplasia, while sixty four samples yield a 95% probability of detecting dysplasia if present (Rubin et al., 1992). A total of two to four samples should be taken from all four quadrants from every ten centimeters of colon (Itzkowitz & Harpaz, 2004). Careful examination and sampling of the rectosigmoid region is crucial as this area has a predominance of neoplasia in UC (Choi, 1993). These specimens should be collected in individual jars to assist in localizing the specimen back to the colonic segment if further monitoring is warranted. The ideal time for surveillance screening with random biopsy sampling should be when the patient is in a state of clinical remission. Active inflammation creates difficulty in distinguishing reactive epithelium from dysplasia (Eaden & Mayberry, 2002). Nonetheless, even with extensive biopsies of the colon, it is still only a small fraction of the entire colon that is sampled (approximately 1%) (Itzkowitz & Harpaz, 2004). Given that dysplasia is most often unifocal in nature, it is still quite possible to miss the one location that has high grade dysplasia or carcinoma. Another complicating factor is that despite consensus recommendations regarding biopsy sampling, surveys of gastroenterologists' biopsy practices in the United States and United Kingdom demonstate poor adherence to these recommendations, further lowering the probability of detecting dysplasia (Bernstein et al., 1995; Eaden et al., 2000c). As newer endoscopic modalities like chromoendoscopy and narrow band imaging are being developed, more targeted biopsies will be possible with the goal of overall improved surveillance of the entire colon.

5.5 Anatomic factors complicating surveillance

Adequate surveillance is also limited by anatomic factors. Presence of either psuedopolyps or strictures has been reported to increase the risk of CRC by two fold and four fold respectively (Rutter et al., 2004c). Other reports found up to 24% of strictures may be malignant (Gumaste et al., 1992). Additionally, strictures throughout the colon may limit the endoscopists ability to adequately maneuver around them limiting the comprehensiveness of the surveillance examination.

6. Assessment, cost and safety, and hurdles to successful screening program

The key features of any surveillance program include (1) a disease with a high prevalence in the selected patient population; (2) a screening test that is highly sensitive and specific, (3) low cost, (4) safe, and (5) acceptable to both the patient and the practitioner. The early detection of disease should then enable early treatment of the disease to ideally prolong survival (Wilson, & Jungner, 1968). The prevalence of UC associated CRC, and the knowledge that dysplastic changes occur in the colon prior to symptoms provides the background for instituting a screening program. However, the costs, risks and associated hurdles all need to be evaluated for the program to be effective.

6.1 Assessment of surveillance programs

Evaluating the success of surveillance programs has been challenging for numerous reasons. The timeframe needed to assess the impact on patients requires approximately fifteen to twenty years (Eaden & Mayberry, 2000). Also, patient compliance over this prolonged period of time is challenging, necessitating multiple visits for follow up colonoscopies. Another confounder is varying treatment recommendations from physicians. As discussed previously, adherence to guideline recommendations is variable. There are some centers that recommend early colectomy for dysplasia resulting in overall lower rates of cancer but at a significant morbidity cost. Finally, randomization is impractical given the ethical issues related to placing high risk patients in control arms (Eaden & Mayberry, 2000). While some studies of screening endoscopies found earlier cases of cancer, this was only in a minority of patients with a high cost-to-benefit ratio (Axon, 1994; Collins et al., 1987; Gyde, 1990). Conversely, a small US study attributed early cancer detection to surveillance with a five year survival rate of 77% in the surveillance group compared to 36% in the control group (Choi, 1993). Other studies that did not find any significant benefit in detection of CRC still found a much lower mortality in the screened group due to associated clinical reviews of their disease and management (Connell et al., 1993; Karlen et al., 1998a). However, a Cochrane meta-analysis failed to show a benefit for surveillance screening colonoscopies to prevent CRC-related death (Rutter et al., 2006).

6.2 Safety and cost effectiveness of surveillance

The overall morbidity associated with surveillance colonoscopy is extremely low. The overall complication rate after 379 surveillance colonoscopies was one silent perforation, or 0.26% (Koobatian & Choi, 1994). Similar findings were noted in a British study of 811 surveillance colonoscopies (Lennard-Jones et al., 1990). Using decision analysis to provide indirect evidence of CRC screening effectiveness, Provenzale et al found life expectancy increased 1.2 years with screening (Provenzale et al., 1995). The overall cost of the surveillance program is difficult to estimate. The costs of the surveillance program need to include not only the medical costs, but also the patients time undergoing the test, travel, lost earnings, and, the more difficult to assess, patient anxiety and discomfort (Eaden & Mayberry, 2000). One US study using a hypothetical scenario of a screening system that found all cancerous lesions in 1000 patients over a ten year period estimated the cost for each cancer found or prevented to be $200,000 (based on cost data from 1983). However, this price does not account for the patient costs or potential complications when performing the numerous colonoscopies. In this study, an estimated 9,775 colonoscopies were performed to locate or prevent a cancer. However, with a perforation rate of 0.2 to 0.4 roughly three patients would need emergent treatment for perforated colon adding to the overall screening cost (Collins et al., 1987; Eaden & Mayberry, 2000; Katzka et al., 1983). A more recent study comparing endoscopic cancer screening tests found a theoretically lower cost. Using an estimated risk of UC related CRC of 1%, and with performingcolonoscopies every two years, they found that 1.4 to 2 cancers per 100 endoscopies would be detected. The overall cost of the procedure alone was $71,000 per cancer detected (Sonnenberg & El-Serag, 1997). Unfortunately, these numbers are only hypothetical costs of the procedures alone in a 100% successful screening system.

6.3 Hurdles to successful screening surveillance program

Crucial to any screening program is the ability of the endoscopist to accurately biopsy the colon and the pathologist to accurately diagnose dysplasia. Discussed early in this chapter, the interobserver variability amongst pathologists can limit the successful diagnosis of dysplasia and appropriate treatment recommendations. Furthermore, despite consensus guidelines published by both European and US societies, there still remains significant variability amongst gastroenterologists' compliance with these recommendations. In one study of US gastroenterologists, only 19% correctly defined dysplasia. Within this group 48% accurately defined high grade dysplasia and only 16% defined low grade dysplasia. When choosing treatment options, nearly one third of gastroenterologists recommended continued surveillance despite a diagnosis of high grade dysplasia (Bernstein et al., 1995). In a British study, only 53% of gastroenterologists recommended colectomy for high grade dysplasia (Eaden et al., 2000b). A more recent study of both colorectal surgeons and gastroenterologists from New Zealand similarly found poor knowledge of the definition of dysplasia, with only 20% responding correctly. In this group, the colorectal surgeons defined dysplasia correctly more often and understood the significance of low grade dysplasia as well (Geary et al., 2004). Despite clear recommendations from the American Gastroenterological Association to perform four quadrant biopsies every ten cm for a total of thirty to forty biopsies, only 41% of gastroenterologists followed this recommendation. 52% of the gastroenterologists only took two to four biopsies and 6% did not follow any protocol. Overall, 73% of the gastroenterologists performed less than thirty biopsies per colonoscopy (van Rijn et al., 2009) . In assessing the overall adequacy of surveillance, 33% of patients received inadequate surveillance for CRC (Reddy et al. 2005; Obrador et al., 2006). In 2009, Kottachchi et al. performed a retrospective study after the publication of the Canadian Association of Gastroenterology screening guidelines and found that the overall adherence improved with 74% of patients receiving follow up surveillance appropriately (Kottachchi et al., 2009). Ultimately, the overall education and continued education in association with consensus guidelines is crucial to adequate screening.

6.4 Patient adherence

Another major hurdle to successful surveillance is patient acceptance of the surveillance process. Multiple aspects of the screening program can create challenges for patients to comply with the screening. Close follow up colonoscopies require patients to repeat bowel preparations, return to clinic, and find a chaperone to take them home. All of these steps are potential pitfalls for patient compliance. Unfortunately, most of these steps cannot be altered to improve patient compliance. However, studies evaluating patient compliance in routine CRC screening found a positive association between knowledge and screening behavior (Vernon, 1997). The lack of knowledge is most prominent among minorities and those of low socioeconomic status (Beeker et al., 2001; Lipkus et al., 1996; Price, 1993). Patients need counseling regarding the importance of CRC surveillance as well as the understanding of the predictive value of the colonoscopy to effectively rule out potential cancer.

Unfortunately, if patients do not adhere to the surveillance recommendations negative consequences may occur (Connell et al., 1994; Lindberg et al., 1996).

Barriers to screening
Definition of dysplasia
Differentiating subtypes of dysplasia
Appropriate number of biopsies
Adherence to guidelines
Surveillance
Treatment
Patient specific barriers
Lack of knowledge
Preferences
Non-compliance with recommendations

Table 9. Barriers to screening

7. Newer imaging modalities

Given that up to 1/3 of dysplasia is not detected on endoscopic examination, better diagnostic modalities are needed in place of just random biopsies. Without improved diagnostic techniques, a negative exam from random biopsies could convey a false sense of reassurance. Newer modalities attempt to delineate those lesions that are subtle but present at the layer of the mucosa, or even deeper providing the endoscopist with both subsurface analysis and instant histologic analysis. Such newer techniques combining both random biopsies with more focused examination would theoretically provide a more thorough and accurate screening process. Newer modalities are sometimes used alone or in combination and include chromoendoscopy with pancolonic dye spraying, autofluorescene, confocal laser endomicroscopy, narrow band imaging, and optical coherence tomography.

7.1 Chromoendoscopy

Chromoendoscopy is a technique that has already been used in Europe and Asia, and more recently in the US, to help identify non-polypoid flat and depressed potentially neoplastic lesions (Soetkino et al., 2006). Chromoendoscopy involves applying mucosal stain or pigment by injecting dye down an endoscopic spray catheter. Indigo carmine is one type of dye which coats the colonic mucosal surface enabling the endoscopist to visualize subtle disruptions in the normal contours of the mucosa. Another dye, methylene blue, is avidly absorbed by non-inflamed mucosa and poorly taken up by inflamed mucosa and dysplastic lesions. The dyes improve the detection of subtle colonic lesions enabling increased sensitivity of screening colonoscopy. Additionally, chromoendoscopy can differentiate neoplastic from non-neoplastic lesions based on the crypt architecture utilizing the modified pit pattern classification (Rutter, 2010). This is further improved when using a magnifying colonoscope (Kudo et al., 2001). These techniques enable the endoscopist to obtain targeted biopsies after pancolonic dye spraying, improving overall sensitivity of the exam (Kiesslich et al., 2003; Marion et al., 2008; Mastumoto et al., 2003; Rutter et al., 2004a).

Chromoendoscopy is also able to provide a more accurate determination of extent of disease as well as degree of inflammation (Kiesslich et al., 2003). The superiority of focused biopsies utilizing methylene blue was supported in a study noting a three fold increase in dysplasia detection compared to random biopsies alone (Kiesslich et al., 2003). In comparing the diagnostic yield to standard colonoscopy, panchromoendoscopy with indigo carmine dye increased the diagnostic yield of dysplasia 3.5 to 4.5 fold (Rutter et al., 2004a). A different study compared 350 patients with long standing UC undergoing surveillance using chromoendoscopy and a high magnification colonoscope to 350 matched UC control patients undergoing standard white light colonoscopy and found that the enhanced screening technique yielded more dysplastic lesions. However, this enhanced detection was at the cost of significantly longer extubation times (average of 24 minutes compared to 13 minutes in the control group) (Hurlstone et al., 2005).

7.2 Autofluorescene imaging

A different imaging enhanced modality, autofluorescene imaging, in a small study showed improved detection of dysplastic lesions compared to routine endoscopy (van den Brock et al., 2008). The sensitivity for detecting dysplastic lesions ranged from 87% to 100% after local sensitization (Kiesslich et al., 2008). However, current guidelines do not currently incorporate this method into their screening recommendations and more studies are needed to assess its overall utility and cost effectiveness.

7.3 Confocal laser endomicroscopy

A newer method, confocal laser endomicroscopy, allows subsurface analysis of intestinal mucosa and analysis of the underlying histology during the endoscopy (Kiesslich et al., 2008). This is attached to a standard endoscope and used in conjunction with a system fluorescent contrast agent or topical agent sprayed on mucosa. The images provide real-time information regarding cellular and vascular changes. The sensitivity reached 97.4% with a specificity of 99.4% and an accuracy of 99.2% (Kiesslich et al., 2007). This method can be used in conjunction with chormoenedoscopy which will help identify circumscript lesions, while the laser endomicroscopy is able to predict the intraepithelial neoplasias (Kiesslich et al., 2008). In a study comparing the combination of panchromoendoscopy and endomicroscopy compared to conventional colonoscopy, the combined modality found significantly more intraepithelial neoplasia (19 versus 3 p value 0.007) but had an 11 minute longer average extubation time (42 minutes versus 31 minutes). This technique provided a 4.75 fold increase in detected dysplastic lesions while needing 50% fewer biopsy specimens (Kiesslich et al., 2007).

7.4 Narrow band imaging, optical coherence tomography

Other modalities like narrow band imaging which uses optical technology to visualize microvascular structures of the mucosal layers has not been shown to be superior to standard colonoscopy (Dekker et al., 2007). Another method, optical coherence tomography, utilizes an optical analog of ultrasound to allow for cross-sectional images of the luminal gastrointestinal tract. This too does not yet provide satisfactory resolution to enhance surveillance over routine colonoscopy (Kiesslich et al., 2008).

Given that all these techniques are still relatively new, it has not been proven yet if the increased sensitivity in locating dysplastic lesions in fact prolongs survival. Also, as white light endoscopy technology continues to improve, it is unclear how many additional lesions will still be found when newer white light endoscopes are studied in comparison to chromoendoscopy (Farraye et al., 2010).

8. Chemoprevention

In the non-UC population, chemoprevention using cox-2 inhibitors or aspirin has been evaluated with success (Arber & Levin, 2008). In UC, chemoprevention is of particular interest for its potential to reduce the risk of CRC. Similar to sporadic CRC, the presumed initial insult is chronic inflammation. As a result, chemoprevention in UC has also focused on anti-inflammatory agents. Aminosalicylates, corticosteroids, folic acid, immunomodulators, and UDCA have all been studied.

8.1 Ursodeoxycholic acid (UDCA)

As mentioned earlier, UC patients with associated PSC are at the highest risk of CRC. UDCA is already used to treat the cholestatic affects of primary sclerosing cholangitis. Retrospective analysis of patients already taking UDCA and with concomitant UC found a strong decreased incidence of colonic dysplasia with an odds ratio of 0.18 (95% CI 0.05-0.61) (Tung et al., 2001). This was confirmed in a prospective study out of Mayo Clinic showing a similar reduction in dysplasia and cancer (Pandi et al., 2003). Unfortunately though, there have been conflicting studies performed showing no chemopreventive effects from the UDCA (Shetty et al., 1999; Wolf et al., 2005). UDCA has also been evaluated in patients with UC with no associated PSC. A small study in Sweden found potential benefits after two years of treatment with UDCA; in the ten patients who took UDCA, none developed high grade dysplasia or cancer (Sjoqvist et al., 2004). The underlying mechanism of UDCA is unknown, but it may decrease bile acids like deoxycholic acid which may have carcinogenic potential.

8.2 Aminosalicylates

Aminosalicylates are used for maintenance therapy in many patients with UC for prolonged periods of time. Studies in England have shown a 75 to 90% reduction in the incidence of CRC (Eaden et al., 2000a). Both mesalazine and sufasalazine have chemoprotective effects with dose response effect. Mesalazine was somewhat superior and reduced cancer by 81% at doses > 1.2 grams daily (Moody et al., 1996; Rubin et al., 2006b; van Staa et al., 2005). Also, the longer the duration of mesalazine use, the more pronounced the effect (van Staa et al., 2005). Other studies have noted 60% to 72% risk reduction rates of CRC with the use of mesalamine. This benefit was separate from the risk reduction associated with surveillance colonoscopy (Rubin et al., 2006b; Velayos et al., 2006). Unfortunately, this benefit is lost with cessation of the drug as noted in a retrospective study with only 3% of patients on mesalamine developing CRC compared to 31% of patients who stopped or could not comply with treatment (Moody et al., 1996). Similar to the UDCA, there are some conflicting studies which did not achieve risk reductions of CRC with any statistical significance (Bernstein et al., 2003; Lindberg et al., 2001; Ullman et al., 2008). A large meta-analysis of the studies using mesalamine showed a preventative effect for CRC with mesalamine use (OR 0.51; 95% CI, 0.37-0.69) and for CRC plus dysplasia (OR 0.51; 95% CI, 0.38-0.69). However, mesalamine did not lower the overall risk of dysplasia (OR 1.18; 95% CI, 0.41-3.43) (Velayos et al., 2005). Given this understanding of mesalamine being protective against CRC but not specifically for dysplasia, it is unclear when mesalamine treatment provides the greatest chemopreventive benefits in the dysplasia-carcinoma sequence. In one retrospective study of high and low dose mesalamine in patients with no dysplasia, indefinite dysplasia, and low grade dysplasia, the largest benefit was found in patients taking high dose mesalamine (>2grams per day) and no dysplasia or indefinite for dysplasia (Ullman et al., 2008). Based on this study it is hypothesized that the most benefit is found early on in the dysplasia-carcinoma sequence prior to any significant dysplastic changes. The underlying mechanism of action of the anti-neoplastic effects has been postulated to be its potential anti-inflammatory activity, promotion of apoptosis of CRC tissue with no effect on normal mucosa, or improved DNA replication fidelity in CRC cells.

8.3 Corticosteroids and Nonsteroidal anti-inflammatory drugs (NSAID)

Continuing with the anti-inflammatory hypothesis to reduce CRC risk, corticosteroids have been evaluated given their known anti-inflammatory effects. While not the primary end-point, most studies have found no chemoprotective effect with the use of corticosteroids. However, some studies found a 60% risk reduction with the use of oral prednisone for greater than one year (OR 0.4; 95% CI 0.2 to 0.8) (Velayos et al., 2006). However, regardless of the potential treatment benefit, the toxicity associated with chronic steroid use limits the benefits of this potential treatment. While NSAID use has been show to be chemoprotective in sporadic CRC, its use in UC related CRC is less clear. A recent study of patients with a history of IBD and NSAID use did not achieve statistical significance (OR 0.47; 95% CI, 0.12-1.86). The results, however, were suggestive of a potential risk reduction, but no definitive recommendations can be made (Samadder et al., 2011).

8.4 Immunomodulators and biologic agents

Since immunomodulators are the cornerstone of therapy for many patients with UC, their potential risk reduction benefits have been evaluated. In patients who were free of dysplasia neither 6-mercaptopurine (6-MP) nor azathioprine (AZA) showed any protection on progression to CRC after eight years (Matula et al., 2005). Among patients with extensive colitis and prolonged use of AZA, there was still no reduced cancer risk (Connell et al., 1994). Even in high risk patients with associated PSC, use of AZA did not provide any chemopreventive benefits (Tung et al., 2001). Similarly, 6-MP did not find any CRC risk reduction, but importantly, it also did not show any increased risk of cancer in the setting of prolonged use (Korelitz et al., 1999). Given the lack of evidence supporting CRC risk reduction with immunomodulators, they cannot be recommended as chemoprophylaxis.

8.5 Supplements (folic acid, calcium, and multivitamins)

In sporadic CRC, folic acid deficiency has been associated with spontaneous CRC formation (Freudenheim et al., 1991). Patients with UC are predisposed to folate deficiency from both poor nutritional intake and intestinal losses associated with inflammation in active disease. Despite this, current studies encorporating folic acid supplementation have been suggestive of a potential benefit but did not achieve any statistically significant reduction (Lashner et al., 1989; Lashner et al., 1996). However, the potential benefit may be confounded due to many patients already taking multivitamins or eating bread that is fortified with folic acid.

Additionally, supplementing with calcium or multivitamins has also not been shown to reduce overall cancer risk in UC (Farraye et al., 2010).

8.6 Statins

More recently, statin therapy has been evaluated as a possible chemopreventive agent. In a case control study based in Israel of a colorectal cancer registry, patients on long term statin use had a reduced risk of developing CRC. In this study, patients with IBD had an overall 1.9 fold increased risk of developing CRC. This was attenuated though with long term statin use (OR 0.07; 95% CI 0.01-0.78) (Samadder et al., 2011). Statin use for five years was found to have a large risk reduction of 94% in patients with IBD (Poynter et al., 2005).

Agents	Chemoprotective benefit
Aminosalicylates	Likely chemoprotective
UDCA	Chemoprotective with comorbid PSC Potentially chemoprotective with UC alone
Statins	Potentially chemoprotective
Corticosteroids	Toxicity outweights any benefit
NSAID	Unclear
Immunomodulators	No effect
Folic acid	Unclear
Calcium	No effect
Multivitamin	No effect

Table 10. Chemoprotective effects of different agents

9. Conclusion

Patients with UC are at increased risk of CRC relative to the general population. The overall risk is still unclear and ranges from a mild to significantly increased risk relative to the general population. Specific patient risk factors including extent of disease, duration of disease, severity of inflammation, age of onset, family history, and associated PSC all increase the risk of CRC. With this increased risk, UC related cancer screening is recommended. More specific recommendations are still needed to help analyze the individual UC patient's risk profile when determining appropriate screening intervals. Additionally, both gastroenterologists and pathologist need continued training on current guidelines and definitions for dysplasia. With improved adherence to guidelines, and correct interpretation of dysplasia, more appropriate treatment can be initiated. The ultimate goal in UC patients is to lower their risk for CRC to that of the general population.

10. References

Ahmadi, A., Polyak, S., & Draganov, P. Colorectal cancer surveillance in inflammatory bowel disease: The search continues. *World Journal of Gastroenterology*. Vol.15, No.1, January 2009, pp. 61-66

Arber, N., & Levin, B. Chemoprevention of colorectal neoplasia: the potential for personalized medicine. *Gastroenterology*. Vol.134, No.4, (April 2008), pp. 1224-37

Askling, J., Dickman, P., Karlén, P., Broström, O., Lapidus, A., Löfberg, R., & Ekbom, A. Family history as a risk factor for colorectal cancer in inflammatory bowel disease. *Gastroenterology*. Vol.120, No.6, (May, 2001) pp. 1356-62

Aust, De., Terdiman, JP., Willenbucher, RF., Chang, CG., Molinaro-Clark, A., Baretton, GB., Loehrs, U., &Waldman, FM. The APC/beta-catenin pathway in ulcerative colitis-related colorectal carcinomas: a mutational analysis. *Cancer*. Vol.94, No.5, (March, 2002), pp. 1421-27

Axon, AT. Cancer surveillance in ulcerative colitis-a time for reappraisal. *Gut*. Vol.35, No.5, (May 1994), pp. 587-589

Baars, J., Looman, C., Steyerberg, E., Beukers, R., Tan, A., Weusten, B., Kuipers, E., van der Woude, C., The risk of inflammatory bowel disease-related colorectal carcinoma is limited: results from a nationwide nested case-control study. *American Journal of Gastroenterology*. Vol.106, No.2, (February 2011), pp. 319-28

Beeker, C., Kraft, JM., Souhwell, BG., & Jorgensen, CM., Colorectal cancer screening in older men and women: qualitative research findings and implications for intervention. *Journal of Community Health*. Vol.25, No.3, (June 2000), pp. 263-78

Befrits, R., Ljung, T., Jaramillo, E., & Rubio, C. Low-grade dysplasia in extensive, long-standing inflammatory bowel disease: a follow-up study. *Diseases of Colon & Rectum*. Vol.45, No.5, (May 2007), pp. 574-83

Bernstein, CN., Blanchard, JF, Metge, C., & Yogendran, M. Does the use of 5-aminosalicylates in inflammatory bowel disease prevent the development of colorectal cancer. *American Journal of Gastroenterology*. Vol.98, No.12, (December 2003), pp. 2784-88

Bernstein, CN., Shanahan, F. & Weinstein, WM. Are we telling patients the truth about surveillance colonoscopy in ulcerative colitis. *Lancet*. Vol.343, No.8889, (January 1994), pp. 71-4

Bernstein, CN., Weinstein, WM ., Levine, DS., & Shanahan, F. Physicians perceptions of dysplasia and approaches to surveillance colonoscopy in ulcerative colitis. Vol.90, No.12, (December 1995), pp. 2106-14

Blackstone, MO., Riddell, RH., Rogers, BH., & Levin, B. Dysplasia-associated lesion or mass (DALM) detected by colonoscopy in long-standing ulcerative colitis: an indication for colectomy. *Gastroenterology*. Vol.80, No.2, (February 1981) pp. 366-74

Brackmann, S., Anderson, SN., Aamodt, G., Roald, B., Langmark, F., Clausen, OP., Aadland, E., Fausa, O., Rydning, A., & Vatn, MH. Two distinct groups of colorectal cancer in inflammatory bowel disease. *Inflammatory Bowel Diseases*. Vol.15, No.1, (January 2009), pp. 9-16

Brentnall, TA., Crispin, DA., Rabinovitch, PS., Haggitt, RC., Rubin, CE., Stevens, AC., & Burmer, GC. Mutations in the p53 gene: an early marker of neoplastic progression in ulcerative colitis. *Gastroenterology*. Vol. 107, No.2, (August 1994), pp. 369-78

Broomé, U., Löfberg, R., Beress, B., & Eriksson, L. Primary sclerosing cholangitis and ulcerative colitis: evidence for increased neoplastic potential. *Hepatology*. Vol.22, No.5, (November 1995), pp. 1404-8

Burner, GC., Rabinovitch, PS., Haggitt, RC., Crispin, DA., Brentnall, TA., Kolli, VR., Stevens, AC., & Rubin, CE. Neopplastic progression in ulcerative colitis: histology, DNA content, and loss of a p53 allele. *Gastroenterology*. Vol.103, No.5 , (November 1992), pp. 1602-10

Cairns, S., Scholefield, J., Steele, R., Dunlop, M., Thomas, H., Evans, G., Eaden, J., Rutter, M., Atkin, W., Saunders, B., Lucassen, A., Jenkins, P., Fairclough, P., & Woodhouse, C. Guidelines for colorectal cancer screening and surveillance in moderate and high risk groups (update from 2002). *Gut*. Vol.59, No.5, (May 2010), pp. 666-89

Choi, PM. Predominance of rectosigmoid neoplasia in ulcerative colitis and its implication on cancer surveillance. *Gastroenterology*. Vol.104, No.2, (February 1993), pp. 666-67

Collins, R., Feldman, M., & Fordtran, J. Colon cancer dysplasia and surveillance in patients with ulcerative colitis. *New England Journal of Medicine*. Vol.316, (June 1987), pp. 1654-58

Collins, R., Lennard-Jones, JE., Williams, CB., Talbot, IC., Price, AB., & Wilkinson, KH. Factors affecting the outcome of endoscopic surveillance for cancer in ulcerative colitis. *Gastroenterology*. Vol.107, No.4, (1994), pp. 934-44

Connell, WR., Kramm, MA., Dickson, M., Balkwill, AM., Ritchie, JK., & Lennard-Jones, JE. Long-term neoplasia of malignancy after azathioprine treatment in inflammatory bowel disease. *Lancet*. Vol.343, No.8908, (May 1994), pp.1249-52

Crohn, B., Rosenberg, H., The sigmoidoscopic picture of chronic ulcerative colitis (non-specific). *American Journal of Medical Science*. Vol.170. (1925), pp. 220-7

Dekker, E., van den Broek, FJ., Reitsma, JB., Hardwick, JC., Offerhaus, GJ., van Deventer, SJ., Hommes, DW., & Fockens, P. Narrow-band imaging compared with conventional colonoscopy for the detection of dysplasia in patients with longstanding ulcerative colitis. *Endoscopy*. Vol.39, No.3 (March 2007), pp. 216-21

Dixon, MF., Brown., LJ., Gilmour, HM., Price, AB., Smeeton, NC., Talbot, IC., & Williams, GT. Observer variation in the assessment of dysplasia in ulcerative colitis. *Histopathology*. Vol.13, No.4, (October 1988), pp.385-397

Dorer, R., & Odze, RD. AMACR immunostaining is useful in detecting dysplastic epithelium in Barrett's esophagus, ulcerative colitis, and Crohn's disease. *American Journal of Pathology*. Vol.30, No.7, (July 2006) pp. 871-77

Eaden, J., & Mayberry, J. Colorectal cancer complicating ulcerative colitis: a review. *The American Journal of Gastroenterology*. Vol.95, No.10, (October 2000), pp. 2710-2719

Eaden, J., & Mayberry, JF. Guidelines for screening and surveillance of asymptomatic colorectal cancer in patients with inflammatory bowel disease. *Gut*. Vol.51, (October 2002) pp. Supplement 5:V10-2

Eaden, J., Abrams, K, McKay, H. Denley, H. & Mayberry, J. Inter-observer variation between general and specialist gastrointestinal pathologists when grading dysplasia in ulcerative colitis. *Journal of pathology*. Vol.194, No.2, (June 2001), pp. 152-57

Eaden, J., Abrams, KR., & Mayberry, JF. The risk of colorectal cancer in ulcerative colitis: a meta-analysis. *Gut*. Vol.48, No.4, (April 2001), pp. 526-35

Eaden, J., Abrams, KR., Ekbom, A., Jackson, E., & Mayberry, JF. Colorectal cancer prevention in ulcerative colitis: a case-control study. *Alimentary Pharmacology & Therapeutics*. Vol.14, No.2, (February 2000), pp. 145-53

Eaden, J., Ward, BA., & Mayberry, JF. How gastroenterologists screen for colon cancer in ulcerative colitis: an analysis of performance. *Gastrointestinal Endoscopy*. Vol.51, No.2, (February 2000), pp. 123-128

Ekbom, A., Helmick, C., Zack, M., & Adami HO. Ulcerative colitis and colorectal cancer. A population-based study. *New England Journal of Medicine*. Vol.323, No.18, (November 1990), pp. 1228-33

Engelsgjerd, M., Farraye, FA., & Odze, RD. Polypectomy may be adequate treatment for adenoma-like dysplastic lesions in chronic ulcerative colitis. *Gastroenterology*. Vol.117, No.6, (December 1999) pp. 1288-94; discussion 1488-91

Farraye, FA., Odze, R., Eaden, J., & Itzkowitz, S. AGA technical review on the diagnosis and management of colorectal neoplasia in inflammatory bowel disease. *Gastroenterology*, Vol.138, (February 2010), pp. 746-74

Fleisher, AJ.,Esteller, M., Harpaz, N., Leytin, A., Rashid, A., Xu, Y., Liang, J., Stine, OC., Yin, J., Zou, TT., Abraham, JM., Kong, D., Wilson, KT., James, SP., Herman, JG., & Melzer, SJ. Microsatellite instability in inflammatory bowel disease-associated neoplastic lesions is associated with hypermethylation and diminished expression of the DNA mismatch repair gene, hMLH1. *Cancer Research*. Vol.60, No.17, (September 2000), pp. 4864-8

Freudenheim, JL., Graham, S. Marshal, JR. Haughey, BP., Cholewinski, S., & Wilkinson, G. Folate intake and carcinogenesis of the colon and rectum. *International Journal of Epidemiology*. Vol, 20, No.2, (June 1991), pp. 368-74

Friedman, S., Odze, RD., & Farraye, FA. Management of neoplastic polyps in inflammatory bowel disease. *Inflammatory Bowel Diseases*. Vol.9, No.4, (July 2003), pp.260-6

Geary, RB., Wakeman, CJ., Barclay, ML. Chapman, BA., Collett, JA., Burt, MJ., & Frizelle, FA. Surveillance for dysplasia in patients with inflammatory bowel disease: a national survey of colonoscopic practice in New Zealand. *Diseases of Colon & Rectum*. Vol.47, No.3, (March 2004), pp. 314-22

Goldman, H. Significance and detection of dysplasia in chronic colitis. *Cancer*. Vol.78, No.11, (December 1996), pp. 2261-63

Gorfine, S., Bauer, J., Harris, M., & Kreel, I. Dysplasia complicating chronic ulcerative colitis: is immediate colectomy warranted. *Diseases of Colon & Rectum*. Vol.43, No.11, (November 2000), pp. 1575-81

Greenstein, AJ. Sachar, DB., Smith, H., Pucillo, A., Papatestas, AE., Kreel, I., Geller, SA., Janowitz, HD., & Aufses, AH. Cancer in universal and left-sided ulcerative colitis: factors determining risk. *Gastroenterology*. Vol.77, No.2, (August 1979), pp. 290-94

Guindi, M., & Riddell, R. The pathology of epithelial pre-malignancy of the gastrointestinal tract. *Best Practice & Research Clinical Gastroenterology*. Vol.15, No.2, (April 2001), pp. 191-210

Gumaste, V., Sachar, DB., & Greenstein, AJ. Benign and malignant colorectal strictures in ulcerative colitis. *Gut*. Vol.33, No.7, (July 1992), pp. 938-41

Gupta, R., Harpaz, N., Itzkowitz, S., Hossain, S., Matula, S., Kornbluth, A., Bodian, C., & Ullman, T. Histologic inflammation is a risk factor for progression to colorectal neoplasia in ulcerative colitis: a cohort study. *Gastroenterology*. Vol.133, No.4, (October 2007), pp.1099-1341

Gyde, SN. Screening for colorectal cancer in ulcerative colitis: dubious benefits and high costs. *Gut*. Vol.31, No.10, (October 1990), pp. 1089-92

Gyde, SN., Prior, P., Allan, RN., Stevens, A., Jewell, DP., Truelove, SC., Löfberg, R., Brostrom, O., & Hellers, G. Colorectal cancer in ulcerative colitis: a cohort study of primary referrals from three centres. *Gut*. Vol.29, No.2, (February 1988), pp. 206-17

Haskall, H. Andrews, CW., Reddy, SI., Dendrinos, K., Farraye, FA., Stucchi, AF., Becker, JM., & Odze, RD. Pathologic features and clinical significance of "backwash" ileitis in ulcerative colitis. *American Journal of Surgical Pathology*. Vol.29, No.11, (November 2005), pp. 1472-81

Hata, K., Watanabe, T., Kazama, S., Suzuki, K., Shinozaki, M., Yokoyama, T., Matsuda, K., Muto, T., & Nagawa, H. Earlier surveillance colonscopy programme improves survival in patients with ulcerative colitis associated colorectal cancer: results of a 23-year surveillance programme in Japanese population. *British Journal of Cancer*. Vol.89, No.7, (October 2003), pp. 1232-1236

Hsieh, CJ., Klump, B., Holzmann, K., Borchard, F., Gregor, M., & Porschen, R. Hypermethylation of the p16ink4a promoter in colectomy specimens of patients with long-standing and extensive ulcerative colitis. *Cancer Research*. Vol.58, No.17, (September 1998), pp. 3942-5

Hurlstone, DP., Sanders, DS., Lobo, AJ., McAlindon, ME., & Cross, SS. Indigo carmine-assisted high-magnification chromoscopic colonoscopy for the detection and characterization of intraepithelial neoplasia in ulcerative colitis: a prospective evaluation. *Endoscopy*. Vol.37, No.12, (December 2005), pp. 1186-92

Hussain, SP., Amstad, P., Raja, K., Ambs, S., Nagashima, M., Bennett, WP., Shields, PG., Ham, AJ., Swenberg, JA., Marrogi, AJ., & Harris, CC. Increased p53 mutation load in noncancerous colon tissue from ulcerative colitis: a cancer-prone chronic inflammatory disease. *Cancer Research*. Vol.60, No.13 (July, 2000), pp. 3333-37

Ilyas, T., & Talbot, IC. p53 expression in ulcerative colitis: a longitudinal study. *Gut*. Vol.37. No.6, (December 1995), pp. 802-4

Issa, JP., Ahuja, N., Toyota, M., Bronner, MP., & Brentnall TA. Accelerated age-related CpG island methylation in ulcerative colitis. *Cancer Research*. Vol.61, No.9, (May 2001), pp. 3573-7

Itzkowitz, S. Colon carcinogenesis in inflammatory bowel disease: applying molecular genetics to clinical practice. *Journal Clinical Gastroenterology*. Vol.36, (May-June 2003) pp. s70-s74

Itzkowitz, S., & Harpaz, N., Diagnosis and management of dysplasia in patients with inflammatory bowel diseases. *Gastroenterology*. Vol.126, No.6, (May 2004), pp. 1634-48

Itzkowitz, S., & Present, DH. Consensus conference: colorectal cancer screening and surveillance in inflammatory bowel disease. *Inflammatory Bowel Diseases*. Vol.11, No.3, (March 2005), pp. 314-21

Itzkowitz, S., & Ullman T. The world isn't flat. *Gastrointestinal Endoscopy*. Vol.60, No.3, (September 2004), pp. 426-27

Itzkowitz, S., & Yio, X. Inflammation and cancer IV. colorectal cancer in inflammatory bowel disease: the role of inflammation. *American Journal of Physiology Gastrointestinal Liver Physiology*. Vol.287, (July 2004), pp. G7-G17

Jess, T., Loftus, E., Velayos, F., Harmsen, S., Zinsmeister, A., Smyrk, T., Schleck, C., Tremaine, W., Melton, LJ., Munkholm, P., & Sandborn, W. Risk of intestinal cancer in inflammatory bowel disease: a population-based study from Olmsted county, Minnesota. *Gastroenterology*. Vol.130, No.4, (April 2006), pp. 1039-46

Karlén, P., Kornfeld, D., Broström, O., Löfberg, R., Persson, P-G., & Ekbom, A. Is colonoscopic surveillance reducing colorectal cancer mortality in ulcerative colitis? A population based case control study. *Gut*. Vol.42, No.5, (May 1998), pp. 711-4

Karlén, P., Young, E., Broström, O., Löfberg, R., Tribukait, B., Ost, K., Bodian, C., & Itzkowitz, S. Sialyl-Tn antigen as a marker of colon cancer risk I nulcerative colitis: relation to dysplasia and DNA aneuploidy. *Gastroenterology*. Vol.115, No.6, (December 1998), pp. 1395-404

Katzka, I., Brody, RS., Morris, E., & Katz, S. Assessment of colorectal cancer risk in patients with ulcerative colitis: experience from a private practice. *Gastroenterology*. Vol.85, No.1, (July 1983), pp. 22-9

Kiesslich, R., & Neurath, MF. What new endoscopic imaging modalities will become important in the diagnosis of IBD. *Inflammatory Bowel Diseases*. Vol.14, No.S2, (October 2008), pp. Supplement 2:S172-6

Kiesslich, R., Fritsch, J., Holtmann, M., Koehler, H., Stolte, M., Kanzler, S., Nafe, B., Jung, M., Galle, PR., & Neurath, MF. Chromoscopy-guided endomicroscopy increases the diagnostic yield of intraepithelial neoplasia in ulcerative colitis. Vol.132, No.3, (March 2007), pp. 874-82

Kiesslich, R., Fritsch, J., Holtmann, M., Koehler, H., Stolte, M., Kanzler, S., Nafe, B., Jung, M., Galle, PR., & Neurath, MF. Methylene blue-aided chromoendoscopy for the detection of intraepithelial neoplasia and colon cancer in ulcerative colitis. *Gastroenterology*.Vol.123, No.4, (April 2003), pp.880-8

Koobatian, GJ. & Choi, PM. Safety of surveillance colonoscopy in long-standing ulcerative colitis. *American Journal of Gastroenterology*. Vol.89, No.9, (September 1994), pp. 1472-5

Korelitz, BI., Mirsky, FJ., Fleisher, MR., Warman, JI., Wisch, N., & Gleim, GW. Malignant neoplasms subsequent to treatment of inflammatory bowel disease with 6-mercaptopurine. *American Journal of Gastroenterology*. Vol.94, No.11, (November 1999), pp. 3248-53

Kottachichi, D., Yung, D., & Marshall, J. Adherence to guidelines for surveillance colonoscopy in patients with ulcerative colitis at a Canadian quaternary care hospital. *Canadian Journal of Gastroenterology*. Vol.23, No.9, (September 2009), pp. 613-17).

Kudo, S., Rubio, CA., Teizeira, CR., Kashida, H., & Kogure, E. Pit pattern in colorectal neoplasia: endoscopic magnifying view. *Endoscopy*. Vol.33, No.4, (April 2003), pp. 367-73

Lakatos, PL., & Lakatos, L. Risk for colorectal cancer in ulcerative colitis: changes, causes and management strategies. *World Journal of Gastroenterology*. Vol.14, No.25, (July 2008), pp. 3937-47

Langholz, E., Munkholm, P., Davidsen, M., & Binder, V. colorectal cancer risk andmortality in patients with ulcerative colitis. *Gastroenterology*. Vol.103, No.5, (November 1992), pp. 1444-51

Lashner, B., Provencher, KS., Seidner, DL., Knesebeck, A., & Brzezinski, A.The effect of folic acid supplementation on the risk for cancer or dysplasia in ulcerative colitis. *Gastroenterology*. Vol.112. No.1, (January 1997), pp. 29-32

Lashner, B., Shapiro, B., Husain, A., & Goldblum, J. Evaluation of the usefulness of testing for p53 mutations in colorectal cancer surveillance for ulcerative colitis. *American Journal of Gastroenterology*. Vol.94, No.2, (February 1999), pp. 456-462

Lashner, B., Turner, B., Bostwick, D., Frank, P., & Hanauer, S. Dysplasia and cancer complicating strictures in ulcerative colitis. *Digestive Diseases and Sciences*. Vol.35, No.3, (March 1990), pp. 349-52

Lennard-Jones, JE., Melville, DM., Morson, BC., Ritchie, JK. & Williams, CB. Precancer and cancer in extensive ccolitis: findings among 401 patients over 22 years. *Gut*. Vol.31, No.7, (July 1990), pp. 800-6

Lim, Ch., Dixon, MF., Vail, A., Forman, D., Lynch, DA., & Axon, AT. Ten year follow up of ulcerative colitis patients with and without low grade dysplasia. *Gut*. Vol.52, No.8, (August 2003), pp. 1127-32

Lindberg, B., Broome, U., & Persson, B., Proximal colorectal dysplasia or cancer in ulcerative colitis. The impact of primary sclerosing cholangitis and sulfasalazine: results from a 20-year surveillance study. *Diseases of Colon & Rectum*. Vol.44, No.1, (January 2001), pp. 77-85

Lindberg, B., Persson, B., Veress, B., Ingelman-Sundberg, H., & Granqvist, S. Twenty years' colonoscopic surveillance of patients with ulcerative colitis. *Scandinavian Journal of Gastroenterology*. Vol.31, No.12, (December 1996), pp.1195-1205

Lipkus, IM., Rimer, BK., Lyna, PR>, Pradhan, AA., Conaway, M., & Woods-Powell, CT. Colorectal screening patterns and perceptions of risk among African-American users of a community health center. *Journal of Community Health*. Vol.21, No.6, (December 1996), pp. 409-27

Löfberg, R., Broström, O., Karlén, P., Tribukait B, & Ost, A. Colonoscopic surveillance in long-standing total ulcerative colitis-a 15 year follow-up study. *Gastroenterology*. Vol.99, No.4, (October 1990), pp. 1021-31

Loftus, E., Aguilar, H., Sandborn, W., Tremaine, W., Krom, R., Zinsmeister, A., Graziadei, I., & Wiesner, R. Risk of colorectal neoplasia in patients with primary sclerosing cholangitis and ulcerative colitis following orthotopic liver transplantation. *Hepatology*. Vol. 27, No.3, (March 1998), pp. 685-690

Loftus, E., Aguilar, H., Sandborn, W., Tremaine, W., Mahoney, DW., Zinsmeister, AR., Offord, KP., & Melton, LJ Risk of colorectal neoplasia in patients with primary sclerosing cholangitis. *Gastroenterology*. Vol.110, No.2, (1996) pp. 432-40

Marion, JF., Waye, JD., Present, DH., Israsel, Y., Bodian, C., Harpaz, N., Chapman, M., Itzkowtiz, S., Steinlauf, AF., Abreu, MT., Ullman, TA., Aisenber, J., & Mayer, L. Chromoendoscopy-targeted biopsies are superior to standard colonoscopic surveillance for detecting dysplasia in inflammatory bowel disease patients: a prospective endoscopic trial. *American Journal of Gastroenterology*. Vol.103, No.9, (September 2008), pp. 2342-9

Mathy, C., Schneider, K., Chen, YY., Varma, M., Terdiman, JP., & Mahadevan, U. Gross versus microscopic pancolitis and the occurrence of neoplasia in ulcerative colitis. *Inflammatory Bowel Diseases*. Vol.9, No.6, (November 2003), pp. 351-5

Matsumoto, T., Nakamura, S., Jo, Y., Yao, T. & Lida, M. Chromoscopy might improve diagnostic accuracy in cancer surveillance for ulcerative colitis. *American Journal of Gastroenterology*. Vol.98, No.8, (August 2003), pp. 1827-33

Matula, S., Croog, V., Itzkowtiz, S., Harpaz, N., Bodian, C., Hossain, S., & Ullman, T. Chemoprevention of colorectal neoplasia in ulcerative colitis: the effect of 6-mercaptopurine. *Clinical Gastroenterology & Hepatology*. Vol.3, No.10, (October 2005), pp. 1015-21

Melville, DM., Jass, JR., Morson, BC., Pollock, DJ, Richman, PI, Shepherd, NA., Ritchie, JK., Love, SB., & Lennard-Jones, JE. Observer study of the grading of dysplasia in ulcerative colitis: comparison with clinical outcome. *Human Pathology*. Vol.20, No.10, (October 1989) pp. 1008-14

Moody, GA., Jayanthi, V., Probert, CS., Mac Kay, H., & Mayberry, JF. Long-term therapy with suphasalazine protects against colorectal cancer in ulcerative colitis: a restrospective study of colorectal cancer risk and compliance with treatment in Leicestershire. *European Journal of Gastroenterology & Hepatology*. Vol.8, No.12, (December 1996), pp. 1179-83

Mpofu, C., Watson, AJ., & Rhodes, JM. Strategies for detecting colon cancer and/or dysplasia in patients with inflammatory bowel disease (Review). *The Cochrane Database of Systemic Reviews*. Vol.2, (2004), pp. 1-14

Munkholm, P. Review article: the incidence and prevalence of colorectal cancer in inflammatory bowel disease. *Alimentary Pharmacology & Therapeutics*. Vol.18, (September 2003), pp. Supplement 2:1-5

Nguyen, GC., Frick, KD., & Dassopoulos, T. Medical decision analysis for the management of unifocal, flat, low-grade dysplasia in ulcerative colitis. *Gastrointestinal Endoscopy*. Vol.69, No.7, (June 2009), pp. 1299-1310

Nuako, KW, Ahlquist, DA., Sandborn, WJ., Mahoney, DW., Siems, DM., & Zinsmeister, AR. Primary sclerosing cholangitis and colorectal carcinoma in patients with chronic ulcerative colitis: a case control study. *Cancer*. Vol.82, No.5, (March 1998) pp. 822-26

Nuako, KW., Ahlquist, DA., Mahoney, DW., Schaid, DJ., Siems, DM., & Lindor, NM. Familial predisposition for colorectal cancer in chronic ulcerative colitis: a case control-study. *Gastroenterology*. Vol.115, No.5, (November 1998), pp.1079-83

Nugent, FW., Haggit, RC., & Gilpin, PA. Cancer surveillance in ulcerative colitis. *Gastroenterology*. Vol.100, No.5, (May 2002), pp. 615-20

Obrador, A., Ginard, D., & Barranco, L. Review article: colorectal cancer surveillance in ulcerative colitis - what should we be doing. *Alimentary Pharmacology & Therapeutics*. Vol.24, (October 2006), pp. Supplement 3:56-63

Odze, RD. Adenomas and adenoma-like DALMs in chronic ulcerative colitis: a clinical, pathological, and molecular review. *American Journal of Gastroenterology*. Vol.94, No.7, (July 1999), pp. 1746-50

Odze, RD. What are the guidelines for treating adenoma-like DALMs in UC. *Inflamatory Bowel Diseases*. Vol.14., (October 2008), pp. Suppl 2: S243-4

Odze, RD., Farraye, FA., Hecht, JL., & Hornick, JL. Long-term follow-up after polypectomy treatment for adenoma-like dysplastic lesions in ulcerative colitis. *Clinical Gastroenterology & Hepatology*. Vol.2, No.7, (July 2004), pp. 534-41

Odze, RD., Goldblum, J., Noffsinger, A., Alsaigh, N., Rybicki, LA., & Fogt, F. Interobserver variability in the diagnosis of ulcerative colitis-associated dysplasia by telepathology. *Modern Pathology*. Vol.15, No.4, (April 2002), pp. 379-86

Pandi, DS., Loftus, EV., Kremers, WK., Keach, J., & Lindor, KD. Ursodeoxycholic acid as a chemopreventive agent in patients with ulcerative colitis and primary sclerosing cholangitis. *Gastroenterology*. Vol.125, No.4, (April 2003), pp. 889-93

Pinczowski, D., Ekbom, A., Baron, J., Yuen, J., & Adami, HO. Risk factors for colorectal cancer in patients with ulcerative colitis: a case-control study. *Gastroenterology*. Vol.107, No.1, (July 1994), pp. 117-20

Poynter, JN., Gruber, SB., Higgins, PD., Almog, R., Bonner, JD., Rennert, HS., Low, M., Greenson, JK., & Rennert, G. Statins and risk of colorectal cancer. *New England Journal of Medicine*. Vol.352, No.21, (May 2005), pp. 2184-92

Price, JH. Perceptions of colorectal cancer in socioeconomically disadvantaged population. *Journal Community Health*. Vol.18, No.6, (December 1993), pp. 347-62

Provenzale, D., Kowdley, KV., Arora, S., & Wong, JB. Prophylactic colectomy or surveillance for chornic ulcerative colitis? A decision analysis. *Gastroenterology*. Vol.109, No.4, (October 1995), pp. 188-96

Ransohoff, DF. Colon cancer in ulcerative colitis. *Gastroenterology*. Vol.94, No.4, (April 1988), pp. 1089-91

Reddy, SI., Friedman, S., Telford, J., Strate, L., Ookubo, R., & Banks, P. Are patients with inflammatory bowel disease receiving optimal care. *American Journal of Gastroenterology*. Vol.100, No.6, (June 2005), pp. 1357-61

Riddell, RH., Goldman, H., Ransohoff, DF., Appelman, HD., Fenoglio, CM., Haggitt, RC., Ahren, C., Correa, P., Hamilton, SR., Morson, BC., & et al. Dysplasia in inflammatory bowel disease: standardized classification with provisional clinical applications. *Human Pathology*. Vol.14, No.11, (November 1983), pp. 931-68

Rubin, CE., Haggitt, RC., Burmer, GC., Brentnall, TA., Stevens, AC., Levine, DS., Dean, PJ., Kimmey, M., Perera, DR., & Rabinovitch, PS. DNA aneuploidy in colonic biopsies predicts future development of dysplasia in ulcerative colitis. *Gastroenterology*. Vol.103, No.5, (November 1992), pp. 1611-20

Rubin, DT., Huo D., Rothe, J., Hetzel, JT., Sedrak, M., Yadron, N., Bunnag, A., Hart, J., & Turner, JR. Increased inflammatory activity is an independent risk factor for dysplasia and colorectal cancer in ulcerative colitis: a case-control analysis with blinded prospective reviews of pathology. *Gastroenterology*. Vol.130, (2006), pp. Supplement A2

Rubin, DT., LoSavio, A., Yadron, N., Huo, D., & Hanauer, SB. Aminosalicylate therapy in the prevention of dysplasia and colorectal cancer in ulcerative colitis. *Clinical Gastroenterology & Hepatology*. Vol.4, No.11, (November 2006), pp.1346-50

Rubin, PH., Friedman, S., Harpaz, N., Goldstein, E., Weiser, J., Schiller, J., Wayne, JD., Present, DH. Colonoscopic polypectomy in chronic colitis: conservative management after endoscopic resection of dysplastic polyps. *Gastroenterology*. Vol.117, No.6, (1999), pp. 1295-1300

Rutter, M. A practical guide and review of colonoscopic surveillance and chromoendoscopy in patients with colitis. *Frontline Gastroenterology*. Vol.1, (July 2010), pp.126-129

Rutter, M., Saunders, B., Wilkinson, K., Rumbles, S., Schofield, G., Kamm, M., Williams, C., & Forbes, A. Most dysplasia in ulcerative colitis is visible at colonoscopy. *Gastrointestinal Endoscopy*. Vol.60, No.3, (September 2004), pp. 334-9

Rutter, M., Saunders, B., Wilkinson, K., Rumbles, S., Schofield, G., Kamm, M., Williams, C., Price, A., Talbot, I., & Forbes, A. Cancer surveillance in longstanding ulcerative colitis endoscopic appearances help predict cancer risk. *Gut*. Vol.53, No.12, (December 2004), pp. 1813-16

Rutter, M., Saunders, B., Wilkinson, K., Rumbles, S., Schofield, G., Kamm, M., Williams, C., Price, A., Talbot, I., & Forbes, A. Severity of inflammation is a risk factor for colorectal neoplasia in ulcerative colitis. *Gastroenterology*. Vol.126, No.2, (February 2004), pp. 451-59

Rutter, M., Saunders, B., Wilkinson, K., Rumbles, S., Schofield, G., Kamm, M., Williams, C., Price, A., Talbot, I., & Forbes, A. Thirty-year analysis of a colonoscopic surveillance program for neoplasia in ulcerative colitis. *Gastroenterology*. Vol.130, No.4, (April 2006), pp. 1030-8

Rutter, M., Saunders, BP., Schofield, G., Forbes, A., Price, AB., & Talbot, IC. Pancolonic indigo carmine dye spraying for the detection of dysplasia in ulcerative colitis. *Gut*. Vol.53, No.2, (February 2004), pp. 256-60

Samadder, NJ., Mukherjee, B., Huang, SC., Ahn, J., Rennert, H., Greenson, J., Rennert, G., & Gruber, S. Risk of colorectal cancer in self-reported inflammatory bowel disease and modification of risk by statin and NSAID use. *Cancer*. Vol.117, (April 2011), pp. 1640-8

Sato, F., Harpaz, N., Shibata, D., Xu, Y., Yin, J., Mori, Y., Zou, TT., Wang, S., Desai, K., Leytin, A., Selaru, F., Abraham, JM., & Melzer, S. Hypermethylation of p14^{ARF} gene in ulcerative colitis-associated colorectal carcinogenesis. *Cancer Research*. Vol.62, No.4 , (February 2002), pp. 1148-51

Schlemper, RJ., Riddell, RH., Kato, Y., Borchard, F., Cooper, HS., Dwasey, SM., Dixon, MF., Fenoglio-Preiser, CM., Fléjou, JF., Geboes, K., Hattori, T., Hirota, T., Itabashi, M., Iwafuchi, M., Iwashita, A., Kim, YI., Kirchner, T., Klimpfinger, M., Koike, M., Lauwers, GY., Lewin, KJ., Oberhuber, G., Offner, F., Price, AB., Rubio, CA., Shimizu, M., Shimoda, T., Sipponen, P., Solcia, E., Stolte, M., Watanabe, H., &Yamabe, H. The Vienna classification of gastrointestinal epithelial neoplasia. *Gut*. Vol.47, No.2, (August 2000), pp. 251-55

Sharan, R., & Schoen, RE. Cancer in inflammatory bowel disease. An evidence-based analysis and guide for physicians and patients. *Gastrointestinal Clinics of North America*. Vol.31, No.1, (March 2002), pp. 237-54

Shetty, K., Rybicki, L., Brezinksi, A., Carey, WD., & Lashner, BA. The risk for cancer or dysplasia in ulcerative colitis patients with primary sclerosing cholangitis. *American Journal of Gastroenterology*. Vol.94, No.6, (June 1999), pp. 1643-9

Sjoqvist, U., Tribukait., B. Ost, A., Einarsson, C., Oxelmark, & Löfberg, R. Ursodeoxycholic acid treatment in IBD-patientes with colorectal dysplasia and/or DNA-anueploidy: a prospective, double-blind randomized controlled pilot study. *Anticancer Research*. Vol.24, No.5B, (September-October 2004), pp. 3121-27

Söderlund, S., Granath, F., Broström, O., Karlén, P., Löfberg, R., & Askling, J. Inflammatory bowel disease confers a lower risk of colorectal cancer to females than to males. *Gastroenterology*. Vol.138, No.5, (May 2010), pp. 1697-703

Soetikno, R., Friedland, S., Kaltenbach, T., Chayama, K., Tanaka, S., Nonpolypoid (flat and depressed) colorectal neoplasm. *Gastroenterology*. Vol.130, No.2, (February 2006), pp. 566-76

Soetikno, R., Lin, O., Heidenreich, P., Young, H., & Blackstone, M. Increased risk of colorectal neoplasia in patients with primary sclerosing cholangitis and ulcerative colitis: a meta-analysis. *Gastrointestinal Endoscopy*. Vol.56, No.1, (July 2002), pp. 48-54

Sonnenberg, A., & El-Serag, HB. Economic aspects of endoscopic screening for intestinal precancerous conditions. *Gastroinestinal Endoscopy Clinics of North America*. Vol.7, No.1, (January 1997), pp. 165-84

Tahara, T., Inoue, N., Hisamatsu, T., Kashiwagi, K., Takaishi, H., Kamai, T., Watanabe, M., Ishii, H., & Hibi, T. Clinical significance of microsatellite instability in the inflamed mucosa for the prediction of colonic neoplasms in patients with ulcerative colitis. *Journal of Gastroenterology & Hepatology*. Vol.20, No.5, (May 2005), pp.710-15

Thomas, T., Abrams, KA., Robinson, RJ. & Mayberry, JF. Meta-analysis: cancer risk of low-grade dysplasia in chronic ulcerative colitis. *Alimentary Pharmacology & Therapeutics*. Vol.25, No.6, (March 2007), pp. 657-68

Torres, C., Antonioli, D., & Odze RD. Polypoid dysplasia and adenomas in inflammatory bowel disease: a clinical, pathologic, and follow-up study of 89 polyps from 59 patients. *American Journal of Surgical Pathology*. Vol.22, No.3, (March 1988), pp. 275-84

Tung, BY., Emond, MJ., Haggitt, RC., Bronner, MP., Kimmey, MB., Kowdley, KV., & Brentnall, TA. Ursodiol use is associated with lower prevalence of colonic neoplasia in patients with ulcerative colitis and primary sclerosing cholangitis. *Annals of Internal Medicine*. Vol.134, No.2, (January 2001), pp. 89-95

Ullman, T, Loftus, EV., Kakar, S., Burgart, LJ., Sandborn, WJ. & Tremaine, WJ. The fate of low grade dysplasia in ulcerative colitis. *American Journal of Gastroenterology*. Vol.97, No.4, (April 2002), pp. 922-27

Ullman, T., & Itzkowitz, S. Intestinal inflammation and cancer. *Gastroenterology*. Vol.140, No.6, (May 2011), pp. 1807-16

Ullman, T., Croog, V., Harpaz, N., Hossain, S., Kornbluth, A., Bodian, C., & Itzkowtiz, S. Progression to colorectal neoplasia in ulcerative colitis: effect of mesalamine. *Clinical Gastroenterology & Hepatology*. Vol.6, No.11, (November 2008), pp. 1225-30

Umetani, N., Sasaki, S., Watanabe, T., Shinozaki, M., Matsuda, K., Ishigami, H., Ueda, E., & Muto, T. Genetic alterations in ulcerative colitis-associated neoplasia focusing on APC, K-ras gene and microsatellite instability. *Japanese Journal of Cancer Research*. Vol.90, No.10, (October 1999), pp. 1081-7

van den Broek, FJ., Fockens, P., van Eeden, S., Reitsma, JB., Hardwick, JC., Stokkers, PC., & Dekker, E. Endoscopic tri-modal imaging for surveillance in ulcerative colitis: randomized comparison of high-resolution endoscopy and autofluorescene imaging for neoplasia detection; and evaluation of narrow-band imaging for classification of lesions. *Gut*. Vol.57, No,8, (August 2008), pp. 1083-9

van Rijn, AF., Fockens, P., Siersema, P., & Oldenburg, B. Adherence to surveillance guidelines for dysplasia and colorectal carcinoma in ulcerative and Crohns colitis patients in the Netherlands. *World Journal of Gastroenterology*. Vol.15, No.2, (January 2009), pp. 226-230

van Staa, TP., Card, T., Logan, RF., & Leufkens, HG. 5-aminosalicylate therapy use and colorectal cancer risk in inflammatory bowel disease: a large epidemiological study. *Gut*. Vol.54, No.11, (November 2005), pp. 1573-78

Velayos, FS., Loftus, EV., Jess, T., Harmsen, WS., Bida, J., Zinsmeister, AR., Tremaine, WJ., & Sandborn, WJ. Predictive and protective factors associated with colorectal cancer in ulcerative colitis: a case-control study. *Gastroenterology*. Vol.130, No.7, (June 2006), pp. 1941-49

Velayos, FS., Terdiman, JP., & Walsh, JM. Effect of 5-aminosalicylate use on colorectal cancer and dysplasia risk: a systemic review and metaanalysis of observational studies. *American Journal of Gastroenterology*. Vol.100, No.6, (June 2005), pp. 1345-53

Vera, A., Gunson, BK., Ussatoff, V., Nightingal, P., Candinas, D., Radley, S., Mayer, AD., Buckels, JA., McMaster, P., Neuberger, J., & Mirza, DF. Colorectal cancer in patients with inflammatory bowel disease after liver transplantation for primary sclerosing cholangitis. *Transplantation*. Vol.75, No.12, (June 2003), pp. 1983-88

Vernon, SW. Participation in colorectal cancer screening: a review. *Journal of National Cancer Institute*. Vol.89, No.19, (October 1997) pp. 1406-22

Vieth, M., Behrens, H., & Stolte, M. Sporadic adenoma in ulcerative colitis: endoscopic resection is an adequate treatment. *Gut*. Vol.55, No.8, (August 2006), pp. 1151-55

Wilson, JM., Jungner, G. Principles and practice of screening for disease. *World Health Organization Chronicles*. Vol.22, No.11, (1968), pp. 1-163

Wolf, JM., Rybicki, LA, & Lashner, BA. The impact of ursodeoxycholic acid on cancer, dysplasia and mortality in ulcerative colitis patients with primary sclerosing cholangitis. *Alimentary Pharmacology & Therapy*. Vol.22, No.9, (November 2005), pp. 783-8

Woolrich, AJ., DaSilva, MD., & Korelitz, BL. Surveillance in the routine management of ulcerative colitis: the predictive value of low-grade dysplasia. *Gastroenterology*. Vol.103, No.2, (August 1992), pp. 431-38

Yashiro, M., Carethers, JM., Laghi, L., Saito, K., Slezak, P., Jaramillo, E., Rbio, C., Koizumi, K., Hirakawa, K., & Boland, CR. Genetic pathways in the evolution of morphologically distinct colorectal neoplasms. *Cancer Research*. Vol.61, No.6, (March 2001), pp. 2676-83.

6

Ulcerative Colitis and Colorectal Cancer: Aneuploidy and Implications for Improved Screening

Jens K. Habermann[1], Gert Auer[2], Thomas Ried[3] and Uwe J. Roblick[1]
[1]University of Lübeck,
[2]Karolinska Institutet,
[3]National Cancer Institute,
[1]Germany
[2]Sweden
[3]USA

1. Introduction

Patients with ulcerative colitis (UC) have a significantly increased lifetime risk for the development of colorectal carcinomas. Ulcerative colitis can therefore be considered a bona fide premalignant condition. It is therefore recommended that patients with UC participate in surveillance programs to screen for early signs of malignancy. However, reliable endoscopic sampling and histopathological evaluation is difficult. The diagnostic dilemma is underlined by the fact that despite screening programs about half of the patients with an ulcerative colitis-associated carcinoma (UCC) are diagnosed at an already advanced tumor stage reflecting poor prognosis. For these reasons, it should be obvious that additional markers with high prognostic impact in the individual risk assessment are of high clinical demand.

While genetic and genomic changes during carcinogenesis have been thoroughly studied in sporadic colorectal cancers, less is known about the development of UCCs. This chapter will therefore focus on the role of genomic instability during colitis-associated carcinogenesis and how ploidy assessment might help to improve individual risk stratification regarding imminent colorectal cancer risk and survival prognosis.

2. Pathogenesis of sporadic and ulcerative colitis-associated colorectal cancer

The normal colonic epithelium (mucosa) is a highly dynamic system: Stem cells are located at the basis of epithelial crypts (Wright 2000). They are a source of constantly proliferating cell populations that - while differentiating - migrate to the surface of the colonic crypts from where they are shed into the lumen. The intestinal epithelium is thus renewed every five to six days. Mucosal cells are prone to genetic damage due to the highly toxic and mechanically stressful intra-luminal environment. The rapid clearance of mucosal cells however prevents these cells from being a source of malignant transformation. However, a high proliferative rate in a toxic environment could also easily accelerate malignant transformation once regulatory mechanisms for cell homeostasis are bypassed. Most colorectal tumors are caused by acquired genetic lesions of single mucosal cells that harbour a growth advantage and - through clonal expansion - rise to invasive carcinomas. Whether these genetic aberrations occur predominantly in stem cells, migrating cells, or mucosal cells at the crypt surface has not been conclusively clarified (Shih et al. 2001; Lamprecht and Lipkin 2002; Bach, Renehan, and Potten 2000). Genetic aberrations can become evident either on the subchromosomal or chromosomal level and target regulatory mechanisms required for the genetic equilibrium such as cell cycle regulation, cellular signalling pathways, proliferation, differentiation, growth inhibition, and apoptosis signalling. Vogelstein and colleagues defined a model of colorectal carcinogenesis in which a non-random accumulation of genetic aberrations can be correlated with morphologic changes of the colon epithelium: the transition from normal mucosa via adenomatous polyp to colorectal cancer and eventually distant metastasis (Fearon and Vogelstein 1990). However, in ulcerative colitis macroscopically visible pre-malignant lesions such as adenomas are missing and the detection of dysplastic lesions and/or dysplasia associated lesion or mass (DALM) are difficult to identify clinically (Riddell 1998).

2.1 Colorectal cancer risk in ulcerative colitis

Three of ten ulcerative colitis patients will eventually develop cancer after a longstanding colitis (Bernstein et al. 2001). Ulcerative colitis can therefore be considered a bona fide premalignant condition. Therefore, it is recommended that patients with UC participate in surveillance programs in order to screen for early signs of malignancy (Daperno et al. 2004). Ulcerative colitis-associated colorectal carcinomas (UCC) do not develop through the adenoma-carcinoma-sequence (Willenbucher 1996). Instead, epithelial dysplasias have been defined as precursor lesions and are meant to be the most predictive feature of intensive and expensive surveillance programs today (Collins, Feldman, and Fordtran 1987). However, reliable endoscopic sampling and histopathological evaluation is difficult (Eaden et al. 2001; Riddell 1998; Lynch et al. 1993). Additionally, a review of 12 surveillance studies with 92 detected carcinomas in 1,916 patients revealed that about half of them were advanced Dukes´ C and D malignancies and only 12% were early stage carcinomas (Lynch et al. 1993).

2.1.1 Tumor dissemination

Metastases are one of the hallmarks of solid tumor malignancy. Once a primary tumor has been detected and surgically removed, the survival of the patient greatly depends on the occurrence of local or distant metastases. Rather than the primary carcinoma itself, it is mainly the metastatic disease that leads to death. The ability of tumor cells to metastasize depends on the acquisition of certain characteristics that allow local or distant spread via the lymphatic or venous system. Early detection of metastasis is important for treatment interventions, however, has proved to be difficult (Calaluce, Miedema, and Yesus 1998).

2.1.2 Local invasion

One of the necessary characteristics of metastasizing tumor cells is the ability to invade the basement membrane. Laminins are major components of the basement membranes that belong to a family of heterotrimeric glycoproteins. They are composed of at least α, β and γ subunits that can form 12 or more isoforms (Iivanainen, Morita, and Tryggvason 1999). The various isoforms have different tissue specific biological functions, such as cell adhesion, migration, proliferation, as well as growth and differentiation (Tryggvason 1993). The laminin-5 isoform (α3: β3: γ2), also known as kalinin, nicein, epiligrin, and ladsin, plays an important role for epithelial cell adhesion to the basement membrane (Carter, Ryan, and Gahr 1991). In order to invade surrounding tissue, tumor cells attach to the basement membrane by binding to laminin receptors from laminin implemented in the basement membrane. This mimics a physiological process: for example, non-neoplastic cells such as inflammatory and endothelial cells regularly cross the basement membrane. These processes are controlled by regulatory mechanisms and it remains unclear how tumor cells can bypass those mechanisms. One possible mechanism is the ability of tumor cells to express laminin themselves. That would enable the attachment to the basement membrane independent from available receptors of the basement membrane laminin. Interestingly, there is much evidence that shows increased expression of the laminin-5 γ2 gene has been found in invasively growing malignant cells at the epithelial-stromal junction, i. e., at the invasion front of different tumors and colorectal cancers (Pyke et al. 1994; Pyke et al. 1995; Sordat et al. 1998).

3. Aneuploidy and cancer risk stratification in ulcerative colitis

Aneuploidy is a consistent genetic alteration of the cancer genome (Duesberg et al. 1998; Lengauer, Kinzler, and Vogelstein 1998; Ried et al. 1999). When the first quantitative measurements of the DNA content of cancer cells were performed, aneuploidy was defined as a variation in nuclear DNA content in the population of cancer cells within a tumor (Caspersson 1979). With increased resolution of cytogenetic techniques, such as chromosome banding, comparative genomic hybridization (CGH), spectral karyotyping (SKY), and multicolor fluorescence *in situ* hybridization, it has become clear that in addition to nuclear aneuploidy, specific non-random chromosomal imbalances (heretofore referred to as chromosomal aneuploidy) exist (Caspersson et al. 1970; Kallioniemi et al. 1992; Schrock et al. 1996; Speicher, Gwyn Ballard, and Ward 1996). Indeed, despite genetic instability in cancer genomes, cancer cell populations as a whole display a surprisingly conserved, tumor-specific pattern of genomic imbalances (Ried et al. 1999; Knuutila et al. 1998; Forozan et al. 1997). At early steps in the sequence of malignant transformation during human tumorigenesis, *e.g.*, in pre-invasive dysplastic lesions, chromosomal aneuploidy can be the first detectable genetic aberration found (Hittelman 2001; Hopman et al. 1988; Heselmeyer et al. 1996; Solinas-Toldo et al. 1996). This suggests that there is both an initial requirement for the acquisition of specific chromosomal aneuploidy and a requirement for the maintenance of these imbalances despite genomic and chromosomal instability. This would be consistent with continuous selective pressure to retain a specific pattern of chromosomal copy number changes in the majority of tumor cells (Bomme et al. 1994; Ried et al. 1999; Nowak et al. 2002; Desper et al. 2000). Additionally, in cell culture model systems in which cells are exposed to different carcinogens, chromosomal aneuploidy is the earliest detectable genomic aberration (Barrett et al. 1985; Oshimura and Barrett 1986). The conservation of these tumor specific patterns of chromosomal aneuploidy suggests that they play a fundamental biological role in tumorigenesis.

3.1 Chromosomal aneuploidy in sporadic colorectal cancer

The progression of colorectal cancer is defined by the sequential acquisition of genetic alterations (Fearon and Vogelstein 1990). At the cytogenetic level, many of these aberrations can be visualized as specific chromosomal gains and losses. These aneuploidies result in a recurrent pattern of genomic imbalances, which is specific and conserved for these tumors (Ried et al. 1996). For instance, one of the earliest acquired genetic abnormalities during colorectal tumorigenesis are copy number gains of chromosome 7 (Bomme et al. 1994). These trisomies can already be observed in benign polyps, and can emerge in otherwise stable, diploid genomes. At later stages, e.g., in high-grade adenomas or in invasive carcinomas, additional specific cytogenetic abnormalities become common, such as gains of chromosome and chromosome arms 8q, 13, and 20q, and losses that map to 8p, 17p, and 18q. For a comprehensive summary see the "Mitelman Database of Chromosome Aberrations in Cancer" at http://cgap.nci.nih.gov/Chromosomes/Mitelman. This chromosomal aneuploidy is accompanied by specific mutations in oncogenes and tumor suppressor genes, including e.g. APC and TP53 (Vogelstein and Kinzler 2004). It is therefore well established that both, chromosomal aneuploidy and specific gene mutations, are required for tumorigenesis.

3.2 Chromosomal aneuploidy in ulcerative colitis-associated colorectal cancer

Unlike sporadic colorectal tumors, UCCs do not follow the adenoma–carcinoma sequence, and the sequential acquisition of chromosomal aneuploidy and gene mutations is less well established. It was therefore questioned if the pattern of chromosomal gains and losses in UCC are similar to that described for sporadic carcinomas. A similar pattern would indicate that the final distribution of genomic imbalances is the product of continuous selection, and that this distribution is independent of whether a carcinoma occurs spontaneously or as a result of, for example, chronic inflammation. Recent reports suggested that in general, genomic imbalances observed in UCC cluster on the same chromosomes as those in sporadic colorectal carcinomas (Kern et al. 1994; Holzmann et al. 2001; Willenbucher et al. 1997; Loeb and Loeb 1999; Aust et al. 2000). Our analyses comprises the largest sample collection of UCCs from one clinical center and supports these findings: all 19 UCC specimens showed chromosomal imbalances by comparative genomic hybridization (CGH) as follows: the most common DNA gains were mapped to chromosomes or chromosome arms 20q (84% of all cases), 7 (74%), 8q (74%), 13q (74%), 11p and 12 (both 42%), 5p and 18p (both 37%), and 17q (31%). Recurrent losses occurred on 8p (58%), 18q (47%), and 5q (26%) (Habermann et al. 2003). These results show that chromosomal imbalances observed in UCC mainly cluster on the same chromosomes as described for sporadic colorectal cancer. For instance, Ried et al reported DNA gains that frequently mapped to chromosomes or chromosome arms 7, 8q, 13q, and 20 in sporadic colorectal carcinomas (Ried et al. 1996). However, it also becomes clear that sporadic colorectal carcinomas have fewer genomic imbalances than UCCs (**Figure 1**). Our previous analyses of sporadic colorectal carcinomas revealed an average number of DNA copy alterations (ANCA, calculated as the number of chromosomal copy number changes divided by the number of cases) of 5.6, which was elevated to 13.3 in UCC. This number exceeds that observed in primary liver metastases from colorectal carcinomas, for which the ANCA had been determined to be 11.7 (Platzer et al. 2002). This high degree of genomic instability is also supported by measurements of the nuclear DNA content, which invariably revealed gross aneuploidy. We also observed a large number of localized high-level copy number increases (amplifications). Amplifications have been described as a reflection of advanced disease and poor prognosis in other malignancies (Blegen et al. 2001). Some of the amplifications occurred in regions known to be affected in colorectal carcinomas, such as chromosome arms 6p, 8q, 13q, 17q, and 20q, and for which the target genes are either known or likely candidates have been identified (http://www.helsinki.fi/cmg/cgh_data.html). For instance, the frequent gain of chromosome 8 and amplifications that map to band 8q24 target the *MYC* oncogene. Candidates on chromosome 20 include the nuclear co-receptor activator gene *NCOA3* and a member of the aurora kinase family. Another correlation is the coincidental overexpression of laminin-5 and gain of chromosome band 1q25-q31, the map position of the *LAMC2* gene (laminin-5). Laminin-5 plays a crucial role for invasive capacities of metastasizing cells but it has not been elucidated how increased expression levels are produced. Genomic amplification could be one molecular mechanism leading to laminin-5 overexpression.

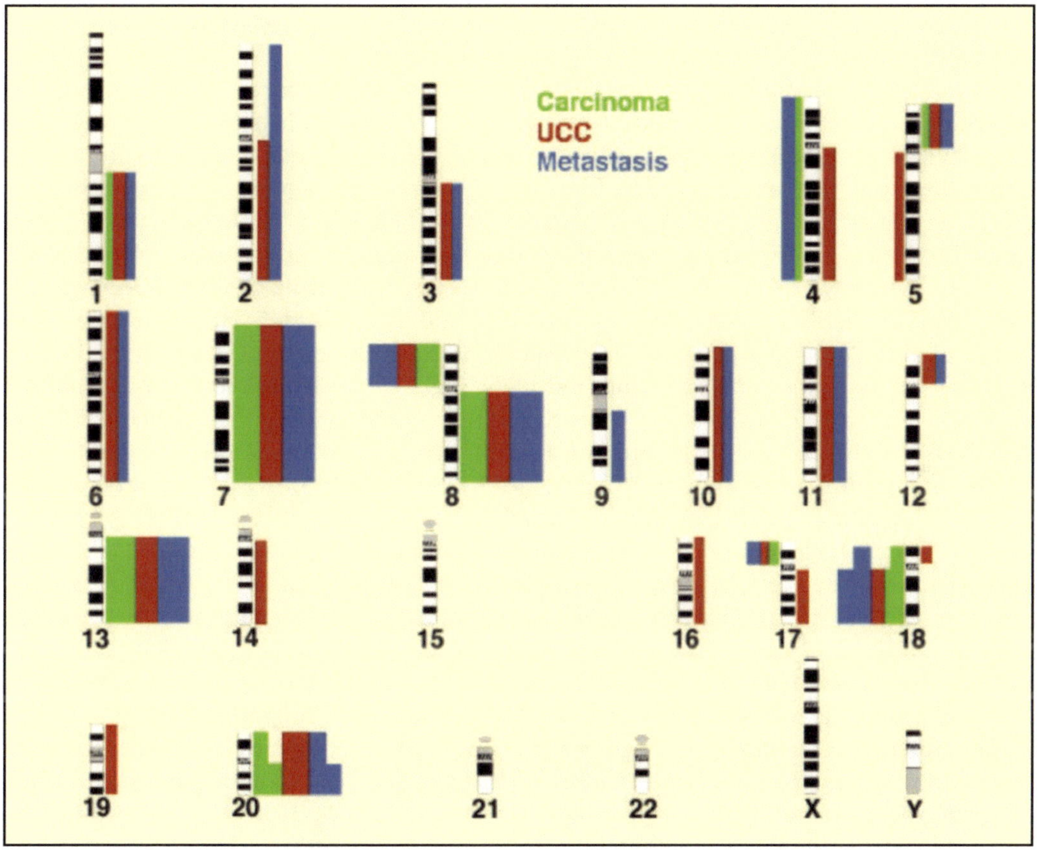

Fig. 1. Comparison of genomic imbalances in sporadic colorectal carcinoma (SCC), ulcerative colitis-associated colorectal cancer (UCC), and liver metastasis of SCC. Bars on the left side of the chromosome ideogram denote a loss of sequence in the tumor genome, bars on the right side a gain of sequence in the tumor genome. The number of alterations per chromosome is normalized to 10 cases for each tumor type. Only ratios greater than 2 have been considered. Figure modified from (Habermann et al. 2003)

The CGH profile for UCC analyzed in our cohort is in concordance with the relatively high ANCA value and severe aneuploidy observed. In comparison, sporadic colon carcinomas show aneuploidy in only 70%–80% of the cases, combined with an overall lower ANCA value. The surprisingly high level of ANCA values in UCC could be a reflection of a generally increased genetic instability in UCC, due to the long latency of inflammatory disease before overt tumors develop; however, the data presented here and in the literature clearly indicate that the tumor cell population as an entity selects for a distribution of genomic imbalances that is similar to sporadic carcinomas. Therefore, the tissue origin of the tumor cell, and not the mode of tumor induction, seems to define the similarity between sporadic colorectal cancers and UCC. This is in striking contrast to hereditary colorectal carcinomas arising in the background of mismatch repair deficiency, where neither aneuploidy nor specific chromosomal imbalances are observed (Ghadimi et al. 2000; Schlegel et al. 1995).

3.3 Nuclear aneuploidy and prognosis in sporadic and UC-associated colorectal cancer

The strikingly conserved pattern of chromosomal aneuploidy in sporadic and UC-associated colorectal carcinomas can be reflected by nuclear DNA aneuploidy. Hereby, flow and/or image cytometry might serve as reliable tools with excellent clinical applicability also for high-throughput clinical diagnostics. Interestingly, reported frequencies of aneuploidy in UCCs vary inconsistently between 28.6% and 100% (Holzmann et al. 1998; Fozard et al. 1986). This rather astonishing range could be due to different ploidy assessment techniques, e.g., flow cytometry versus image cytometry, different standardization methodologies, as well as varying definitions of the terms "diploidy" and "aneuploidy" (Holzmann et al. 1998; Fozard et al. 1986; Klump et al. 1997; Clausen et al. 2001; Levine et al. 1991). In addition, a major drawback of the above mentioned studies might be the overall low number of UCC cases analyzed, varying from single case studies up to 17 individual UCC patients (Clausen et al. 2001; Makiyama et al. 1995; Burmer, Rabinovitch, and Loeb 1991). The latter study by Burmer et al found aneuploidy in 88% of cases investigated, however, did not distinguish between carcinomas and nonmalignant dysplastic lesions within these 17 UCC patients (Burmer, Rabinovitch, and Loeb 1991). Against this background, we had compiled 31 UCCs in order to evaluate the frequency of aneuploidy and its association to clinical parameters and survival and in comparison to 257 sporadic colorectal carcinomas. We performed nuclear DNA ploidy measurement by means of image cytometry which allows for simultaneous assessment of histomorphology and/or cytopathology. Histograms were classified according to Auer (**Figure 2**) (Auer, Caspersson, and Wallgren 1980).
UCCs presented aneuploidy at significantly higher frequency than sporadic colorectal carcinomas (100% versus 74.6%; $P < 0.0006$) (Gerling et al. 2010). In addition, we performed a logistic regression analysis comprising age, sex, UICC stage, T- and N-status, histologic tumor grading, underlying inflammation, and DNA ploidy status. Out of these features, logistic regression yielded two parameters to be of significant prognostic value for 5-year survival subsequent to operation for colorectal cancer. Those two significant parameters were age and DNA ploidy status indicating that patients of higher age at diagnosis and patients with aneuploid tumor cell populations have a poor survival prognosis. Additional logistic regression analysis comprising these two significant parameters only, confirmed age (odds ratio [OR], 1.05; 95% CI, 1.02–1.09; $P = 0.003$) and DNA ploidy (OR, 4.07; 95% CI, 1.46

-11.36; $P = 0.007$) to be independent prognostic parameters. According to the OR of 4.07, DNA ploidy seemed to be the main influencing feature. This was further supported by Kaplan-Meier-Plots showing that diploid SCCs had a more favorable 5-year survival (88.2%) than aneuploid SCCs (69.0%) and UCCs (73.1%) ($P = 0.074$). Thus, aneuploidy proved to be the strongest independent prognostic marker for R0-resected colorectal cancer patients overall (Gerling et al. 2010).

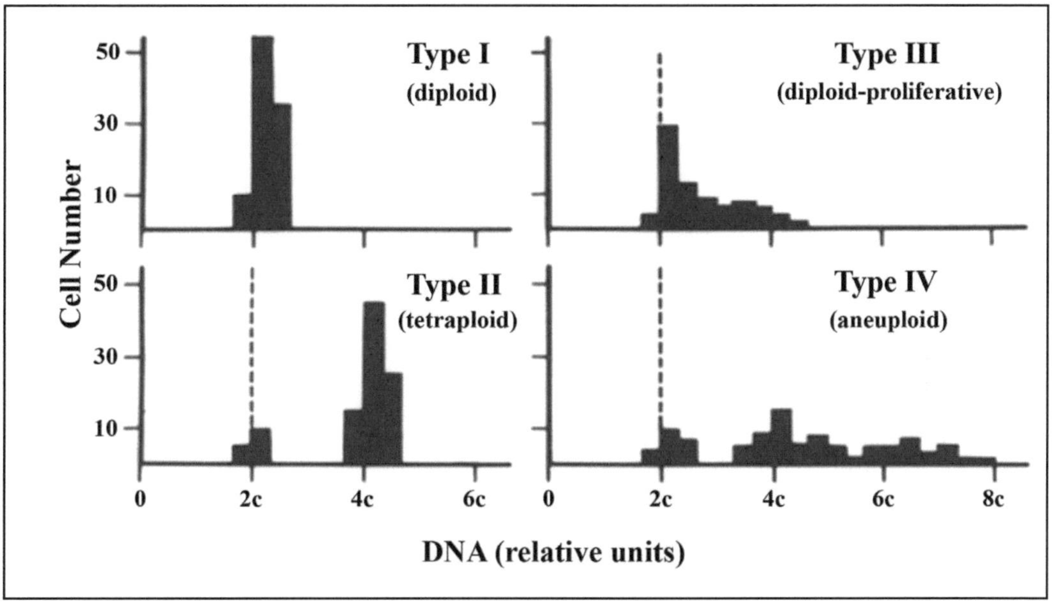

Fig. 2. DNA Histogram types according to Auer. Histograms characterized by a single peak in the diploid or near-diploid region (1.5–2.5 c) were classified as type I. The total number of cells with DNA values exceeding the diploid region (>2.5 c) was <10%. Type II histograms showed a single peak in the tetraploid region (3.5– 4.5 c) or peaks in both the diploid and tetraploid regions (>90% of the total cell population). The number of cells with DNA values between the diploid and tetraploid region and those exceeding the tetraploid region (>4.5 c) was <10%. Type III histograms represented highly proliferating near-diploid cell populations and were characterized by DNA values ranging between the diploid and the tetraploid regions. Only a few cells (<5%) showed more than 4.5 c. The DNA histograms of types I, II, and III thus characterize euploid cell populations. Type IV histograms showed increased (>5%) and/or distinctly scattered DNA values exceeding the tetraploid region (>4.5 c). These histograms reflect aneuploid populations of colon mucosa nuclei with decreased genomic stability

Furthermore, we also showed that diploid tumors at advanced stages (UICC stage III/IV) do present similar survival as compared with aneuploid sporadic and UC-associated carcinomas at early tumor stages (**Figure 3**). This finding might point to the conclusion that the presence of aneuploid tumor cell populations might influence patient's prognosis more dominantly than does tumor stage. This is in line with the finding that the most pronounced difference in prognosis can be observed between diploid SCCs at early stages and aneuploid colorectal carcinomas at advanced stages. Furthermore, UCCs at advanced stages show a prognosis inferior to that of their sporadic counterpart at the same tumor stage.

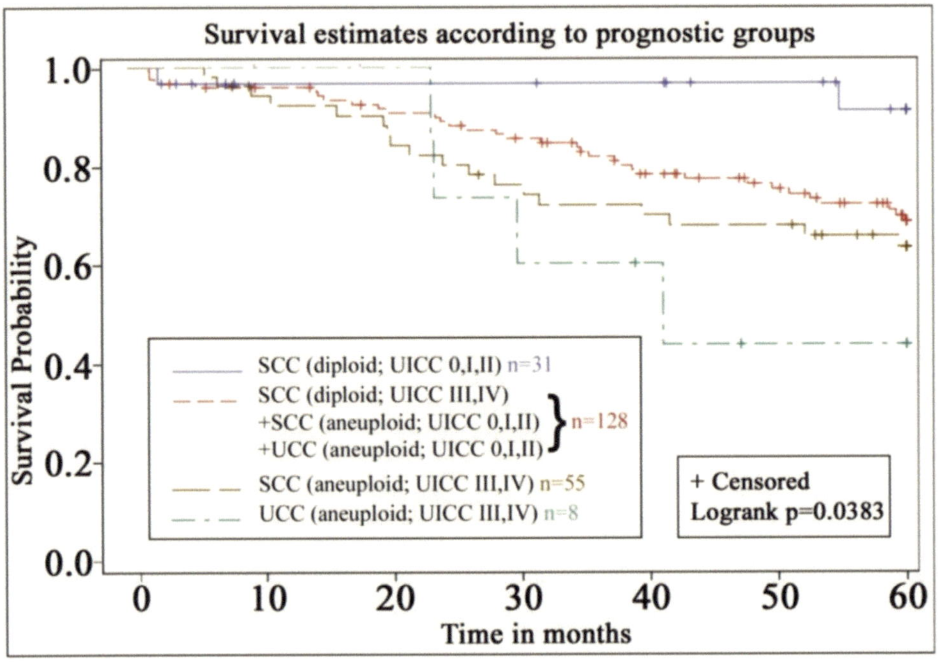

Fig. 3. Kaplan-Meier survival estimates of significant prognostic groups according to UICC stage, ploidy status, and underlying inflammatory disease. SCC, sporadic colorectal cancer; UCC, ulcerative colitis-associated colorectal cancer. Modified from (Gerling et al. 2010)

3.4 Aneuploidy and colorectal cancer risk in ulcerative colitis

The significantly higher frequency of aneuploidy in UCCs than in sporadic colorectal cancer might indicate the dominance of genomic instability not only at the time when malignancy is overt but also for the development of malignant properties. In order to evaluate aneuploidy as a potential predictive marker in patient risk assessment, we analyzed two groups (Habermann et al. 2001): eight patients with ulcerative colitis-associated colorectal carcinomas (UCC), and 16 ulcerative colitis (UC) patients without malignancy but comparable risk factors (duration of disease, extent of inflammation, epithelial dysplasia). A total of 683 paraffin-embedded mucosal biopsies were retrospectively evaluated for inflammatory activity, grade of dysplasia, ploidy status, laminin-5 γ2 chain and cyclin A expression. In all biopsies, mild or moderate inflammatory activity was present in 78% while low-grade or high-grade dysplasia was found in 5.5%. There was, however, no difference in inflammatory activity and dysplasia between patient groups (Habermann et al. 2001).

It is a known fact that dysplasia is absent in 20% - 30% of colectomy specimens containing UCC (Dobbins 1977). A review of 12 surveillance studies with 92 detected carcinomas in 1,916 patients revealed that only 12% were early carcinomas detected by surveillance (Lynch et al. 1993). In our study, only two cancer patients had a distinct high-grade dysplastic lesion prior to the final diagnosis. One of them was underestimated in the original routine histopathological diagnosis. The tumor stages of the eight UCCs were as follows: one Dukes' A, three Dukes' B, two Dukes' C and two Dukes' D. One of the most important findings of this study was the detection of highly aneuploid epithelial cell populations scattered over the colon and rectum in premalignant biopsies of all eight UCC patients (**Figure 4**). These lesions could be observed up to 11 years prior to the final cancer diagnosis (average 7.8 years). They were found in macro- and microscopically unsuspicious mucosa, could even be detected in regenerative epithelium, and were not related to dysplasia. This DNA aneuploidy occurred more frequently in biopsies (75%) of UC patients with a subsequent UCC than in those without subsequent malignancy (14%, $p = 0.006$). The carcinoma samples of the eight UCC patients also exhibited highly aneuploid DNA distribution patterns. Löfberg et al. reported aneuploid biopsies in 25% of high-risk patients at least once during 10 years of observation (Lofberg et al. 1992). In other studies, aneuploidy has been repeatedly observed by flow-cytometry in non-dysplastic mucosa of high-risk patients (Rubin et al. 1992). The results of our study support the above-mentioned observations. Genomic instability, represented by DNA aneuploidy, could initiate the process of malignant transformation in colitis as an early event.

Little is known about laminin-5 $\gamma 2$ chain immunoreactivity in precancerous lesions of malignant human tumors. Previous data from our group had shown various degrees of cytoplasmic laminin-5 $\gamma 2$ chain immunoreactivity in 96% of primary colon carcinomas, whereas staining was absent in stromal cells and adjacent normal colonic mucosa. There was also an interrelationship between a strong staining pattern and a worse clinical outcome (Lenander et al. 2001). In the present study, seven of the eight UCC specimens had a moderate or strong $\gamma 2$ chain expression, which was observed predominantly in malignant cells at the invasive front. An interesting finding in patient group A was the detection of immunoreactivity in biopsy specimens up to 13 years prior to the subsequent carcinoma (average 8 years). The overall expression of laminin-5 was significantly more frequent throughout the entire observation period in UC biopsies of patients with a subsequent UCC (20%) than in those without subsequent UCC (5%, $p = 0.002$). Laminin-5 $\gamma 2$ chain positive cells were distributed over the whole colon and rectum and were not correlated with dysplasia ($r = 0.357$) or inflammatory activity ($r = 0.142$), but interestingly, related to aneuploidy: in the UCC group as many as 26 of 37 of the laminin-5 immunopositive biopsies were aneuploid. In the non-malignancy group, only 2 of 8 immunopositive biopsies showed aneuploidy and the rarely occurring laminin-5 positive cells were generally localized close to the basement membrane, mainly in flat, regenerative epithelium. Thus, the observation of laminin-5 immunoreactivity years prior to a UCC might not just represent the ability of cells to invade but also to wound healing. In fact, strong laminin-5 expression has also been observed in migrating keratinocytes in healing skin wounds (Larjava et al. 1993). The observed phenomenon could thus be affected by the underlying inflammatory disease (Haapasalmi et al. 1995; Thorup et al. 1998). Laminin-5 $\gamma 2$ chain overexpression in repeated biopsies might be related to upregulated regenerative processes in ulcerative colitis. However, since normal regenerative processes and wound healing generally occur in diploid cell populations, the combined analysis of ploidy and laminin-5 $\gamma 2$ chain expression may allow identification of premalignant populations with invasive capacity. The present data strongly indicate an increased risk of progression to invasive properties in genetically unstable cells.

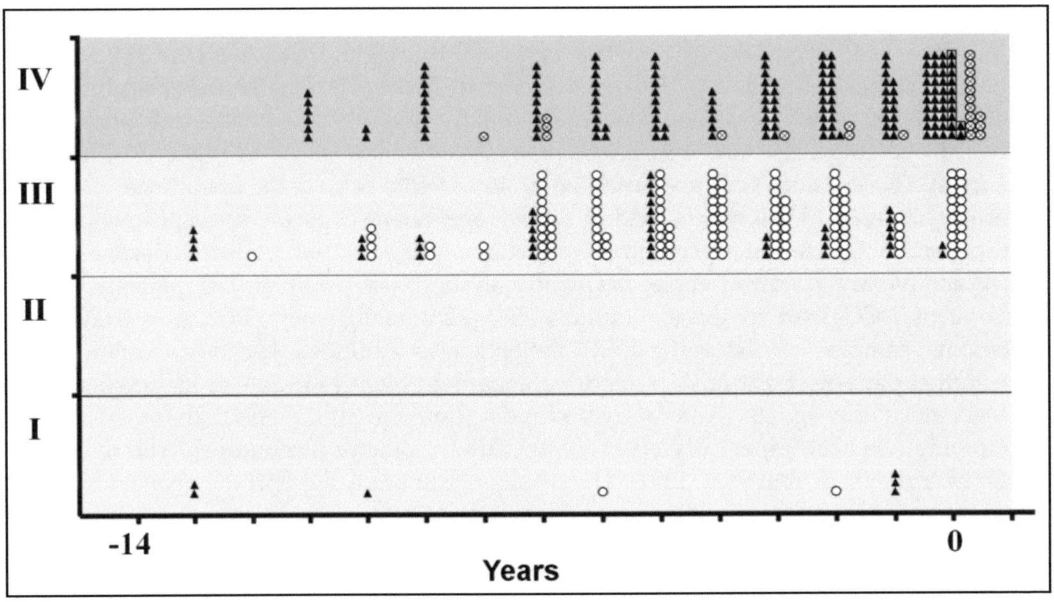

Fig. 4. DNA histogram types in biopsies of 8 patients with (▲) and 16 patients without UCC (O). Aneuploid biopsies defined six patients without UCC to be at increased UCC risk (⊗). The carcinoma specimens are framed ([▲]). The endpoint of the study is represented by year 0 on the x-achsis. Modified from (Habermann et al. 2001)

However, aneuploidy may be reversible over time once cells are not longer exposed to the inducing agent or carcinogen (Auer et al. 1982; Ono et al. 1984). Thus, it is reasonable to suggest that the genomic instability reflected by aneuploidy has to be followed by multiple cellular alterations in order to reach malignant properties. One of the decisive steps in this transformational process is the ability of genomically altered cells to proliferate, which is compulsory for clonal expansion (Wang et al. 2002). In the present study, six out of eight UCC specimens exhibited an increased cyclin A expression pattern. In addition, cyclin A expression was found in 98% of all biopsies, with a higher number of immunopositive cells in biopsies of the UCC group ($p = 0.014$), as well as being mainly observed in aneuploid populations: in the UCC group as many as 12 of 13 biopsies with increased cyclin A staining were aneuploid, whereas in the non-malignancy group only one of four biopsies with similar staining intensity showed aneuploidy. Thus in the UCC group, increased cyclin A expression was significantly correlated to aneuploidy ($r = 0.791$). However, there was no significant correlation with inflammatory activity ($r = 0.178$), grade of dysplasia ($r = 0.485$) or laminin-5 immunopositivity ($r = 0.140$). Since cyclin A expression indicates whether a cell is committed to pass through the cell cycle and divide, i.e. participate in clonal expansion, the fraction of cyclin A positive cells may be used to estimate the risk of aneuploid populations to progress to malignancy. At the study's conclusion and establishment of a risk profile, based on the three parameters discussed above, it was discovered that six out of the 16 patients in group B could be identified as high-risk patients. Of these six patients, one patient developed an invasive carcinoma after the endpoint of the study. By fitting a logistic regression model, DNA-cytometry, laminin-5 positivity and increased cyclin A expression were confirmed as significant predictors for malignant transformation.

4. Conclusions

Genomic aneuploidy occurs early and is commonly found in precancerous biopsies of ulcerative colitis patients who subsequently develop an ulcerative colitis-associated colorectal carcinoma (UCC). The assessment of DNA ploidy could therefore become a basic element in future surveillance programs in ulcerative colitis. The complementary detection of laminin-5 positivity and increased cyclin A expression in aneuploid lesions - indicating invasive potential and clonal expansion - seems to be the most powerful combination to predict imminent malignant transformation for an individual patient. Moreover, genomic aneuploidy in UCC tumors correlates with specific chromosomal gains and losses, which are similar to that seen in sporadic colorectal carcinomas. However, the frequency of aneuploidy in UCC is significantly higher than in the sporadic counterpart and is an indpendent poor prognosis factor for the affected patients.

5. Future perspectives

The analysis of DNA ploidy measurements in premalignant ulcerative colitis lesions could profoundly improve individual risk assessment for imminent colorectal cancer development. However, large multicentric prospective studies are warranted to corroborate the value for improved screening and prognostication in ulcerative colitis by means of ploidy assessment. For this purpose we have initiated the *North German Tumor Biobank of Colorectal Cancer* (Acronym: ColoNet; www.northgermantumorbankcrc.de) that currently comprises the catchment areas of the universities and clinics of Hamburg, Lübeck, Rostock, Greifswald, Bad Oldesloe, Berlin-Buch and associated private practices in northern Germany. Within this network, we will investigate the potential benefit of ploidy measures for individual risk and prognosis assessment in ulcerative colitis and associated colorectal carcinomas.

6. Acknowledgements

We thank all members of the Auer lab, the Ried lab, the Laboratory for Surgical Research and all colleagues of the Department of Surgery, Department of Pathology and Unit of Gastroenterology at the University of Lübeck who made these studies possible. Furthermore we gratefully acknowledge the intramural funding of the National Institutes of Health, the Karolinska Institutet, the University of Lübeck and the Werner and Clara Kreitz Foundation, the Ad Infinitum Foundation, the Swedish Cancer Society, the Cancer Society Stockholm, the Swedish Research Council, the King Gustav V Jubilee Fund, the Wallenberg Consortium North, and the Knut and Alice Wallenberg Foundation. These studies were performed in connection with the Surgical Center for Translational Oncology - Lübeck (SCTO-L) and were based on sample collections of the *North German Tumorbank of Colorectal Cancer* (DKH #108446).

7. References

Auer, G., J. Ono, M. Nasiell, T. Caspersson, H. Kato, C. Konaka, and Y. Hayata. 1982. Reversibility of bronchial cell atypia. *Cancer Res* 42 (10):4241-7.

Auer, G. U., T. O. Caspersson, and A. S. Wallgren. 1980. DNA content and survival in mammary carcinoma. *Anal Quant Cytol* 2 (3):161-5.

Aust, D. E., R. F. Willenbucher, J. P. Terdiman, L. D. Ferrell, C. G. Chang, D. H. Moore, 2nd, A. Molinaro-Clark, G. B. Baretton, U. Loehrs, and F. M. Waldman. 2000. Chromosomal alterations in ulcerative colitis-related and sporadic colorectal cancers by comparative genomic hybridization. *Hum Pathol* 31 (1):109-14.

Bach, S. P., A. G. Renehan, and C. S. Potten. 2000. Stem cells: the intestinal stem cell as a paradigm. *Carcinogenesis* 21 (3):469-76.

Barrett, J. C., M. Oshimura, N. Tanaka, and T. Tsutsui. 1985. Role of aneuploidy in early and late stages of neoplastic progression of Syrian hamster embryo cells in culture. *Basic Life Sci* 36:523-38.

Bernstein, C. N., J. F. Blanchard, E. Kliewer, and A. Wajda. 2001. Cancer risk in patients with inflammatory bowel disease: a population-based study. *Cancer* 91 (4):854-62.

Blegen, H., B. M. Ghadimi, A. Jauho, A. Zetterberg, E. Eriksson, G. Auer, and T. Ried. 2001. Genetic instability promotes the acquisition of chromosomal imbalances in T1b and T1c breast adenocarcinomas. *Anal Cell Pathol* 22 (3):123-31.

Bomme, L., G. Bardi, N. Pandis, C. Fenger, O. Kronborg, and S. Heim. 1994. Clonal karyotypic abnormalities in colorectal adenomas: clues to the early genetic events in the adenoma-carcinoma sequence. *Genes Chromosomes Cancer* 10 (3):190-6.

Burmer, G. C., P. S. Rabinovitch, and L. A. Loeb. 1991. Frequency and spectrum of c-Ki-ras mutations in human sporadic colon carcinoma, carcinomas arising in ulcerative colitis, and pancreatic adenocarcinoma. *Environ Health Perspect* 93:27-31.

Calaluce, R., B. W. Miedema, and Y. W. Yesus. 1998. Micrometastasis in colorectal carcinoma: a review. *J Surg Oncol* 67 (3):194-202.

Carter, W. G., M. C. Ryan, and P. J. Gahr. 1991. Epiligrin, a new cell adhesion ligand for integrin alpha 3 beta 1 in epithelial basement membranes. *Cell* 65 (4):599-610.

Caspersson, T. O. 1979. Quantitative tumor cytochemistry--G.H.A. Clowes Memorial Lecture. *Cancer Res* 39 (7 Pt 1):2341-5.

Caspersson, T., L. Zech, C. Johansson, and E. J. Modest. 1970. Identification of human chromosomes by DNA-binding fluorescent agents. *Chromosoma* 30 (2):215-27.

Clausen, O. P., S. N. Andersen, H. Stroomkjaer, V. Nielsen, T. O. Rognum, L. Bolund, and S. Koolvraa. 2001. A strategy combining flow sorting and comparative genomic hybridization for studying genetic aberrations at different stages of colorectal tumorigenesis in ulcerative colitis. *Cytometry* 43 (1):46-54.

Collins, R. H., Jr., M. Feldman, and J. S. Fordtran. 1987. Colon cancer, dysplasia, and surveillance in patients with ulcerative colitis. A critical review. *N Engl J Med* 316 (26):1654-8.

Daperno, M., R. Sostegni, A. Lavagna, L. Crocella, E. Ercole, C. Rigazio, R. Rocca, and A. Pera. 2004. The role of endoscopy in inflammatory bowel disease. *Eur Rev Med Pharmacol Sci* 8 (5):209-14.

Desper, R., F. Jiang, O. P. Kallioniemi, H. Moch, C. H. Papadimitriou, and A. A. Schaffer. 2000. Distance-based reconstruction of tree models for oncogenesis. *J Comput Biol* 7 (6):789-803.

Dobbins, W. O., 3rd. 1977. Current status of the precancer lesion in ulcerative colitis. *Gastroenterology* 73 (6):1431-3.

Duesberg, P., C. Rausch, D. Rasnick, and R. Hehlmann. 1998. Genetic instability of cancer cells is proportional to their degree of aneuploidy. *Proc Natl Acad Sci U S A* 95 (23):13692-7.

Eaden, J., K. Abrams, H. McKay, H. Denley, and J. Mayberry. 2001. Inter-observer variation between general and specialist gastrointestinal pathologists when grading dysplasia in ulcerative colitis. *J Pathol* 194 (2):152-7.

Fearon, E. R., and B. Vogelstein. 1990. A genetic model for colorectal tumorigenesis. *Cell* 61 (5):759-67.

Forozan, F., R. Karhu, J. Kononen, A. Kallioniemi, and O. P. Kallioniemi. 1997. Genome screening by comparative genomic hybridization. *Trends Genet* 13 (10):405-9.

Fozard, J. B., P. Quirke, M. F. Dixon, G. R. Giles, and C. C. Bird. 1986. DNA aneuploidy in ulcerative colitis. *Gut* 27 (12):1414-8.

Gerling, M., K. F. Meyer, K. Fuchs, B. W. Igl, B. Fritzsche, A. Ziegler, F. Bader, P. Kujath, H. Schimmelpenning, H. P. Bruch, U. J. Roblick, and J. K. Habermann. 2010. High Frequency of Aneuploidy Defines Ulcerative Colitis-Associated Carcinomas: A Comparative Prognostic Study to Sporadic Colorectal Carcinomas. *Ann Surg*.

Ghadimi, B. M., D. L. Sackett, M. J. Difilippantonio, E. Schrock, T. Neumann, A. Jauho, G. Auer, and T. Ried. 2000. Centrosome amplification and instability occurs exclusively in aneuploid, but not in diploid colorectal cancer cell lines, and correlates with numerical chromosomal aberrations. *Genes Chromosomes Cancer* 27 (2):183-90.

Haapasalmi, K., M. Makela, O. Oksala, J. Heino, K. M. Yamada, V. J. Uitto, and H. Larjava. 1995. Expression of epithelial adhesion proteins and integrins in chronic inflammation. *Am J Pathol* 147 (1):193-206.

Habermann, J. K., M. B. Upender, U. J. Roblick, S. Kruger, S. Freitag, H. Blegen, H. P. Bruch, H. Schimmelpenning, G. Auer, and T. Ried. 2003. Pronounced chromosomal instability and multiple gene amplifications characterize ulcerative colitis-associated colorectal carcinomas. *Cancer Genet Cytogenet* 147 (1):9-17.

Habermann, J., C. Lenander, U. J. Roblick, S. Kruger, D. Ludwig, A. Alaiya, S. Freitag, L. Dumbgen, H. P. Bruch, E. Stange, S. Salo, K. Tryggvason, G. Auer, and H. Schimmelpenning. 2001. Ulcerative colitis and colorectal carcinoma: DNA-profile, laminin-5 gamma2 chain and cyclin A expression as early markers for risk assessment. *Scand J Gastroenterol* 36 (7):751-8.

Heselmeyer, K., E. Schrock, S. du Manoir, H. Blegen, K. Shah, R. Steinbeck, G. Auer, and T. Ried. 1996. Gain of chromosome 3q defines the transition from severe dysplasia to invasive carcinoma of the uterine cervix. *Proc Natl Acad Sci U S A* 93 (1):479-84.

Hittelman, W. N. 2001. Genetic instability in epithelial tissues at risk for cancer. *Ann N Y Acad Sci* 952:1-12.

Holzmann, K., B. Klump, F. Borchard, C. J. Hsieh, A. Kuhn, V. Gaco, M. Gregor, and R. Porschen. 1998. Comparative analysis of histology, DNA content, p53 and Ki-ras mutations in colectomy specimens with long-standing ulcerative colitis. *Int J Cancer* 76 (1):1-6.

Holzmann, K., M. Weis-Klemm, B. Klump, C. J. Hsieh, F. Borchard, M. Gregor, and R. Porschen. 2001. Comparison of flow cytometry and histology with mutational screening for p53 and Ki-ras mutations in surveillance of patients with long-standing ulcerative colitis. *Scand J Gastroenterol* 36 (12):1320-6.

Hopman, A. H., F. C. Ramaekers, A. K. Raap, J. L. Beck, P. Devilee, M. van der Ploeg, and G. P. Vooijs. 1988. In situ hybridization as a tool to study numerical chromosome aberrations in solid bladder tumors. *Histochemistry* 89 (4):307-16.

Iivanainen, A., T. Morita, and K. Tryggvason. 1999. Molecular cloning and tissue-specific expression of a novel murine laminin gamma3 chain. *J Biol Chem* 274 (20):14107-11.

Kallioniemi, A., O. P. Kallioniemi, D. Sudar, D. Rutovitz, J. W. Gray, F. Waldman, and D. Pinkel. 1992. Comparative genomic hybridization for molecular cytogenetic analysis of solid tumors. *Science* 258 (5083):818-21.

Kern, S. E., M. Redston, A. B. Seymour, C. Caldas, S. M. Powell, S. Kornacki, and K. W. Kinzler. 1994. Molecular genetic profiles of colitis-associated neoplasms. *Gastroenterology* 107 (2):420-8.

Klump, B., K. Holzmann, A. Kuhn, F. Borchard, M. Sarbia, M. Gregor, and R. Porschen. 1997. Distribution of cell populations with DNA aneuploidy and p53 protein expression in ulcerative colitis. *Eur J Gastroenterol Hepatol* 9 (8):789-94.

Knuutila, S., A. M. Bjorkqvist, K. Autio, M. Tarkkanen, M. Wolf, O. Monni, J. Szymanska, M. L. Larramendy, J. Tapper, H. Pere, W. El-Rifai, S. Hemmer, V. M. Wasenius, V. Vidgren, and Y. Zhu. 1998. DNA copy number amplifications in human neoplasms: review of comparative genomic hybridization studies. *Am J Pathol* 152 (5):1107-23.

Lamprecht, S. A., and M. Lipkin. 2002. Migrating colonic crypt epithelial cells: primary targets for transformation. *Carcinogenesis* 23 (11):1777-80.

Larjava, H., T. Salo, K. Haapasalmi, R. H. Kramer, and J. Heino. 1993. Expression of integrins and basement membrane components by wound keratinocytes. *J Clin Invest* 92 (3):1425-35.

Lenander, C., J. K. Habermann, A. Ost, B. Nilsson, H. Schimmelpenning, K. Tryggvason, and G. Auer. 2001. Laminin-5 gamma 2 chain expression correlates with unfavorable prognosis in colon carcinomas. *Anal Cell Pathol* 22 (4):201-9.

Lengauer, C., K. W. Kinzler, and B. Vogelstein. 1998. Genetic instabilities in human cancers. *Nature* 396 (6712):643-9.

Levine, D. S., P. S. Rabinovitch, R. C. Haggitt, P. L. Blount, P. J. Dean, C. E. Rubin, and B. J. Reid. 1991. Distribution of aneuploid cell populations in ulcerative colitis with dysplasia or cancer. *Gastroenterology* 101 (5):1198-210.

Loeb, K. R., and L. A. Loeb. 1999. Genetic instability and the mutator phenotype. Studies in ulcerative colitis. *Am J Pathol* 154 (6):1621-6.

Lofberg, R., O. Brostrom, P. Karlen, A. Ost, and B. Tribukait. 1992. DNA aneuploidy in ulcerative colitis: reproducibility, topographic distribution, and relation to dysplasia. *Gastroenterology* 102 (4 Pt 1):1149-54.

Lynch, D. A., A. J. Lobo, G. M. Sobala, M. F. Dixon, and A. T. Axon. 1993. Failure of colonoscopic surveillance in ulcerative colitis. *Gut* 34 (8):1075-80.

Makiyama, K., M. Tokunaga, M. Itsuno, W. Zea-Iriarte, K. Hara, and T. Nakagoe. 1995. DNA aneuploidy in a case of rectosigmoid adenocarcinoma complicated by ulcerative colitis. *J Gastroenterol* 30 (2):258-63.

Nowak, M. A., N. L. Komarova, A. Sengupta, P. V. Jallepalli, M. Shih Ie, B. Vogelstein, and C. Lengauer. 2002. The role of chromosomal instability in tumor initiation. *Proc Natl Acad Sci U S A* 99 (25):16226-31.

Ono, J., G. Auer, T. Caspersson, M. Nasiell, T. Saito, C. Konaka, H. Kato, and Y. Hayata. 1984. Reversibility of 20-methylcholanthrene-induced bronchial cell atypia in dogs. *Cancer* 54 (6):1030-7.

Oshimura, M., and J. C. Barrett. 1986. Chemically induced aneuploidy in mammalian cells: mechanisms and biological significance in cancer. *Environ Mutagen* 8 (1):129-59.

Platzer, P., M. B. Upender, K. Wilson, J. Willis, J. Lutterbaugh, A. Nosrati, J. K. Willson, D. Mack, T. Ried, and S. Markowitz. 2002. Silence of chromosomal amplifications in colon cancer. *Cancer Res* 62 (4):1134-8.

Pyke, C., J. Romer, P. Kallunki, L. R. Lund, E. Ralfkiaer, K. Dano, and K. Tryggvason. 1994. The gamma 2 chain of kalinin/laminin 5 is preferentially expressed in invading malignant cells in human cancers. *Am J Pathol* 145 (4):782-91.

Pyke, C., S. Salo, E. Ralfkiaer, J. Romer, K. Dano, and K. Tryggvason. 1995. Laminin-5 is a marker of invading cancer cells in some human carcinomas and is coexpressed with the receptor for urokinase plasminogen activator in budding cancer cells in colon adenocarcinomas. *Cancer Res* 55 (18):4132-9.

Riddell, R. H. 1998. How reliable/valid is dysplasia in identifying at-risk patients with ulcerative colitis? *J Gastrointest Surg* 2 (4):314-7.

Ried, T., K. Heselmeyer-Haddad, H. Blegen, E. Schrock, and G. Auer. 1999. Genomic changes defining the genesis, progression, and malignancy potential in solid human tumors: a phenotype/genotype correlation. *Genes Chromosomes Cancer* 25 (3):195-204.

Ried, T., R. Knutzen, R. Steinbeck, H. Blegen, E. Schrock, K. Heselmeyer, S. du Manoir, and G. Auer. 1996. Comparative genomic hybridization reveals a specific pattern of chromosomal gains and losses during the genesis of colorectal tumors. *Genes Chromosomes Cancer* 15 (4):234-45.

Rubin, C. E., R. C. Haggitt, G. C. Burmer, T. A. Brentnall, A. C. Stevens, D. S. Levine, P. J. Dean, M. Kimmey, D. R. Perera, and P. S. Rabinovitch. 1992. DNA aneuploidy in colonic biopsies predicts future development of dysplasia in ulcerative colitis. *Gastroenterology* 103 (5):1611-20.

Schlegel, J., G. Stumm, H. Scherthan, T. Bocker, H. Zirngibl, J. Ruschoff, and F. Hofstadter. 1995. Comparative genomic in situ hybridization of colon carcinomas with replication error. *Cancer Res* 55 (24):6002-5.

Schrock, E., S. du Manoir, T. Veldman, B. Schoell, J. Wienberg, M. A. Ferguson-Smith, Y. Ning, D. H. Ledbetter, I. Bar-Am, D. Soenksen, Y. Garini, and T. Ried. 1996. Multicolor spectral karyotyping of human chromosomes. *Science* 273 (5274):494-7.

Shih, I. M., T. L. Wang, G. Traverso, K. Romans, S. R. Hamilton, S. Ben-Sasson, K. W. Kinzler, and B. Vogelstein. 2001. Top-down morphogenesis of colorectal tumors. *Proc Natl Acad Sci U S A* 98 (5):2640-5.

Solinas-Toldo, S., C. Wallrapp, F. Muller-Pillasch, M. Bentz, T. Gress, and P. Lichter. 1996. Mapping of chromosomal imbalances in pancreatic carcinoma by comparative genomic hybridization. *Cancer Res* 56 (16):3803-7.

Sordat, I., F. T. Bosman, G. Dorta, P. Rousselle, D. Aberdam, A. L. Blum, and B. Sordat. 1998. Differential expression of laminin-5 subunits and integrin receptors in human colorectal neoplasia. *J Pathol* 185 (1):44-52.

Speicher, M. R., S. Gwyn Ballard, and D. C. Ward. 1996. Karyotyping human chromosomes by combinatorial multi-fluor FISH. *Nat Genet* 12 (4):368-75.

Thorup, A. K., J. Reibel, M. Schiodt, T. C. Stenersen, M. H. Therkildsen, W. G. Carter, and E. Dabelsteen. 1998. Can alterations in integrin and laminin-5 expression be used as markers of malignancy? *Apmis* 106 (12):1170-80.

Tryggvason, K. 1993. The laminin family. *Curr Opin Cell Biol* 5 (5):877-82.

Vogelstein, B., and K. W. Kinzler. 2004. Cancer genes and the pathways they control. *Nat Med* 10 (8):789-99.

Wang, Y., M. C. Wu, J. S. Sham, W. Zhang, W. Q. Wu, and X. Y. Guan. 2002. Prognostic significance of c-myc and AIB1 amplification in hepatocellular carcinoma. A broad survey using high-throughput tissue microarray. *Cancer* 95 (11):2346-52.

Willenbucher, R. F. 1996. Inflammatory bowel disease. *Semin Gastrointest Dis* 7 (2):94-104.

Willenbucher, R. F., S. J. Zelman, L. D. Ferrell, D. H. Moore, 2nd, and F. M. Waldman. 1997. Chromosomal alterations in ulcerative colitis-related neoplastic progression. *Gastroenterology* 113 (3):791-801.

Wright, N. A. 2000. Epithelial stem cell repertoire in the gut: clues to the origin of cell lineages, proliferative units and cancer. *Int J Exp Pathol* 81 (2):117-43.

7

Carcinogenesis in Ulcerative Colitis

Adam Humphries[1], Noor Jawad[2], Ana Ignjatovic[3], James East[3] and Simon Leedham[3,4]
[1]London Research Institute, Histopathology Lab, Cancer Research UK,
[2]Blizard Institute of Cell and Molecular Science, Bart's and The London School of Medicine and Dentistry, Queen Mary, University of London,
[3]Translational Gastroenterology Unit, John Radcliffe Hospital, Oxford,
[4]Wellcome Trust Centre for Human Genetics, University of Oxford, Oxford UK

1. Introduction

Crohn's disease (CD) and Ulcerative Colitis (UC) are collectively referred to as inflammatory bowel disease (IBD). Ulcerative Colitis was originally described in the medical journals in 1859, but it was not until 1925 that the first case-report of a colitis-associated colorectal cancer (CACRC) was published by Crohn and Rosenborg (reviewed in (Greenstein, 2000)). Since then it has become clear that IBD ranks as a high-risk condition for the development of colorectal cancer (CRC), with a standardized incidence ratio of 2.4 (95% CI 0.6-6.0) in patients with extensive or pan UC. This risk is associated with longer disease duration, earlier age of onset (Ekbom et al., 1990), the greater the severity of inflammation (Rutter et al., 2004) and the presence of concomitant inflammatory conditions such as primary sclerosing cholangitis (PSC) (Claessen et al., 2009). This suggests that the acquired cancer risk is a consequence of the inflammatory process itself, resulting from repeated cycles of ulceration and epithelial regeneration. Moreover, the molecular and histopathology of colitis-associated colorectal cancer (CACRC) is distinct from that of sporadic colorectal cancer (SCRC), and understanding this is crucial to enable the development of effective and beneficial screening programmes for patients with long-standing ulcerative colitis (UC).

2. Tumorigenesis of colon cancer in ulcerative colitis

2.1 Stem cells, inflammation and field cancerisation

It is generally thought that most cancers arise as a result of a single, mutated stem cell, as these are the only cells that have sufficient life span to acquire the multiple oncogenic mutations required for tumorigenesis. There is now good evidence to support this in mice. Deletion of *Apc* in the intestinal stem cells resulted in large numbers of intestinal macro-adenomas; however when *Apc* was deleted in non-stem cells, adenomas were significantly fewer and only able to reach a very small size (Barker et al., 2009). In this section the processes by which the progeny of a mutated stem cell can come to form a dysplastic lesion and the pro-oncogenic effects of chronic inflammation will be summarised.

2.1.1 Inflammation and the stem cell niche

Inflammatory bowel disease is characterised by the presence of an inflammatory mucosal infiltrate. Infiltrating leucocytes and activated mesenchymal myofibroblasts secrete a large number of pro-inflammatory cytokines, growth factors and morphogens that can all have profound effects on the stem cell niche. At present there is little evidence for a direct effect of inflammation on the mammalian intestinal stem cell niche however this is a research area of great interest. A recent study by Ren et al (Ren et al., 2010) in Drosophila intestine demonstrated that the evolutionary conserved Hippo (Hpo) signalling pathway is important for regulating intestinal stem cell proliferation and survival, and that dysregulation of this pathway with increased stem cell proliferation occurs with mucosal inflammation. Importantly disruption of the Hpo pathway has been associated with a number of human cancers, thus suggesting one possible mechanism whereby inflammation may be driving tumorigenesis in IBD through a direct effect on the stem cell niche.

2.1.2 Crypt fission and clonal expansion

In order to understand how a single, mutated stem cell can result in a cancer we need to look at the dynamics of the normal colonic crypt. There are thought to be a small number of clonally related stem cells located at the base of each crypt within a niche (Williams et al., 1992; Campbell et al., 1996; Yatabe et al., 2001; Barker et al., 2007). The number of stem cells within the niche is tightly controlled. However with random loss or gain of stem cells from the niche, a single stem cell and its progeny can stochastically expand within the niche until all the stem cells within the niche are derived from the same lineage (Yatabe et al., 2001) – this process is termed *niche succession* (Figure 1). In the normal human crypt this is thought to be a slow process, with successive niche succession cycles occurring around every 8-9 years (Humphries & Wright, 2008; Graham et al., 2011). As a consequence of the niche succession process the progeny of that stem cell lineage will then take over the whole crypt, and this is termed *monoclonal conversion* (Figure 1). In order for the normal gut to grow during childhood or to replace crypts that die, often as a result of inflammation – *epithelial restitution*, there has to be a mechanism for crypts to expand, and this is achieved via the process of *crypt fission* whereby a single parent crypt divides to form two daughter crypts (Figure 1). Although all these processes are slow in the normal colon, they have the potential to be up-regulated, either due to inflammation or an oncogenic mutation arising in a stem cell, and it is by the process of crypt fission that mutated crypts are then able to expand and grow within the epithelium to form a dysplastic lesion (Park et al., 1995; Wong et al., 2002; Greaves et al., 2006 ; Humphries & Wright 2008).

We have discussed the processes of niche succession and monoclonal conversion as inherent properties of the stem cell niche. Now imagine that a stem cell gains a selective advantage, potentially an oncogenic mutation induced by the dysregulation of normal inhibitory pathways of stem cell proliferation due to chronic inflammation, then the process of niche succession and clonal conversion will take place rapidly with the result mutant cells occupying the whole crypt. The mutant clone is then able to expand further within the epithelium by crypt fission, perhaps gaining further mutations as it grows. Niche succession and crypt fission are likely to be the initial mechanisms behind clonal expansion in CACRC. Crypt fission has been shown to be responsible for the expansion spread of individual crypts in the colon (Greaves et al., 2006), small intestine (Gutierrez-Gonzales et al., 2009) and stomach (McDonald et al., 2008), and this process is a histological feature of colitis and dysplasia (Park et al., 1995; Wong et al., 2002). Chen et al (Chen et al., 2005) used a fluorescent in-situ hybridisation technique to demonstrate the spread of *TP53* mutations into the daughter crypts of a crypt in the process of fission in UC.

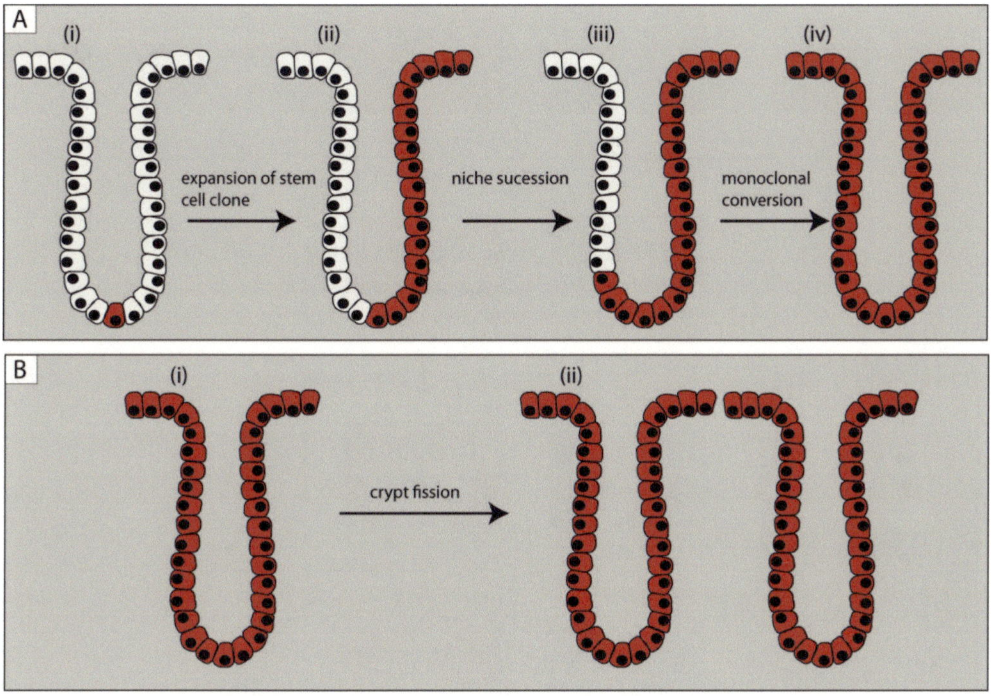

Fig. 1. Expansion of a mutated stem cell within the colonic crypt and epithelium
(A): a stem cell (highlighted in red) within the niche is able to expand within the niche via niche succession (i-iii), subsequently all the progeny of that stem cell lineage take over the crypt - monoclonal conversion (iv). If the stem cell has gained a selective advantage via an oncogenic mutation, then this can happen rapidly. (B): The mutated crypt (i) then clonally expands within the epithelium by dividing from the bottom up to produce two daughter crypts - crypt fission (ii)

2.2 The carcinogenesis pathway in CACRC is distinct to that of SCRC

There is accumulating histopathological, genetic and functional evidence to suggest that SCRC and CACRC are separate diseases. Clinically the two conditions have a number of distinguishing features: CACRC arises in a younger population, often from flat, not polypoid dysplasia and has a more proximal distribution, there is a greater frequency of mucinous or signet cell histology, and a higher incidence of multiple synchronous lesions in CACRC (Itzkowitz & Yio, 2004). From a histological perspective, sporadic tumours tend to follow the adenoma-carcinoma sequence. The stepwise accumulation of genetic mutations in onco- and tumour suppressor genes that underpins this histological progression is well established and has significantly altered worldwide clinical practice (Vogelstein et al., 1988). However CACRC progresses through low (LGD) and high-grade dysplasia (HGD) to carcinoma, and this carcinogenesis pathway is less well explored with significantly differences in the requirement and timing of genetic and epigenetic alterations (Figure 2).

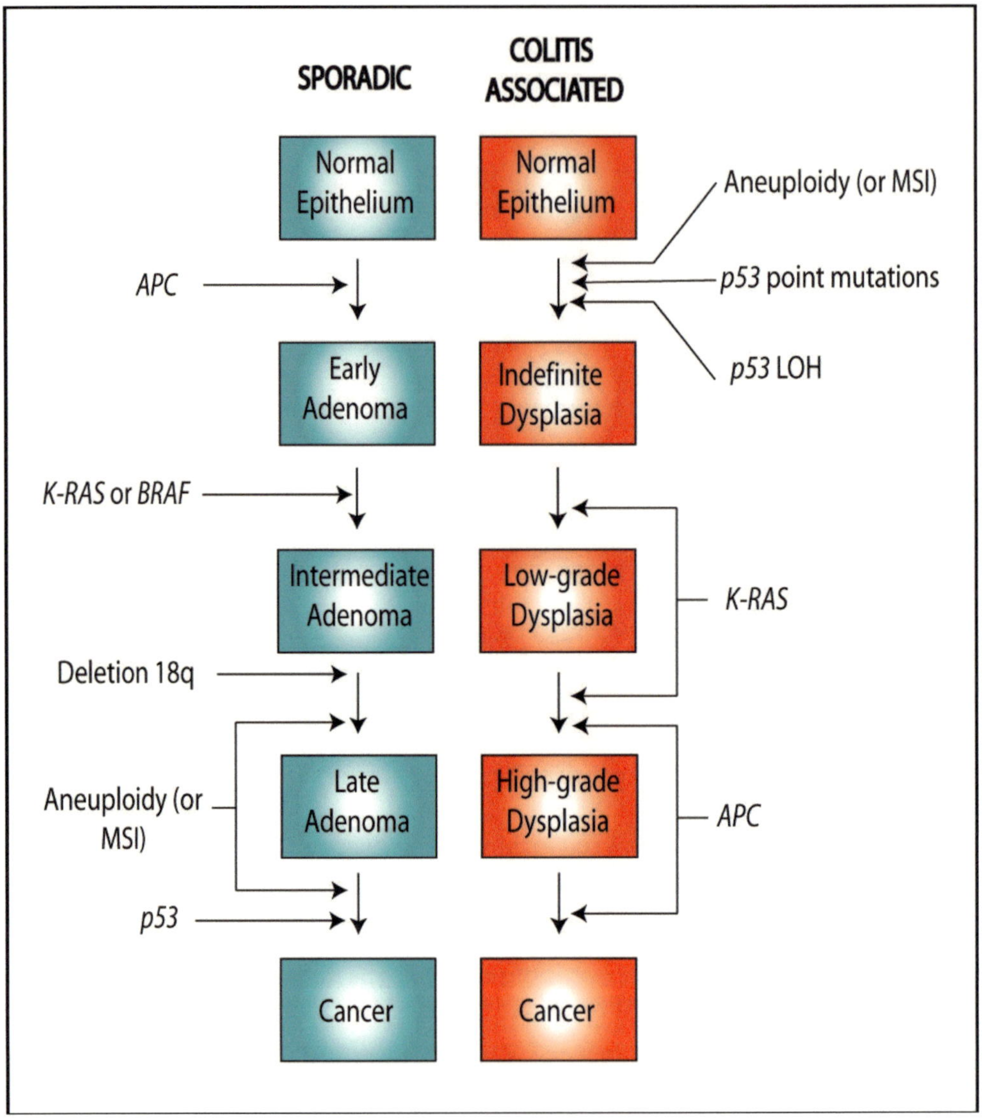

Fig. 2. Comparison of CACRC and SCRC carcinogenesis pathways

Both types of cancer show multi-step development with sequential mutation in tumour suppressor and oncogenes. The main difference between the pathways is in the timing of these mutations: APC is the initiating mutation in almost all SCRC, but is rarely found in CACRC and when present often occurs late in tumour development. **Abbreviations:** APC, Adenomatous polyposis coli; DCC, deleted in colon cancer; K-RAS, Kirsten-Ras; LOH, loss of heterozygosity; MSI, microsatellite instability.

2.2.1 Canonical Wnt signalling in SCRC and CACRC

Wnts are a large family of secreted glycoproteins with at least 19 known human members that are expressed in species ranging from Drosophila to man. Wnt signalling plays a critical role in the development and homeostasis of the intestinal epithelium, having a central role in maintenance of the stem cell phenotype, control of epithelial cell proliferation and localisation, secretory lineage development and the maturation of Paneth cells (reviewed in (Scoville et al., 2008)). As the main proliferative drive, Wnt signalling is also believed to play a crucial role in the regeneration of the intestinal epithelium following damage. The Adenomatous Polyposis Coli (APC) protein is a component of the canonical Wnt pathway and is responsible for the regulation of the transcription factor *β-catenin*. In the absence of canonical Wnt ligand the APC destruction complex phosphorylates the N-terminal of *β-catenin*, targeting it for ubiquitin-proteosome mediated destruction. Truncation or loss of APC disrupts the *β-catenin* degradation complex and nuclear translocation of the stabilised *β-catenin* causes increased expression of Wnt target genes (reviewed in (Sieber et al., 2000)). Somatic *APC* mutation is the initiating, gate-keeping lesion in sporadic colorectal carcinogenesis (Kinzler and Vogelstein 1996), and is found in 60% of sporadic adenomas (Powell et al., 1992) and 80% of carcinomas (Miyoshi et al., 1992), many of which show abnormal beta catenin expression on immunohistochemical staining (Preston et al., 2003). In contrast, *APC* mutations are rare in CACRC, occurring at a frequency of just 3-6% in the biggest studies (Tarmin et al., 1995; Aust et al., 2002) (Figure 2).

2.2.2 Epithelial restitution and alternative activation of the Wnt pathway

Activation of the Wnt pathway by *APC* or *β-catenin* mutation is uncommon in CACRC, yet Wnt signalling has a key role in the control of epithelial proliferation and is up-regulated in epithelial restitution with increased expression of ligands and Wnt target genes such as *C-MYC* in regenerating epithelium (You et al., 2008). Furthermore in mouse models, activation of the Wnt pathway using R-spondin (Zhao et al., 2007), or knock-out of the Wnt antagonist Dkk-1 (Koch et al., 2011) can prevent the initiation and improve the recovery from DSS-induced colitis. Recent work by Lee et al (Lee et al., 2010) proposes that an alternative, inflammation-induced mechanism of *β-catenin* stabilisation may be responsible for this Wnt activation in colitis. They demonstrated that the PI3 Kinase / Akt pathway phosphorylates *β-catenin* at a specific moiety - serine 552. Whereas N-terminal phosphorylation by the APC destruction complex triggers proteosome mediated destruction, PI3K phosphorylation of this specific amino acid does the opposite, causing nuclear translocation and target gene activation. This mechanism effectively bypasses the destruction complex and explains why *APC* mutation is rarely selected for in CACRC (Figure 3).

Although Wnt signalling may be essential to induce intestinal regeneration in the short term, longstanding inflammation-induced Wnt activation is mitogenic (Kim et al., 2005) and Ashton et al (Ashton et al., 2010) have recently demonstrated one mechanism that illustrates how closely the inflammation and carcinogenesis pathways are entwined. They used mouse models to conditionally delete the downstream c-Myc target focal adhesion kinase (FAK), and found that these animals were unable to regenerate the intestine following tissue damage. However, when FAK was deleted within the adult intestine this abrogated tumour formation caused by Apc loss, mainly mediated by a reduction in phospho-Akt levels. This suggests that FAK is required downstream of Wnt signalling and upstream of P13K/Akt/mTor activation, mediating both intestinal regeneration and neoplastic transformation following Apc loss. It is these potential feedback loops between Wnt target genes and PI3K-mediated Wnt activation that may be responsible for driving tumorigenesis in chronic intestinal inflammation (Figure 3).

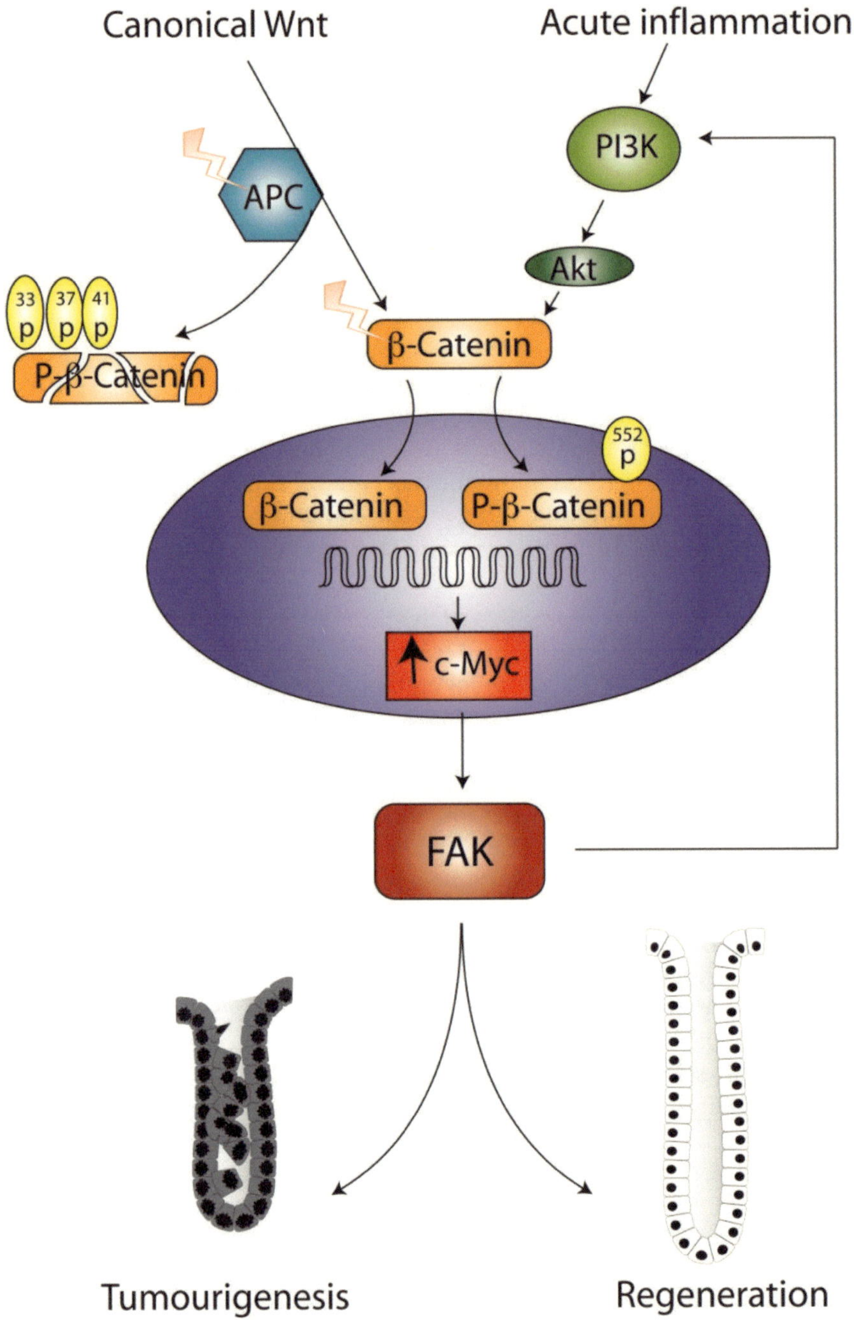

Fig. 3. Wnt activation via APC dependent and alternative inflammation induced mechanisms

In sporadic tumours inactivation of APC or stabilisation of β-catenin occurs by mutation (flashes) inhibiting the destruction complex from N-terminal phosphorylation of β-catenin (P-β-catenin at amino acids 33, 37 and 41) and preventing proteosome mediated breakdown.

However in acute inflammation, PI3K/Akt mediated phosphorylation of serine residue 552 (P-β-catenin at 552) causes nuclear translocation of beta catenin and target gene activation. Downstream of upregulated wnt target genes such as c-Myc, focal adhesion kinase (FAK) is involved in mediating both crypt regeneration and neoplastic transformation. Additionally FAK also activates P13K and this cycle of P13K/Wnt cross-talk may be involved in neoplastic transformation in longstanding colitis.

2.2.3 Genetic instability in CACRC carcinogenesis

It is now becoming clear that the inflammation and restitution processes that underlay chronic inflammatory bowel disease drive CACRC down alternative carcinogenesis pathways to their sporadic counterparts. In SCRC carcinogenesis, chromosomal instability leading to aneuploidy, detectable by both image and flow cytometry, is rare in established precursor lesions before the development of high-grade dysplasia or cancer (Sieber et al., 2002). Yet in ulcerative colitis chromosomal instability (CIN) can be detected in histologically non-dysplastic tissue from high-risk patients by comparative genomic hybridisation (Willenbucher et al., 1997; Rabinovitch et al., 1999) and image or flow cytometry (Keller et al., 2001). These chromosomal abnormalities are diverse and generally found at low-levels (<10% of sampled cells) in pre-dysplastic biopsy samples, suggesting they are *pre-clonal* chromosomal alterations that are infrequent, random and pre-date clonal expansion (Bronner et al., 2008). It has been suggested that CIN occurs as a consequence of the effect of inflammation and reactive oxygen species encouraging telomere shortening, so permitting chromosomal end fusion. This results in cycles of chromatin bridge breakage and fusion, promoting the accumulation of chromosomal aberrations (O'Sullivan et al., 2002).

Mutator phenotype or natural selection

Chen et al. further analysed the genetic instability seen in early lesions in UC using arbitrarily-primed (AP-PCR) and inter-simple-sequence repeat PCR (ISSR-PCR) genetic fingerprinting techniques (Chen et al., 2003, 2005). The identification of DNA fingerprint abnormalities throughout normal and dysplastic areas of the colon allowed the subdivision of patients with IBD into UC progressors: patients with identifiable genomic instability who are likely to progress to dysplasia or cancer, and UC non-progressors: patients with normal DNA fingerprints who are unlikely to progress. The authors proposed that this colon-wide genomic instability in UC progressors provides a field from which dysplasia develops, and is evidence of a *mutator phenotype*. This theory proposes that the initiating mutation arises in one of the genes that maintain genetic stability, leading to an increased mutation rate and resulting in a heterogeneous collection of cells with the only shared mutation in the gene ensuring DNA fidelity (Loeb & Loeb, 1999; Chen et al., 2005). However recent experimental data involving detailed examination of areas of dysplasia in UC does not support this hypothesis. Laser dissection and genetic analysis of individual crypts across colitis associated dysplasia and tumours showed that these lesions can be readily identified as clonal, with a shared initiating tumour suppressor or oncogene mutation demonstrated in each case (Leedham et al., 2009). Thus CACRC appears to follow the somatic mutation theory of carcinogenesis, where initial mutations in key target genes introduce a selective growth advantage to a cell and then the forces of natural selection and evolution act to expand this clone — a so called *selective sweep* (Maley et al., 2004). When a mutation has spread through an entire population it is said to have gone to fixation, as there are no longer any competing alleles. Further mutations within this clone can then expand producing regional selective sweeps and clonal diversity.

Clonal ordering studies utilise the spatial distribution of shared mutations throughout different areas of dysplasia and cancer to make inferences about the timing of mutations and selective sweeps. A recent clonal ordering study of colitis-associated lesions identified *TP53* as the most common single founding mutation, with *K-RAS* mutations the only other detected unique gate-keeping mutation (Leedham et al., 2009). *TP53* mutation is commonly seen in colitis-associated lesions, with the frequency of both point mutations and 17qLOH correlating with malignant progression (Burmer et al., 1992; Brentnall et al., 1994; Hussain et al., 2000). From an evolutionary perspective the high frequency of initiating *TP53* mutations in colitis is not surprising. With chromosomal instability arising in chronically inflamed pre-dysplastic tissues there would be a strong selective pressure for *TP53* mutation as inactivation of this protein would disrupt mitotic checkpoints and permit the survival of stem-cells with gross chromosomal changes.

Clonal expansion and field cancerisation

Slaughter et al. (Slaughter et al., 1953) originally proposed the term *field cancerisation* to explain the presence of multifocal head and neck cancers developing out of a field of precancerous change that had developed as a consequence of carcinogen exposure. The theory was further expanded by Braakhuis et al (Braakhuis et al., 2003), who proposed that the field was in fact a clonally-expanded area of mutated cells. Clonally-expanded mutated patches have been noted in dysplastic (Lyda et al., 1998, 2000) and phenotypically normal mucosa of colitis patients (Chaubert et al., 1994). Using individual crypt genetic analysis Leedham et al (Leedham et al, 2009) were able to demonstrate the presence of oncogenic mutations in non-dysplastic crypts surrounding clonal neoplastic lesions, suggesting that the tumours had arisen from a field of genetically mutant yet non-dysplastic crypts. The presence of tumorigenic mutations in areas of morphologically *non-dysplastic* mucosa has significant clinical implications as at the present time the histological detection of dysplasia is the gold standard biomarker of disease progression in UC. Although endoscopic resection of visible dysplastic lesions may prevent tumour progression in that lesion, this work suggest that fields of clonally expanded genetically mutant, but non-dysplastic, crypts may well be left behind.

2.2.4 DNA methylation

CpG island hypermethylation often starts in normal mucosa as a function of age and is markedly increased in cancer (Issa et al., 2001). Such silencing is clonal and thought to be physiologically irreversible in somatic cells. Neoplastic cells often display aberrant promoter region methylation with epigenetic silencing of multiple genes including genes that regulate critical processes such as cell cycle control, DNA repair, and angiogenesis. In the colon, CpG islands methylated in cancer have been divided into two groups: those that display cancer-restricted methylation (type C), and those that are methylated initially in aging normal epithelial cells (type A). It has been proposed that age-related methylation contributes to an acquired predisposition to colorectal neoplasia because methylation alters the physiology of aging cells and tissues (Issa et al., 2001). This hypothesis predicts that higher levels of age-related methylation are associated with a heightened susceptibility to developing colorectal cancer, and it may be present in conditions of rapid cell turnover that mimic premature aging such as IBD.

Issa et al (Issa et al., 2001), investigated the methylation status of 4 genes in patients with UC versus controls *(ER, MYOD1, CSPG2* and *p16*). All four genes were highly methylated in dysplastic epithelium from patients with colitis-associated HGD or cancer. In addition, three of the four genes (*ER, MYOD* and *p16)* were also highly methylated in the normal appearing (non-dysplastic) epithelium from these same HGD/cancer patients, indicating that methylation precedes dysplasia and is widespread in these patients. These results are consistent with the hypothesis that age-related methylation marks (and may lead to) the field defect that reflects acquired predisposition to colorectal neoplasia. More recently, Kukitsu et al (Kukitsu et al., 2008) identified hypermethylation and subsequent reduced *p16* gene expression in aberrant crypt foci (ACF) in UC. These are the earliest detectable lesions in the CACRC pathway and suggest that aberrant methylation of tumour suppressor genes may also be an early event in CACRC carcinogenesis

3. Who, when and how to screen?

3.1 Who to screen

Patients with colitis are overall thought to be at increased risk of colorectal cancer compared to the general population, which has lead to the development of colonoscopic surveillance programmes. There is no randomised data to confirm that such programmes are effective either in lives saved, cancer prevented or that they are cost effective. However, there is case-control data suggesting that those in surveillance programmes have cancer detected at an earlier stage and are less likely to die from their cancer (Loftus, 2003; Collins et al., 2006; Lutgens et al., 2009).

The level of risk of colorectal cancer in colitis had recently been questioned: a meta-analysis from 2001 (Eaden et al., 2001) suggested that the risk might be as high as 20% at 20 years of disease. However more recent analyses have suggested the risk may much lower: Rutter at al (Rutter et al., 2006) analysed prospectively collected data from six-hundred patients collected over a thirty-year period and found that the CRC risk by colitis duration was 2.5% at 20 years, 7.6% at 30 years, and 10.8% at 40 years. This may reflect a higher risk seen in studies based in referral centres compared to true population-based estimates. Disease extent is also important, with extensive disease conferring the highest risk and proctitis generally being regarded as harbouring no increased risk (Ekbom et al., 1990). Indeed, in the Olmstead county population based study from Minnesota USA (Jess et al., 2006), only patients with extensive colitis were seen to be at increased risk of colorectal cancer.

Other significant risk factors, apart from disease extent, include primary sclerosing cholangitis (even after liver transplant) (Broome et al., 1995; Claessen et al., 2009), a family history of colorectal cancer (Askling et al., 2001), persistent mucosal inflammation (Rutter et al., 2004), strictures, post-inflammatory polyps (Rutter, Saunders et al. 2004) and previous dysplasia. Conversely, patients with no endoscopic or histological evidence of inflammation - mucosal healing - have the same 5-year risk of CRC as the background, non-UC population (Rutter et al., 2004). This recognition that not all patients have the same level of risk has led some guideline writers to move to a surveillance model based on risk stratification, rather than by disease duration as had been done previously. This has been adopted most clearly in the new British Society of Gastroenterology Guidelines 2010 (Cairns et al., 2010) (Figure 3), with very similar UK guidance released for the National Institute for Clinical Excellence in 2011 (NICE, 2011), with those at highest risk now being offered yearly surveillance, and those at lowest risk 5-yearly interval surveillance.

3.2 When to start screening

Most guidelines recommend starting screening at 8-10 years of disease duration (N.B. not from diagnosis, but from when symptoms started). This is based on the relatively low cancer rates seen within 10 years of disease initiation, particularly with population-based estimates, and is consistent with long-term inflammation driving the increased cancer risk in colitis. Nevertheless, some studies have reported relatively high rates of cancer within the 1st decade of disease (Lutgens et al., 2008). However most studies show that the incidence of CRC is low in the first decade (Eadens et al., 2001; Jess et al., 2006; Rutter et al., 2006), and therefore commencing surveillance prior to 8-10 years increases the cost of surveillance programmes with little added benefit.

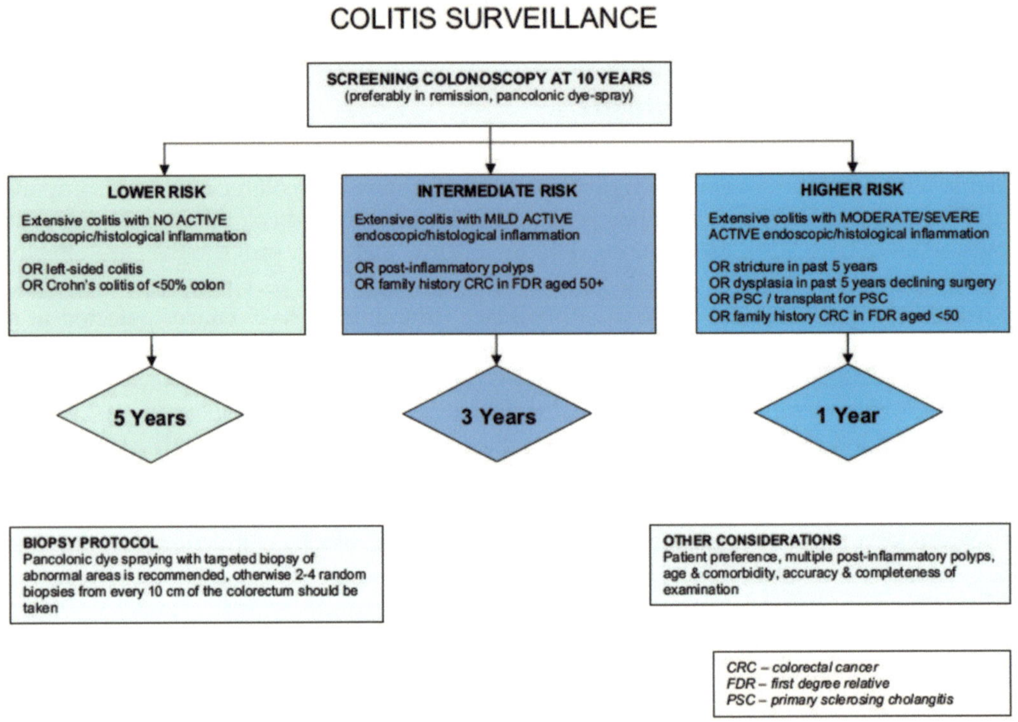

Fig. 4. Updated endoscopic surveillance recommendations from the British Society of Gastroenterology (Cairns et al., 2010)

Patients are now statified according to low, intermediate and high risk risk and advised to undergo 5-yearly, 3-yearly or yearly colonoscopic screening respectively.

3.3 How to screen

3.3.1 Endoscopic screening

Recent guidelines from the United Kingdom and Europe have endorsed the use of chromoendoscopy to enhance dysplasia detection, on the basis of single-centre randomised trials, back-to-back studies and case-control data (see Table 1). This is a paradigm shift away from previous strategies that relied upon large numbers of random biopsies (33 or more) to detect *invisible* or *flat* dysplasia. Recent evidence suggest that much, if not most, dysplasia in colitis is detectable with white light endoscopy (Rutter et al., 2004), probably reflecting better endoscope optics (high resolution instruments) and improved operator experience in detecting subtle, flat lesions. Detection can be further enhanced by the use of chromoendoscopy dye-spray, where dye is sprayed onto the bowel epithelium to highlight subtle mucosal abnormalities; the use of dye-spray increases dysplasia detection by 2-3 fold on a per patient basis, and 4-5 fold on a per lesion basis. However, it remains unclear whether dysplasia detected with dye-spray has the same natural history as that detected with white light endoscopy and multiple random biopsy strategy. Other advanced imaging techniques such as auto-fluorescence endoscopy, narrowed spectrum endoscopy (NBI, FICE, i-Scan), and confocal endomicroscopy remain research based and are not endorsed in any international guideline at present.

Author, Journal, Year	***WLE detection rate***	***Chromo detection rate***
Marion, *Am J Gastro*, 2008	9/102 (8.8%)	17/102 (16.7%)
Kiesslich, *Gastroenterology*, 2007	4/73 (5.5%)	13/84 (15.5%)
Hurlstone, *Endoscopy*, 2005	24/350 (6.9%)	69/350 (19.7%)
Rutter, Gut, 2004	2/100 (2%)	7/100 (7%)
Kiesslich, *Gastroenterology*, 2003	6/81 (7.4%)	11/80 (13.8%)
SUMMARY	**45/706, 6.4%**	**117/716, 16.3%**
	(95% CI 4.6-8.2)	**(95% CI 13.6-19.1)**

WLE, white light endoscopy; Chromo, chromoendoscopy

Table 1. Summary of trials of chromo-endoscopy in UC surveillance
Proportion of patients with at least one dysplastic lesion detected is denoted in brackets. Chromo-endoscopic techniques significantly increase detection of dysplasia in UC screening colonoscopy

3.3.2 Molecular techniques and biomarkers for progression to neoplasia

Biopsies from screening colonoscopies of patients with UC are still routinely processed and only basic histological techniques used to look for evidence of dysplasia or cancer. The interpretation of biopsies in the presence of active inflammation is difficult, therefore combining basic histology with analysis of the molecular pathology or protein expression could enable improved detection of dysplasia. Moreover, a significant proportion of patients with low-grade dysplasia or who are indefinite for dysplasia (ID) do not progress to neoplasia, therefore there is a need for biomarkers that can accurately differentiate the non-progressors from the progressors who require intensive surveillance or more aggressive management. Although there has been much focus from various groups on developing simple techniques that can complement standard histology, these are yet to be translated to everyday clinical practice.

As previously discussed, for over 20 years image cytometry looking for evidence of aneuploidy in biopsy samples has been shown to correlate with dysplasia and identify a sub-group of patients at higher risk of developing dysplasia and cancer (Lofberg et al., 1992; Rubin et al., 1992; Keller et al., 2001) – UC progressors. It is known that patients with UC harbour *TP53* mutations in non-dysplastic mucosa and this may confer susceptibility to the development of CRC (Hussain et al., 2000; Leedham et al., 2009), therefore this offers another potential way of identifying those patients at high risk of CRC that may need intensive endoscopic screening. Immunohistochemical staining of tissue for TP53 and Alpha-methylacyl-CoA racemase (AMACR) - an enzyme involved in fatty acid metabolism that has known altered expression in various cancers including CRC – has recently been shown to be a potential marker for progression to HGD and neoplasia in UC (van Schaik et al., 2011). Using comparative and quantitative proteomics, panels of proteins that are differentially expressed in the dysplastic and non-dysplastic mucosa of UC progressors and non-progressors have been identified (Bronner et al., 2010; May et al., 2011). Specifically S100P - a calcium binding protein, TRAP1 - a mitochondrial heat-shock protein, and CPS1 - a mitochondrial protein involved in urea metabolism, have all been shown to be significantly over-expressed by immunohistochemical staining in both the dysplastic and non-dysplastic (rectal) tissue of UC progressors compared to non-progressors. Immunohistochemistry for rectal CPS1 was able to predict dysplasia or cancer in the colon with 87% sensitivity and 45% specificity (May et al., 2011).

Genomic biomarkers offer perhaps the most promising molecular tool for screening UC patients: Studies have demonstrated that genomic instability can be detected throughout the colon of patients with UC, importantly genomic instability detected in non-dysplastic rectal biopsies, using FISH or array based comparative genomic hybridisation, is able to differentiate UC progressors from non-progressors with a high sensitivity and specificity (Bronner et al., 2008, 2010).

Biomarkers appear to offer the potential to identify those high-risk patients that require colonoscopic screening on only a few rectal biopsies. However, it remains to be seen whether larger studies confirm this and if an affordable, simple, reproducible and reliable technique can be developed for standard clinical use.

3.4 Management of dysplasia in UC

The aim of screening is to detect dysplasia that can then be removed, either endoscopically or by colectomy depending on the type of lesion and histological grade, in order to prevent the development of cancer. The more specific, surgical aspects of how to manage patients once dysplasia has been detected are covered in a separate chapter.

There has been a recent significant practice shift in the management of dysplasia and dysplastic polyps when detected in the colon of patients with UC, with the recent publication of guidelines from the United Kingdom, Europe and the United States (Travis et al., 2008; Cairns et al., 2010; Farraye et al., 2010; NICE, 2011) all advocating a similar, more conservative approach. Where a dysplastic polyp arises in an area proximal to the extent of the colitis, with no evidence of dysplasia in the surrounding flat mucosa, it can be treated in the same way as a sporadic adenoma, usually with complete endoscopic resection. Dysplastic polyps arising in an area of inflammation have been termed dysplasia-associated lesions or masses (DALMs). More recently, the term adenoma-like mass (ALM) or adenoma-like DALMs have been used to describe areas of dysplasia in the inflamed colon that more resemble sporadic adenomas and are thus endoscopically resectable. Previously, if an area of dysplasia was detected within the inflamed colon then colectomy was felt to be mandatory. However, a number of studies have demonstrated that for ALM or adenoma-like DALMs, once endoscopically resected, prognosis is good (Engelsgjerd et al., 1999; Rubin et al., 1999; Odze et al., 2004; Rutter et al.,2004). One such study examining 40 patients undergoing endoscopic resection of dysplastic polyps within inflamed mucosa reported one case of adenocarcinoma after a mean follow-up period of 4.1 years (Odze et al., 2004). This was not significantly different from the frequency of cancer within the surveillance population as a whole (p=1.0, Fisher 's exact test). On the other hand, if the dysplastic polyp cannot be completely excised, urgent re-assessment of resectability by an experienced colonoscopist or urgent surgery is mandatory regardless of the grade of dysplasia. If a dysplastic polyp is arising within a field change of dysplastic tissue in the surrounding flat mucosa colectomy is advised, as complete endoscopic excision of the lesion is not achievable (Mowat et al., 2011).

4. Prevention is better than cure

4.1 Mucosal healing in UC

The management of IBD is fast evolving, with tantalising therapeutic biological agents currently under review and there has been a paradigm shift in the way in which Gastroenterologists manage UC. Traditionally, inducing and maintaining symptom control was the focal aim, however *mucosal healing* is now a key endpoint in the management of IBD. Mucosal healing is defined as the absence of all mucosal ulceration, both macroscopic and microscopic, providing a sigmoidoscopy score of 0, as assessed by the Ulcerative Colitis Disease Activity Index. As previously discussed, severity of inflammation, more extensive disease and longer duration of disease have all been demonstrated to increase the overall risk of CRC (Ekbom et al., 1990; Eaden et al., 2001; Rutter et al., 2004; Bielas et al., 2006; Jess et al., 2006; Rutter et al., 2006). Consequently, mucosal inflammation is clearly associated in CRC development and tailoring treatments towards mucosal healing should, therefore, curtail the risk of CRC development. However serious infections, malignancies - namely lymphomas - and neurological disease all complicate current anti-TNF treatments and long-term immunosuppression in IBD patients (Lees et al., 2009). Long-term follow up data is lacking, especially for combination therapies, but it appears that thiopurines are associated with a 3-5 fold increase in lymphoma risk and there is as much as a 3-fold increased relative risk for anti-TNF therapies (Bewtra & Lewis 2010). Although the absolute risks are low, careful consideration needs to be given when using these therapies and patients require close monitoring and follow up. As long-term studies become available we will be better equipped to assess the chemo-preventative benefits of immunomodulator induced mucosal healing versus the small risks of lymphoproliferative cancer induction.

4.2 Chemo-prevention in UC

4.2.1 5-ASAs

An important aspect of the use of 5-ASAs is not only in the induction and maintenance of remission, but also in the prevention of colonic dysplasia and CRC. Their efficacy may be only partially explained by anti-inflammatory effects, as other more potent anti-inflammatory agents, such as glucocorticoids and azathioprine, have a lower cancer protective effect. Further chemo-preventative effects of 5-ASA compounds are thought to comprise modulation of inflammatory cytokine production (Foutch & Zimmerman 1996), inhibition of cyclo-oxygenase (Allgayer, 2003), inducible NO synthase (Kennedy et al., 1999; Hasko et al., 2001) and nuclear factor KB (Wahl et al., 1998; Greten et al., 2004), as well as activation of peroxisome proliferator activated receptor (PPAR) gamma (Rousseaux et al., 2005; Dubuquoy et al., 2006). In addition, 5-ASA's scavenge oxygen free radicals, have an antimicrobial action and are capable of inhibiting protein phosphatase 2A - which, in turn, can curtail Wnt pathway activity (van Rijn et al., 2006). Despite the notion that these processes could be chemo-preventative, there are no prospective randomised controlled trials to substantiate the protective effect of 5-ASA in cancer chemoprevention in colitis. The most impressive evidence to support their use comes from the meta-analysis by Velayos et al (Rubin et al., 2008): this study showed a significantly reduced risk of the development of cancer or dysplasia in UC patients on long-term 5-ASA treatment, with a pooled odds ratio of 0.51 (95% CI 0.38- 0.69).

4.2.2 Folic acid

It is hypothesised that folic acid deficiency can induce DNA hypomethylation and thus dysregulated expression of oncogenes (Duthie 1999). There are a number of long-term observational studies that demonstrate a significant reduction in colorectal adenoma and cancer rates in patients taking folate supplements (Giovannucci et al., 1998; Terry et al., 2002). However no studies specifically looking at ulcerative colitis or IBD have been undertaken, and a more recent study found no protective effect of folic acid on colorectal adenoma recurrence (Logan et al., 2008).

4.2.3 Ursodeoxycholic acid

Patients with ulcerative colitis and PSC have significantly increased risks of colorectal cancer (Claessen et al., 2009), and treatment with the synthetic bile acid ursodeoxycholic acid has been advocated to treat complications of liver disease in both PSC and other cholestatic liver conditions, however its exact mechanism of action is unclear. There is evidence that the secondary bile acid, deoxycholic acid, promotes colorectal carcinogenesis: Patients with ulcerative colitis and colonic dysplasia or carcinoma have higher faecal bile acid concentrations than do patients with ulcerative colitis but without colonic neoplasia (Hill et al., 1987), and serum levels of deoxycholic acid, which in a steady state are assumed to reflect the amount of deoxycholic acid absorbed from the colon, have also been found to be significantly elevated in men with colonic adenomas compared with controls (Bayerdorffer et al., 1993; Bayerdorffer et al., 1995). A prospective, randomised control trial of ursodeoxycholic acid in patients with ulcerative colitis and PSC, demonstrated significantly lower rates of colorectal dysplasia and cancer in the treatment group, with an odds ratio of 0.26 (95% CI, 0.06–0.92; $P < 0.03$) (Pardi et al., 2003). However other studies have not confirmed this observed reduction (Wolf et al., 2005), and a recent long-term study of patients with UC and PSC taking high dose ursodeoxycholic acid reported an increased rate of colorectal neoplasia (Eaton et al., 2011). Thus this is a controversial area and long-term ursodeoxycholic acid cannot currently be recommended as chemoprevention in patients with ulcerative colitis (Chapman et al., 2010).

4.3 NSAIDs and aspirin chemoprevention of CRC

It is generally thought that carcinogenesis seems to arise as a result of accumulations of genetic and epigenetic modifications in tissue stem cells or progenitors which are pluripotent and capable of self-renewal (Humphries & Wright 2008). A recent study has suggested that NSAIDS are able to provide effective chemoprevention of CRC by targeting stem cells that have accumulated pro-tumorigenic mutations, and can eliminate them by the induction of apoptosis (Qiu et al., 2010). In an *Apc* $^{Min/+}$ mouse model, dietary sulindac, (an NSAID), induced apoptosis in intestinal stem cells with nuclear or phosphorylated β-catenin. Not only that, in human colonic polyps, NSAIDS were shown to induce apoptosis in cells with aberrant Wnt signalling. The tumour-suppressive effect of sulindac in the *Apc* $^{Min/+}$ mouse model was reduced by a deficiency in mitochondrial apoptogenic protein, SMAC. It blocked apoptosis and removal of stem cells with nuclear or phosphorylated β-catenin. This is an exciting prospect for the use of chemical agents or simple dietary changes as anti-cancer therapies in the future.

Studies have demonstrated that the use of aspirin (Baron et al., 2003; Benamouzig et al., 2003; Logan et al., 2008; Cole et al., 2009) and cyclo-oxygenase-2 enzyme (COX-2) inhibitors (Bertagnolli et al., 2006; Arber et al., 2006; Baron et al., 2003) is associated with a 20% reduction in adenoma recurrence, the precursor lesion of most SCRC. However, certain COX-2 inhibitors were taken off the market by the Food and Drug Administration (FDA), in 2004, following several landmark studies showing an increased risk of stroke and myocardial infarction (Kerr et al., 2007) and are thus no longer able to be considered as preventative treatments. Aspirin is still a contender for usage as long-term chemoprevention. A recent meta-analysis pooling long-term follow up data from four randomized, double-blind, placebo-controlled trials of aspirin treatment (Rothwell et al., 2010), demonstrated that regular low dose (75mg) aspirin reduced long-term risk of colon cancer - its overt effect taking 7-8 years; (incidence hazard ratio [HR] 0.76, 95% CI 0.60-0.96, p=0.02; mortality HR 0.65, 0.48-0.88, p=0.005). The median follow follow up was over 18 years. Aspirin doses less than 30mg were less effective than 75mg and greater than 75mg conferred no further advantage. Furthermore, aspirin 75mg reduced cancer risk in the proximal colon by 5%. This was not demonstrated in the distal colon. In addition, 5-year maintenance treatment with aspirin resulted in a 70% decrease in the consequent risk of proximal colon cancer (Rothwell et al., 2010). However, one of several limitations in this study was that CRC was not the primary outcome in any of the included trials. Furthermore, overall mortality was not reported upon, nor was the mortality related to aspirin side effects. What is more, the trials mostly involved men with cardiovascular risk. The underlying CRC carcinogenesis process may vary between patients, particularly those with cardiovascular risk factors. Eberhart et al, (Eberhart et al., 1994) published a prospective cohort study of 1279 patients, and demonstrated that after CRC diagnosis, exclusively in patients who's cancers over expressed COX-2, routine aspirin usage was associated with a decreased cancer-specific and overall mortality.

Although these studies do not specifically look at CRC risk in patients with UC, a previous case-control study (Bansal & Sonnenberg 1996) did demonstrate a protective effect of NSAID in IBD patients similar to that in patients without IBD. However, in the absence of prospective, randomized controlled data the potential side effects of long term aspirin or NSAIDs in IBD patients mean their use as chemo-preventative agents cannot currently be advocated.

5. Conclusions

In this chapter the origins of dysplasia in CACRC have been summarised and the key contrasts to tumorigenesis in SCRC highlighted. UC involves chronic inflammation of the bowel mucosa, so it is logical to think that this is the key mechanism that drives carcinogenesis in these patients. The carcinogenic effect of chronic inflammation is multi-factorial, directly affecting the stem cell niche as well as altering key signalling pathways and promoting genetic and epigenetic instability. Here we have demonstrated how a mutated stem cell can become fixed within a colonic crypt and then drive the progression and clonal expansion of that mutated crypt to form a dysplastic lesion. In SCRC mutations in *APC* are the initial oncognenic change that enables the growth of most adenomas. However, in IBD, dysplasia develops on the background of a field of mutated crypts that have clonally expanded over a significant area of the epithelium, but may appear histologically normal, with mutations in the tumour suppressor *TP53* and the *KRAS* oncogene occurring early in the carcinogenesis pathway. Chromosomal instability is another key early event in the progression to dysplasia in IBD patients, and there is much evidence to suggest that this is a pan-colonic event that precedes dysplasia. Thus dysplasia and cancer in UC may arise from a process of CIN that affects the entire colon, some of these changes select for loss of tumour suppressor genes with subsequent clonal expansion, field cancerisation and evolution to cancer.

In order to improve outcomes of patients with IBD it is now apparent that suppressing chronic inflammation is crucial. As goals of treatment become more aggressive - aimed at mucosal healing rather than just symptom control, and more effective medical treatments become available, we may well see a drop in the colorectal cancer rates over time. An understanding of the molecular pathogenesis of dysplasia and CRC in UC is now crucial for clinicians in order that they may effectively manage the long-term outcomes of these patients. Although many centres operate endoscopic screening programmes aimed at detecting dysplasia in high-risk patients, the evidence that they significantly alter the natural history of colorectal cancer is limited. Also, there appears to have been little appetite to improve histological detection of dysplasia by complementing standard histopathology with more advanced, molecular and immunohistochemical techniques that have been shown to correlate with histological stage progression to neoplasia. Genomic biomarkers and immunohistochemical staining of rectal biopsies appear to be able to distinguish UC-progressors from non-progressors. Therefore we may soon see a move to combined endoscopic and biomarker based screening programmes that are able to identify those patients at high risk of dysplasia that require intensive colonoscopic screening from a simple rectal biopsy.

There is not yet sufficient experimental evidence for effective, safe chemo-preventative treatments aimed at reducing colorectal cancer risk in IBD patients. However, as our understanding of the detailed molecular histopathological pathways of colorectal cancer in inflammatory bowel disease develops, so the likelihood of identifying novel targets and developing regimes that can significantly reduce the incidence of CRC in ulcerative colitis increases.

6. References

Allgayer, H. (2003). Review article: mechanisms of action of mesalazine in preventing colorectal carcinoma in inflammatory bowel disease. *Aliment Pharmacol Ther* 18 Suppl 2: 10-4.

Ashton, G. H., J. P. Morton, et al. (2010). Focal adhesion kinase is required for intestinal regeneration and tumorigenesis downstream of Wnt/c-Myc signaling. *Dev Cell* 19(2): 259-69.

Askling, J., P. W. Dickman, et al. (2001). Colorectal cancer rates among first-degree relatives of patients with inflammatory bowel disease: a population-based cohort study. *Lancet* 357(9252): 262-6.

Arber, N., C. J. Eagle, et al. (2006). Celecoxib for the prevention of colorectal adenomatous polyps. *N Engl J Med* 355(9): 885-95.

Aust, D. E., J. P. Terdiman, et al. (2002). The APC/beta-catenin pathway in ulcerative colitis-related colorectal carcinomas: a mutational analysis. *Cancer* 94(5): 1421-7.

Bansal, P. and A. Sonnenberg (1996). Risk factors of colorectal cancer in inflammatory bowel disease. *Am J Gastroenterol* 91(1): 44-8.

Barker, N., R. A. Ridgway, et al. (2009). Crypt stem cells as the cells-of-origin of intestinal cancer. *Nature* 457(7229): 608-11.

Barker, N., J. H. van Es, et al. (2007). Identification of stem cells in small intestine and colon by marker gene Lgr5. *Nature* 449(7165): 1003-7.

Baron, J. A., B. F. Cole, et al. (2003). A randomized trial of aspirin to prevent colorectal adenomas. *N Engl J Med* 348(10): 891-9.

Bayerdorffer, E., G. A. Mannes, et al. (1995). Unconjugated secondary bile acids in the serum of patients with colorectal adenomas. *Gut* 36(2): 268-73.

Bayerdorffer, E., G. A. Mannes, et al. (1993). Increased serum deoxycholic acid levels in men with colorectal adenomas. *Gastroenterology* 104(1): 145-51.

Benamouzig, R., J. Deyra, et al. (2003). Daily soluble aspirin and prevention of colorectal adenoma recurrence: one-year results of the APACC trial. *Gastroenterology* 125(2): 328-36.

Bertagnolli, M. M., C. J. Eagle, et al. (2006). Celecoxib for the prevention of sporadic colorectal adenomas. *N Engl J Med* 355(9): 873-84.

Bewtra, M. and J. D. Lewis (2010). Update on the risk of lymphoma following immunosuppressive therapy for inflammatory bowel disease. *Expert Rev Clin Immunol* 6(4): 621-31.

Bielas, J. H., K. R. Loeb, et al. (2006). Human cancers express a mutator phenotype. *Proc Natl Acad Sci U S A* 103(48): 18238-42.

Braakhuis, B. J., M. P. Tabor, et al. (2003). A genetic explanation of Slaughter's concept of field cancerization: evidence and clinical implications. *Cancer Res* 63(8): 1727-30.

Brentnall, T. A., D. A. Crispin, et al. (1994). Mutations in the p53 gene: an early marker of neoplastic progression in ulcerative colitis. *Gastroenterology* 107(2): 369-78.

Bronner, M. P., J. N. O'Sullivan, et al. (2008). Genomic biomarkers to improve ulcerative colitis neoplasia surveillance. *Am J Pathol* 173(6): 1853-60.

Bronner, M. P., M. Skacel, et al. (2010). Array-based comparative genomic hybridization in ulcerative colitis neoplasia: single non-dysplastic biopsies distinguish progressors from non-progressors. *Mod Pathol* 23(12): 1624-33.

Broome, U., R. Lofberg, et al. (1995). Primary sclerosing cholangitis and ulcerative colitis: evidence for increased neoplastic potential. *Hepatology* 22(5): 1404-8.

Burmer, G. C., P. S. Rabinovitch, et al. (1992). Neoplastic progression in ulcerative colitis: histology, DNA content, and loss of a p53 allele. *Gastroenterology* 103(5): 1602-10.

Cairns, S. R., J. H. Scholefield, et al. (2010). Guidelines for colorectal cancer screening and surveillance in moderate and high risk groups (update from 2002). *Gut* 59(5): 666-89.
Campbell, F., G. T. Williams, et al. (1996). Post-irradiation somatic mutation and clonal stabilisation time in the human colon. *Gut* 39(4): 569-73.
Chapman, R., J. Fevery, et al. (2010). Diagnosis and management of primary sclerosing cholangitis. *Hepatology* 51(2): 660-78.
Chaubert, P., J. Benhattar, et al. (1994). K-ras mutations and p53 alterations in neoplastic and nonneoplastic lesions associated with longstanding ulcerative colitis. *Am J Pathol* 144(4): 767-75.
Chen, R., P. S. Rabinovitch, et al. (2005). The initiation of colon cancer in a chronic inflammatory setting. *Carcinogenesis* 26(9): 1513-9.
Chen, R., P. S. Rabinovitch, et al. (2003). DNA fingerprinting abnormalities can distinguish ulcerative colitis patients with dysplasia and cancer from those who are dysplasia/cancer-free. *Am J Pathol* 162(2): 665-72.
Claessen, M. M., F. P. Vleggaar, et al. (2009). High lifetime risk of cancer in primary sclerosing cholangitis. *J Hepatol* 50(1): 158-64.
Cole, B. F., R. F. Logan, et al. (2009). Aspirin for the chemoprevention of colorectal adenomas: meta-analysis of the randomized trials. *J Natl Cancer Inst* 101(4): 256-66.
Collins, P. D., C. Mpofu, et al. (2006). Strategies for detecting colon cancer and/or dysplasia in patients with inflammatory bowel disease. *Cochrane Database Syst Rev*(2): CD000279.
Dubuquoy, L., C. Rousseaux, et al. (2006). PPARgamma as a new therapeutic target in inflammatory bowel diseases. *Gut* 55(9): 1341-9.
Duthie, S. J. (1999). Folic acid deficiency and cancer: mechanisms of DNA instability. *Br Med Bull* 55(3): 578-92.
Eaden, J. A., K. R. Abrams, et al. (2001). The risk of colorectal cancer in ulcerative colitis: a meta-analysis. *Gut* 48(4): 526-35.
Eaton, J. E., M. G. Silveira, et al. (2011). High-Dose Ursodeoxycholic Acid Is Associated With the Development of Colorectal Neoplasia in Patients With Ulcerative Colitis and Primary Sclerosing Cholangitis. *Am J Gastroenterol.*
Eberhart, C. E., R. J. Coffey, et al. (1994). Up-regulation of cyclooxygenase 2 gene expression in human colorectal adenomas and adenocarcinomas. *Gastroenterology* 107(4): 1183-8.
Ekbom, A., C. Helmick, et al. (1990). Ulcerative colitis and colorectal cancer. A population-based study. *N Engl J Med* 323(18): 1228-33.
Engelsgjerd, M., F. A. Farraye, et al. (1999). Polypectomy may be adequate treatment for adenoma-like dysplastic lesions in chronic ulcerative colitis. *Gastroenterology* 117(6): 1288-94; discussion 1488-91.
Farraye, F. A., R. D. Odze, et al. (2010). AGA technical review on the diagnosis and management of colorectal neoplasia in inflammatory bowel disease. *Gastroenterology* 138(2): 746-74, 774 e1-4; quiz e12-3.
Foutch, P. G. and K. Zimmerman (1996). Diverticular bleeding and the pigmented protuberance (sentinel clot): clinical implications, histopathological correlation, and results of endoscopic intervention. *Am J Gastroenterol* 91(12): 2589-93.

Giovannucci, E., M. J. Stampfer, et al. (1998). Multivitamin use, folate, and colon cancer in women in the Nurses' Health Study. *Ann Intern Med* 129(7): 517-24.

Graham, T. A., A. Humphries, et al. (2011). Use of methylation patterns to determine expansion of stem cell clones in human colon tissue. *Gastroenterology* 140(4): 1241-1250 e1-9.

Greaves, L. C., S. L. Preston, et al. (2006). Mitochondrial DNA mutations are established in human colonic stem cells, and mutated clones expand by crypt fission. *Proc Natl Acad Sci U S A* 103(3): 714-9.

Greenstein, A. J. (2000). Cancer in inflammatory bowel disease. *Mt Sinai J Med* 67(3): 227-40.

Greten, F. R., L. Eckmann, et al. (2004). IKKbeta links inflammation and tumorigenesis in a mouse model of colitis-associated cancer. *Cell* 118(3): 285-96.

Gutierrez-Gonzalez, L., M. Deheragoda, et al. (2009). Analysis of the clonal architecture of the human small intestinal epithelium establishes a common stem cell for all lineages and reveals a mechanism for the fixation and spread of mutations. *J Pathol* 217(4): 489-96.

Hasko, G., C. Szabo, et al. (2001). Sulphasalazine inhibits macrophage activation: inhibitory effects on inducible nitric oxide synthase expression, interleukin-12 production and major histocompatibility complex II expression. *Immunology* 103(4): 473-8.

Hill, M. J., D. M. Melville, et al. (1987). Faecal bile acids, dysplasia, and carcinoma in ulcerative colitis. *Lancet* 2(8552): 185-6.

Humphries, A. and N. A. Wright (2008). Colonic crypt organization and tumorigenesis. *Nat Rev Cancer* 8(6): 415-24.

Hussain, S. P., P. Amstad, et al. (2000). Increased p53 mutation load in noncancerous colon tissue from ulcerative colitis: a cancer-prone chronic inflammatory disease. *Cancer Res* 60(13): 3333-7.

Issa, J. P., N. Ahuja, et al. (2001). Accelerated age-related CpG island methylation in ulcerative colitis. *Cancer Res* 61(9): 3573-7.

Itzkowitz, S. H. and X. Yio (2004). Inflammation and cancer IV. Colorectal cancer in inflammatory bowel disease: the role of inflammation. *Am J Physiol Gastrointest Liver Physiol* 287(1): G7-17.

Jess, T., E. V. Loftus, Jr., et al. (2006). Risk of intestinal cancer in inflammatory bowel disease: a population-based study from olmsted county, Minnesota. *Gastroenterology* 130(4): 1039-46.

Keller, R., E. C. Foerster, et al. (2001). Diagnostic value of DNA image cytometry in ulcerative colitis. *Dig Dis Sci* 46(4): 870-8.

Kennedy, M., L. Wilson, et al. (1999). 5-aminosalicylic acid inhibits iNOS transcription in human intestinal epithelial cells. *Int J Mol Med* 4(4): 437-43.

Kerr, D. J., J. A. Dunn, et al. (2007). Rofecoxib and cardiovascular adverse events in adjuvant treatment of colorectal cancer. *N Engl J Med* 357(4): 360-9.

Kim, K. A., M. Kakitani, et al. (2005). Mitogenic influence of human R-spondin1 on the intestinal epithelium. *Science* 309(5738): 1256-9.

Kinzler, K. W. and B. Vogelstein (1996). Lessons from hereditary colorectal cancer. *Cell* 87(2): 159-70.

Koch, S., P. Nava, et al. (2011). The wnt antagonist dkk1 regulates intestinal epithelial homeostasis and wound repair. *Gastroenterology* 141(1): 259-268 e8.

Kukitsu, T., T. Takayama, et al. (2008). Aberrant crypt foci as precursors of the dysplasia-carcinoma sequence in patients with ulcerative colitis. *Clin Cancer Res* 14(1): 48-54.

Lee, G., T. Goretsky, et al. (2010). Phosphoinositide 3-kinase signaling mediates beta-catenin activation in intestinal epithelial stem and progenitor cells in colitis. *Gastroenterology* 139(3): 869-81, 881 e1-9.

Leedham, S. J., T. A. Graham, et al. (2009). Clonality, founder mutations, and field cancerization in human ulcerative colitis-associated neoplasia. *Gastroenterology* 136(2): 542-50 e6.

Lees, C. W., A. I. Ali, et al. (2009). The safety profile of anti-tumour necrosis factor therapy in inflammatory bowel disease in clinical practice: analysis of 620 patient-years follow-up. *Aliment Pharmacol Ther* 29(3): 286-97.

Loeb, K. R. and L. A. Loeb (1999). Genetic instability and the mutator phenotype. Studies in ulcerative colitis. *Am J Pathol* 154(6): 1621-6.

Lofberg, R., O. Brostrom, et al. (1992). DNA aneuploidy in ulcerative colitis: reproducibility, topographic distribution, and relation to dysplasia. *Gastroenterology* 102(4 Pt 1): 1149-54.

Loftus, E. V., Jr. (2003). Does monitoring prevent cancer in inflammatory bowel disease? *J Clin Gastroenterol* 36(5 Suppl): S79-83; discussion S94-6.

Logan, R. F., M. J. Grainge, et al. (2008). Aspirin and folic acid for the prevention of recurrent colorectal adenomas. *Gastroenterology* 134(1): 29-38.

Lutgens, M. W., B. Oldenburg, et al. (2009). Colonoscopic surveillance improves survival after colorectal cancer diagnosis in inflammatory bowel disease. *Br J Cancer* 101(10): 1671-5.

Lutgens, M. W., F. P. Vleggaar, et al. (2008). High frequency of early colorectal cancer in inflammatory bowel disease. *Gut* 57(9): 1246-51.

Lyda, M. H., A. Noffsinger, et al. (2000). Microsatellite instability and K-ras mutations in patients with ulcerative colitis. *Hum Pathol* 31(6): 665-71.

Lyda, M. H., A. Noffsinger, et al. (1998). Multifocal neoplasia involving the colon and appendix in ulcerative colitis: pathological and molecular features. *Gastroenterology* 115(6): 1566-73.

Maley, C. C., P. C. Galipeau, et al. (2004). Selectively advantageous mutations and hitchhikers in neoplasms: p16 lesions are selected in Barrett's esophagus. *Cancer Res* 64(10): 3414-27.

May, D., S. Pan, et al. (2011). Investigating neoplastic progression of ulcerative colitis with label-free comparative proteomics. *J Proteome Res* 10(1): 200-9.

McDonald, S. A., L. C. Greaves, et al. (2008). Mechanisms of field cancerization in the human stomach: the expansion and spread of mutated gastric stem cells. *Gastroenterology* 134(2): 500-10.

Miyoshi, Y., H. Nagase, et al. (1992). Somatic mutations of the APC gene in colorectal tumors: mutation cluster region in the APC gene. *Hum Mol Genet* 1(4): 229-33.

Mowat, C., A. Cole, et al. (2011). Guidelines for the management of inflammatory bowel disease in adults. *Gut* 60(5): 571-607.

NICE. Colonoscopic surveillance for prevention of colorectal cancer in people with ulcerative colitis, Crohn's disease or adenomas: NICE guidance 2011.

O'Sullivan, J. N., M. P. Bronner, et al. (2002). Chromosomal instability in ulcerative colitis is related to telomere shortening. *Nat Genet* 32(2): 280-4.

Odze, R. D., F. A. Farraye, et al. (2004). Long-term follow-up after polypectomy treatment for adenoma-like dysplastic lesions in ulcerative colitis. *Clin Gastroenterol Hepatol* 2(7): 534-41.

Pardi, D. S., E. V. Loftus, Jr., et al. (2003). Ursodeoxycholic acid as a chemopreventive agent in patients with ulcerative colitis and primary sclerosing cholangitis. *Gastroenterology* 124(4): 889-93.

Park, H. S., R. A. Goodlad, et al. (1995). Crypt fission in the small intestine and colon. A mechanism for the emergence of G6PD locus-mutated crypts after treatment with mutagens. *Am J Pathol* 147(5): 1416-27.

Powell, S. M., N. Zilz, et al. (1992). APC mutations occur early during colorectal tumorigenesis. *Nature* 359(6392): 235-7.

Preston, S. L., W. M. Wong, et al. (2003). Bottom-up histogenesis of colorectal adenomas: origin in the monocryptal adenoma and initial expansion by crypt fission. *Cancer Res* 63(13): 3819-25.

Qiu, W., X. Wang, et al. (2010). Chemoprevention by nonsteroidal anti-inflammatory drugs eliminates oncogenic intestinal stem cells via SMAC-dependent apoptosis. *Proc Natl Acad Sci U S A* 107(46): 20027-32.

Rabinovitch, P. S., S. Dziadon, et al. (1999). Pancolonic chromosomal instability precedes dysplasia and cancer in ulcerative colitis. *Cancer Res* 59(20): 5148-53.

Ren, F., B. Wang, et al. (2010). Hippo signaling regulates Drosophila intestine stem cell proliferation through multiple pathways. *Proc Natl Acad Sci U S A* 107(49): 21064-9.

Rothwell, P. M., M. Wilson, et al. (2010). Long-term effect of aspirin on colorectal cancer incidence and mortality: 20-year follow-up of five randomised trials. *Lancet* 376(9754): 1741-50.

Rousseaux, C., B. Lefebvre, et al. (2005). Intestinal antiinflammatory effect of 5-aminosalicylic acid is dependent on peroxisome proliferator-activated receptor-gamma. *J Exp Med* 201(8): 1205-15.

Rubin, C. E., R. C. Haggitt, et al. (1992). DNA aneuploidy in colonic biopsies predicts future development of dysplasia in ulcerative colitis. *Gastroenterology* 103(5): 1611-20.

Rubin, D. T., M. R. Cruz-Correa, et al. (2008). Colorectal cancer prevention in inflammatory bowel disease and the role of 5-aminosalicylic acid: a clinical review and update. *Inflamm Bowel Dis* 14(2): 265-74.

Rubin, P. H., S. Friedman, et al. (1999). Colonoscopic polypectomy in chronic colitis: conservative management after endoscopic resection of dysplastic polyps. *Gastroenterology* 117(6): 1295-300.

Rutter, M., B. Saunders, et al. (2004). Severity of inflammation is a risk factor for colorectal neoplasia in ulcerative colitis. *Gastroenterology* 126(2): 451-9.

Rutter, M. D., B. P. Saunders, et al. (2004). Most dysplasia in ulcerative colitis is visible at colonoscopy. *Gastrointest Endosc* 60(3): 334-9.

Rutter, M. D., B. P. Saunders, et al. (2004). Cancer surveillance in longstanding ulcerative colitis: endoscopic appearances help predict cancer risk. *Gut* 53(12): 1813-6.

Rutter, M. D., B. P. Saunders, et al. (2006). Thirty-year analysis of a colonoscopic surveillance program for neoplasia in ulcerative colitis. *Gastroenterology* 130(4): 1030-8.

Scoville, D. H., T. Sato, et al. (2008). Current view: intestinal stem cells and signaling. *Gastroenterology* 134(3): 849-64.

Sieber, O. M., K. Heinimann, et al. (2002). Analysis of chromosomal instability in human colorectal adenomas with two mutational hits at APC. *Proc Natl Acad Sci U S A* 99(26): 16910-5.

Sieber, O. M., I. P. Tomlinson, et al. (2000). The adenomatous polyposis coli (APC) tumour suppressor--genetics, function and disease. *Mol Med Today* 6(12): 462-9.

Slaughter, D. P., H. W. Southwick, et al. (1953). Field cancerization in oral stratified squamous epithelium; clinical implications of multicentric origin. *Cancer* 6(5): 963-8.

Tarmin, L., J. Yin, et al. (1995). Adenomatous polyposis coli gene mutations in ulcerative colitis-associated dysplasias and cancers versus sporadic colon neoplasms. *Cancer Res* 55(10): 2035-8.

Terry, P., M. Jain, et al. (2002). Dietary intake of folic acid and colorectal cancer risk in a cohort of women. *Int J Cancer* 97(6): 864-7.

Travis, S. P., E. F. Stange, et al. (2008). European evidence-based Consensus on the management of ulcerative colitis: Current management. *J Crohns Colitis* 2(1): 24-62.

van Rijn, J. C., J. B. Reitsma, et al. (2006). Polyp miss rate determined by tandem colonoscopy: a systematic review. *Am J Gastroenterol* 101(2): 343-50.

van Schaik, F. D., B. Oldenburg, et al. (2011). Role of immunohistochemical markers in predicting progression of dysplasia to advanced neoplasia in patients with ulcerative colitis. *Inflamm Bowel Dis.*

Vogelstein, B., E. R. Fearon, et al. (1988). Genetic alterations during colorectal-tumor development. *N Engl J Med* 319(9): 525-32.

Wahl, C., S. Liptay, et al. (1998). Sulfasalazine: a potent and specific inhibitor of nuclear factor kappa B. *J Clin Invest* 101(5): 1163-74.

Willenbucher, R. F., S. J. Zelman, et al. (1997). Chromosomal alterations in ulcerative colitis-related neoplastic progression. *Gastroenterology* 113(3): 791-801.

Williams, E. D., A. P. Lowes, et al. (1992). A stem cell niche theory of intestinal crypt maintenance based on a study of somatic mutation in colonic mucosa. *Am J Pathol* 141(4): 773-6.

Wolf, J. M., L. A. Rybicki, et al. (2005). The impact of ursodeoxycholic acid on cancer, dysplasia and mortality in ulcerative colitis patients with primary sclerosing cholangitis. *Aliment Pharmacol Ther* 22(9): 783-8.

Wong, W. M., N. Mandir, et al. (2002). Histogenesis of human colorectal adenomas and hyperplastic polyps: the role of cell proliferation and crypt fission. *Gut* 50(2): 212-7.

Yatabe, Y., S. Tavare, et al. (2001). Investigating stem cells in human colon by using methylation patterns. *Proc Natl Acad Sci U S A* 98(19): 10839-44.

You, J., A. V. Nguyen, et al. (2008). Wnt pathway-related gene expression in inflammatory bowel disease. *Dig Dis Sci* 53(4): 1013-9.

Zhao, J., J. de Vera, et al. (2007). R-spondin1, a novel intestinotrophic mitogen, ameliorates experimental colitis in mice. *Gastroenterology* 132(4): 1331-43.

8

Ulcerative Colitis-Associated Colorectal Cancer Prevention by 5-Aminosalicylates: Current Status and Perspectives

Jean-Marie Reimund et al.*
Université de Caen Basse-Normandie, EA 3919, SFR ICORE, UFR de Médecine, CHU de Caen, 14032 Caen Cedex 5,
CHU de Caen, Service d'Hépato-Gastro-Entérologie et Nutrition, Pôle Reins - Digestif - Nutrition, 14033 Caen Cedex 09
France

1. Introduction

Patients with ulcerative colitis (UC) are at increased risk of developing colorectal cancer. This risk increased mainly with longer duration of colitis, greater anatomic extent, and/or association to primary sclerosing cholangitis (PSC). Recent work highlighted also the carcinogenetic role of long-standing - despite if mild or moderate - mucosal inflammation, bringing an additional argument to support the growing concept of mucosal healing as the final target of current and future treatments (Lichtenstein & Rutgeerts, 2010).

Until now, repeated colonoscopic surveillance with biopsies targeted on visible lesions associated to multiple random biopsies in endoscopically normal-appearing mucosa, remains the major way to detect mucosal dysplasia (a precancerous lesion), thereby decreasing colitis-associated cancer (CAC) mortality in UC patients. Colorectal cancer chemoprevention is a second promising strategy to reduce CAC risk in this patients' population. In particular, most of the available epidemiological data indicate a preventive role for 5-aminosalicylic acid derivatives (5-ASA), despite recent work suggested also a protective role for purine derivatives. Although the main mechanisms by which 5-ASA may reduce CAC risk is not exactly known and remains controversial, some interesting

* Marion Tavernier[1,3], Stéphanie Viennot[2], Inaya Abdallah Hajj Hussein[4], Benoît Dupont[2], Anne-Marie Justum[2], Abdo R. Jurjus[4], Jean-Noël Freund[5] and Mathilde Lechevrel[1]
[1]*Université de Caen Basse-Normandie, EA 3919, SFR ICORE, UFR de Médecine, CHU de Caen, Avenue Côte de Nacre, 14032 Caen Cedex 5, France*
[2]*CHU de Caen, Service d'Hépato-Gastro-Entérologie et Nutrition, Pôle Reins – Digestif – Nutrition, 14033 Caen Cedex 09, France*
[3]*CHU de Caen, Service de Chirurgie Digestive et Viscérale, Pôle Reins – Digestif – Nutrition, 14033 Caen Cedex 09, France*
[4]*American University of Beirut, Department of Human Morphology, Riad El-Solh, Beirut, Lebanon*
[5]*INSERM U682, 3, avenue Molière, 67200 Strasbourg, France*

hypothesis have emerged, resulting from fundamental research in molecular biology and pharmacology. This increased understanding of the putative pathway(s) by which 5-ASA may interfere with CAC development appears also as the starting point for optimising 5-ASA derivatives or identifying new compounds acting more specifically and/or being more efficient in preventing neoplastic transformation of the colonic epithelium in UC patients. These different points will be addressed more precisely in the three next parts.

2. Frequency of colorectal cancer risk in ulcerative colitis and risk factors

Ulcerative colitis is a worldwide distributed inflammatory bowel disease (IBD). In a recent review, Cosnes et al., reported that in the West, its incidence and prevalence has increased in the past 50 years, respectively up to 8-14/10^5 and 120-200/10^5 persons (Cosnes et al., 2011).

2.1 Frequency of colorectal cancer risk in ulcerative colitis

Compared to the general population, patients with UC have an increased risk to develop colorectal cancer (Kulaylat & Dayton, 2010; Viennot et al., 2009). Early data by Ransohoff estimate the risk of CAC at 0.5% per year after 10 years of UC, and 1.0% per year after 20 years of disease (Ransohoff, 1988). Later, a meta-analysis by Eaden et al. reviewing 116 studies representing a total of 54,478 UC patients, placed the risk of CAC in UC at 2% at 10 years, 8% at 20 years, and 18% at 30 years (Eaden et al., 2001). However, more recently published results, in particular those reporting general population data (in comparison to studies performed in reference centres), suggest that the risk may probably not be so high as reported earlier. This has been the case in a large population-based study by Bernstein et al. in Canada (Manitoba district), were the CAC risk was estimate to be 2.75 increased (95% CI: 1.91-3.97) (Bernstein et al., 2001). In a large study from Denmark (22,290 person-years), Winter et al. reported a 30-year cumulative probability of CAC in UC of 2.1%, a risk not statistically different than in the general population (Winther et al., 2004). Finally, Rutter et al. reported a cumulative CAC incidence of 2.5% at 20 years, 7.6% at 30 years, and 10.8% after 40 years following disease onset (Rutter et al., 2006). However, this study has been performed in a reference centre. This change in risk magnitude reflects probably a change in clinical practice such as a more often use of surveillance colonoscopy, a more systematic use of chemoprevention, and the fact that in several countries surgery was more commonly used in UC treatment than before the advent and progresses in total colectomy or coloproctectomy with either ileorectal or ileoanal anastomosis. However, the influence of other factors (e.g. environmental factors) cannot be excluded. Taking together 48 studies critically appraised for study population type, person years at risk, disease localisation in Crohn's disease (CD) and censoring for colectomy, Lutgens et al. found a cumulative risk in all IBD patients in population-based studies of 1%, 2% and 5% after 10, 20 or more than 30 years of disease, with a pooled standardised morbidity ratio (SMR) of 3.6 (95% CI: 3.1-4.1), compared to 1%, 11% and 43%, and a pooled SMR of 8.8 (95% CI: 7.3-11) in reference centres studies (Lutgens et al., 2008). In UC pooled SMR was also higher in reference studies (9.0, 95% CI: 7.4-11.1) compared to 3.7 (95% CI: 3.3-4.3) in population-based studies (Lutgens et al., 2008).

2.2 Factors increasing colorectal cancer risk in ulcerative colitis patients

A number of studies have identified clear risk factors exposing UC patients to CAC risk. Most of these factors are inherent to the disease, although possible genetic factors may contribute to increase this risk. The identification of these factors is of outstanding importance, as it will allow us to better define the patients at high risk, representing the target population for colonoscopic surveillance and chemoprevention.

2.2.1 Age of onset and duration of disease

Patients with disease onset at an early age have been shown to be at higher risk of CAC. For example, Ekbom et al. estimated that patients with UC diagnosed before the age of 15, have a 40% risk of CAC after 35 years of disease onset compared to a 25% risk in patients with UC diagnosed between age 15 and 39 (Ekbom et al., 1990). However, the role of age at UC diagnosis alone remains controversial, as most authors suggest that this increased risk results probably (at least in part) from a longer UC duration. Before 8 to 10 years of UC progression, despite a study by Lutgens et al. reporting early occurring CAC (Lutgens et al., 2008), it is currently assumed that the risk of colorectal cancer is not different than the risk for sporadic colorectal cancer in the general population (Eaden et al., 2001; Rutter et al., 2006; Ekbom et al., 1990). It is only later that it increases by approximately 0.5 to 1% each year, reaching the incidence rates reported in Section 2.1.

2.2.2 Disease extension

Extension of colonic disease is a second really important independent risk factor, CAC occurring principally in UC patients having a history of pancolitis or at least of extended colitis (i.e. colitis beyond the left colonic angle). In these patients, relative risk (RR) is about 14.8 (95% IC: 11.4-18.9) compared to 2.8 (95% IC: 1.6-4.4) in patients with left sided UC and 1.7 (95% CI: 0.8-3.2) when disease is limited to the rectosigmoid. In case of proctitis, CAC risk is virtually not higher than in the general population (Ekbom et al., 1990).

2.2.3 Family history of colorectal cancer

A family history of colorectal cancer increases slightly the CAC risk in UC patients (Nuako et al., 1998; Askling et al., 2001a). By contrast, having a first-degree relative affected by UC does not increase the risk for colorectal cancer among other healthy family members (Askling et al., 2001b).

2.2.4 Presence of backwash ileitis

The presence of reflux (or backwash) ileitis has been suggested by several authors to increase CAC risk (Heuschen et al., 2001). However, it remains controversial as other studies found no relation between backwash ileitis and risk for CAC (Rutter et al., 2006a).

2.2.5 Association with primary sclerosing cholangitis

Until now, the most important risk factor for CAC in UC patients is the presence of concomitant PSC (for review see: Torres et al., 2011), even this association occurs only in a minority of patients. For example, a case-control study performed by Broome et al. reported a cumulative CAC risk of 9% after 10 years, 21% after 20 years and 50% after 25 years in patients having both UC and PSC, compared with 2%, 5% and 10% in patients with only UC

(Broome et al., 1995). More recently, Sokol et al. showed a 25-year cumulative rate of CAC of 23.4% in patients suffering both from IBD [n = 75; final diagnosis: 42 UC, 21 CD, 1 indeterminate colitis, 11 unclassified IBD (uIBD)] and PSC, compared to 0% in patients with IBD alone (n = 150; final diagnosis: 80 UC, 43 CD, 3 indeterminate colitis, 5 uIBD) ($P = 0.002$), despite patients with both IBD and PSC had milder disease and a higher use of 5-ASA ($P < 0.001$) (Sokol et al., 2008). Noteworthy, this risk remains even after liver transplantation for PSC treatment (Loftus et al., 1998).

2.2.6 Chronic inflammation

The impact of chronic inflammation and CAC has long been a matter of debate. In fact, from a theoretical point of view, increasing evidence supported the hypothesis that chronic inflammation contributes to colon carcinogenesis, in particular by generating a favourable microenvironment for cancer initiation, development, and progression. Increase in mucosal pro-inflammatory cytokine or other inflammatory mediators such as reactive oxygen and nitrogen species, or cyclooxygenase-2 (COX-2)-derived prostaglandins production results in alterations of a large number of molecules such as DNA, RNA, proteins or lipids. For example, they induce the formation of adducts to DNA, generating point mutations in genes like the *p53* tumour suppressor gene, which is early mutated in IBD inflamed mucosa (even before neoplastic transformation) (Laurent et al., 2011), and in CpG islands involved in DNA methylation. In addition, the increase in local tissue pro-inflammatory cytokines and prostaglandins inhibits apoptosis and favours cell proliferation, thereby facilitating carcinogenesis. Currently, both clinical and experimental data demonstrate that chronic inflammation represents probably a key factor in CAC pathogenesis. Rutter et al. indirectly suggest this relationship by showing that endoscopic features indicative of previous severe inflammation, such as pseudopolyps, or indicative of chronically active colitis such as shortened or tubular colon and stricture formation are associated with a significant increase in CAC (Rutter et al., 2004a). More direct clinical evidence came from studies by Rutter et al. and Gupta et al. (Rutter et al., 2004b; Gupta et al., 2007). Rutter et al. found that the endoscopically- and histologically-assessed severity of inflammation significantly enhanced the risk of CAC (2.5 and 5.1 respectively) (Rutter et al., 2004b). More recently, a cohort study by Gupta et al. reported a significant link between histological inflammation and progression towards high-grade dysplasia or CAC, with a RR of 2 (Gupta et al., 2007). Finally, Garrity-Park et al. showed an association between myeloperoxydase immunochemistry, TNF-α polymorphism and RUNX3 methylation and CAC (Garrity-Park et al., 2011). In addition to these clinical data, experimental results contribute to clarify the underlying cellular or molecular mechanisms explaining the link between inflammation and colorectal carcinogenesis in UC patients. For example, excessive pro-inflammatory cytokine production increases the expression of COX-2 and 5-lipoxygenase (5-LOX) (Agoff et al., 2000). This effect will result in a decrease in the non-esterified arachidonic acid pool responsible for decreased apoptosis, therefore favouring tumorigenesis (Cao et al., 2000). Inflammatory mediators also influence suppressor gene activity; this has been demonstrated for macrophage inhibiting factor which suppresses *p53* transcriptional activity *in vitro* (Hudson et al., 1999), a result which appears important as *p53* immunopositivity (together with abnormal DNA ploidy) has been suggested to be an important risk factor of developing CAC in longstanding IBD (Gerrits et al., 2011). In addition, recently, experimental data clearly demonstrate the role of TNF-α as a key mediator in inflammation-driven CAC (Popivanova et al., 2008). The authors showed that invalidation of the p55 TNF-α receptor dramatically reduced the colon tumour formation in mice treated by azoxymethane (AOM, a carcinogen instilled intrarectally) in dextran-sulphate (DSS)-induced experimental colitis in mice. Moreover, wild type mice transplanted with bone marrow from TNF-Rp55-deficient mice appear less susceptible to develop colon tumours, whereas transplantation of bone marrow from wild type animals to TNF-Rp55-deficient mice does not significantly increase tumour formation compared to wild-type animals. Finally, etanercept administration (a monoclonal antibody blocking the p75 TNF-α receptor) reduced both tumour size and number in wild type mice both treated with AOM and DSS (Popivanova et al., 2008). Taken together, these results provide a strong rationale for chemoprevention in order to reduce the mucosal inflammation in longstanding UC patients, and appear as relevant arguments in favour of mucosal healing as a new goal for evaluation of therapeutic efficacy.

2.3 Factors suspected to protect from colitis-associated cancer

2.3.1 Folate supplementation

Several experimental and epidemiologic studies have suggested that low folate concentrations increase the risk to develop sporadic colorectal cancer, probably by inducing DNA strand breaks in the *p53* tumour suppressor gene (Giovannucci et al., 1993; Giovannucci et al., 1998; Kim et al., 1997). Despite patients with IBD have an increased risk of folate deficiency (Phelip et al., 2008) - but more probably CD patients than UC patients (Yakut et al., 2010) -, until now only one case-control study (including 6 cases and 61 controls) found a significant protective effect of folate supplementation (Lashner, 1993) and one small 3 months pilot randomized placebo controlled trial reported a decrease in cell proliferation examined by immunohistochemistry in 12 UC patients (Biasco et al., 1997). All other found no effect of folate supplementation, which therefore could not be seriously considered as an effective chemopreventive treatment against CAC (Rutter et al., 2004b; Lashner et al., 1989; Lashner et al., 1997; Pardi et al., 2003).

2.3.2 Ursodeoxycholic acid treatment

Several years ago, ursodeoxycholic acid (UDCA) treatment has been considered as playing a protective role against CAC in patients with both UC and PSC. Harnois et al. found that high-doses of UDCA (13-15 mg/kg body weight/day) increased the 4-year survival of these patients (Harnois et al, 2003). Concerning CAC, Pardi et al, studying 52 patients with UC associated to PSC, reported that UDCA treatment (n = 29 patients, 13-15 mg/kg body weight/day for a median of 42 months) decreased dysplasia or CAC risk compared to placebo (10% *versus* 35% after an average follow-up of 6.5 years; RR = 0.26, 95% CI: 0.07-0.99) (Pardi et al., 2003). However, this result contrasts with studies by Sjöqvist et al. and Wolf et al. which found no protective effect of UDCA (Sjöqvist et al., 2004; Wolf et al., 2005). In addition, higher doses of UDCA (28-30 mg/kg body weight/day) have been recently associated to an increased risk of CAC in UC patients with PSC (Eaton et al., 2011). Therefore, at the present time, the protective role of UDCA remains controversial and it could not be recommended as a chemopreventive treatment, at least at doses higher than 15 mg/kg body weight/day.

3. Chemoprevention by 5-aminosalicylic acids

3.1 5-aminosalicylates basic pharmacology

Sulphasalazine is the original 5-aminosalicylate (5-ASA)-containing medication used in UC. Chemically, named salicylazosulphapyridine (SASP), it combines two molecules with different properties, sulfapyridine (SP), which has a bacteriostatic activity, and 5-ASA (or mesalazine), the moiety having the anti-inflammatory properties. These two compounds were linked together by an azo bond (Azadkahn et al., 1982). After an oral intake, only a small portion of SASP is absorbed in the small intestine and the bulk of the sulphasalazine reaches the colon intact, where colonic bacterial azoreductase enzymes cleave the azo bond with the subsequent liberation of SP and 5-ASA. As SP seems to be responsible for most of the SASP side effects, new approaches for delivering only 5-ASA have emerged, either using pro-drugs (olsalazine, balsalazide) or oral mesalazine formulations "protecting" 5-ASA from release, absorption, and metabolism in the stomach and proximal small bowel by delayed release (Asacol®, Salofalk®, Mesasal®, Claversal®) or controlled release mechanisms (Pentasa®) (Chourasia & Jain, 2003; Sandborn & Hanauer, 2003). Free 5-ASA administered orally undergoes rapid and nearly complete absorption from the distal ileum or colon (actually depending on concentration and local pH), followed by extensive metabolism to N-Acetyl-5-ASA (N-Ac-5-ASA) by the N-acetyl-transferase 1 (NAT 1) in intestinal epithelial cells and the liver (Sandborn & Hanauer, 2003). A mixture of free 5-ASA and N-Ac-5-ASA is excreted in the urine (Mardini et al., 1987; Rijk et al., 1988; Vree et al., 2000). Only 5-ASA is therapeutically active, some placebo-controlled trial in UC patients having shown that the N-Ac-5-ASA metabolite is inactive (van Hogezand et al., 1988).

3.2 Clinical data

In a retrospective case-control study comparing 102 UC patients with CAC to 196 cancer-free UC patients, Pinczowski et al. provided the first evidence for a role of aminosalicylates in CAC prevention (Pinczowski et al., 1994). They found an independent chemoprotective effect for sulfasalazine taken for at least 3 months with an odds ratio of 0.38 (95% CI: 0.2-0.69 after adjusting for disease activity) (Pinczowski et al., 1994). In an other retrospective study by Moody et al., the crude proportion of UC patients developing CAC was of 3% in those taking long-term 5-ASA compared to 31% in those who stopped their treatment or had poor compliance with 5-ASA therapy ($\chi^2 = 20.2$, $P < 0.001$) (Moody et al., 1996). Several years later, Eaden et al. confirmed these findings in a retrospective case-control study: in UC patients, continuous treatment (defined as a treatment for 5 to 10 years) with 5-ASA reduced the CAC risk, at least by 75% [Odds ratio (OR): 0.75, 95% CI: 0.13-0.48] (Eaden et al., 2000). Even after adjustment for other potentially most influential variables, this reduction was the highest in patients taking mesalazine at doses > 1.2 g/day (OR: 0.19; 95% CI: 0.04-0.60), whereas SASP at a dose of 2 g/day or more was not effective (OR: 0.85, 95% CI: 0.32-2.26) (Eaden et al., 2000). Nevertheless, this study had two important drawbacks as cases and controls were not always taken from the same population and as they differed by their ethnic composition. However, more recently, studies by Velayos et al., van Staa et al., and Terdiman et al., brought additional data to reinforce the hypothesis that regular use of 5-ASA may reduce the risk of CAC in UC patients (Velayos et al., 2005; Velayos et al., 2006;

van Staa et al., 2005; Terdiman et al., 2007). Velayos et al. first performed a meta-analysis on 9 (3 cohort and 6 case-control) studies including 334 CAC cases and 140 cases of dysplasia, and found a protective effect of 5-ASA for CAC risk (OR: 0.51, 95% CI: 0.38-0.69), but not for risk of dysplasia (OR: 1.18, 95% CI: 0.41-3.43; but only 2 studies evaluated this outcome) (Velayos et al., 2005). They confirmed these results in a case-control study (188 CAC compared to matched controls) showing a significant decrease in CAC risk in patients taking 5-ASA for 1 to 5 years (OR: 0.4, 95% CI: 0.2-0.9) (Velayos et al., 2006). However, this protective role for 5-ASA use for more than 6 years (6 to 10 years) does not remain statistically significant (6 to 10 years OR: 0.6, 95% CI: 0.3-1.4; > 10 years OR: 0.6, 95% CI: 0.3-1.3) (Velayos et al., 2006). In 2005, van Staa et al. conducted a large population-based study (18,969 patients, 100 with CAC despite 5-ASA use), and distinguished patients considered as 5-ASA regular users (if they had 6 or more 5-ASA prescriptions in the previous 12 months) and non-regular users. Their results could be summarized as followed: (1) regular users had a lower CAC risk (OR: 0.7, 95% CI: 0.44-1.43), (2) this effect does not occur in SASP users, and (3) for mesalazine regular users this protective effect was only statistically significant in patients with 13-30 prescriptions (OR: 0.30, 95% CI: 0.11-0.84). Finally, Terdiman et al. in a stratum-specific case-control study reported a trend towards a reduced CAC risk related to increasing number of mesalamine prescription, but this tendency was not statistically significant ($p = 0.08$) and the authors were not definitively confident regarding the CAC protective properties of 5-ASA treatment (Terdiman et al., 2007).

This doubt was reinforced by additional data published during the last 4 years, and clearly brought some confusion into clinicians' mind concerning the real effect of 5-ASA in CAC prevention, despite they have been considered as protective by several health authorities. Bernstein et al. in a population-based survey in Canada (Manitoba University) among 4,325 UC patients and 4,419 CD patients with colonic disease, found no difference in CAC between patients using 5-ASA for more than 1 or 5 years (OR: 1.02, 95% CI 0.60-1.74 and OR: 1.96, 95% CI 0.84-4.55 respectively), with a similar mean number of 5-ASA prescriptions at 10 vs. 11 ($p = 0.8$) and a similar mean number of dose days at 330 vs. 410 ($p = 0.69$) (Bernstein et al., 2011).

Unfortunately, it would probably not be possible to conduct a prospective double-blinded, placebo-controlled trial to definitively prove or infirm the chemopreventive role of 5-ASA against CAC; regarding the slow CAC increased risk in the general UC population, such a study needed a too important number of patients and a too long period of surveillance. Cost-effectiveness, as well as its impact on clinical practice to prevent CAC, of such a study seems not realistic and will probably never been performed. Therefore, clinicians have to weight the risk/benefit balance of CAC chemoprevention using 5-ASA, and to consider more attentively other strategies increasing their ability to decrease CAC development and morbidity or mortality in UC (and in general colonic IBD) patients (see Chapter 4.).

3.3 Mechanisms of action

As stated above, despite current controversy, clinical data suggest that 5-aminosalicylates may have antineoplastic and potentially chemopreventive properties. It is hypothesized that 5-aminosalicylates may have roughly similar genetic and molecular targets as nonsteroidal anti-inflammatory drugs (NSAIDs), including interactions with ROS production, with the COX and LOX cascade, with the activation of the transcription factor nuclear factor (NF)-κB-dependent effects, and with the peroxisome proliferator-activated receptor-γ (PPAR-γ)-dependent pathway.

3.3.1 Oxidative stress and DNA damage: role in UC-associated CRC carcinogenesis

Oxidative stress is a common consequence of inflammatory and immune activation. Several experimental data have shown that oxidative stress, by affecting both DNA damage and DNA repair processes, and by activating key genes are involved in several inflammatory and carcinogenetic pathways, contributing particularly to epithelial cells neoplastic transformation (Hussain et al., 2003; Boland et al., 2005). In aerobic cells, reactive oxygen species (ROS) are generated as a byproduct of normal mitochondrial activity. However, inflammation induces an increased mitochondrial oxidative metabolism resulting in an enhanced ROS production [e.g. superoxide anion radical (•O_2^-), hydrogen peroxide (H_2O_2), hydroxyl radical (•OH), as well as nitric oxide (NO)] (Boland et al., 2005). These ROS cause major damage to cellular macromolecules, including DNA alterations. Increased expression of ROS and NO [or NO-synthase (NOS), the enzyme which drives NO production from arginine] has been reported in inflamed mucosa from UC or CD patients (Hussain et al., 2000; Oshitani et al., 1993; Rachmilewitz et al., 1995; Kimura et al., 1998; Hofseth et al., 2003). The role of oxidative stress in CAC development has also been suggested. D'Inca et al. reported increased levels of 8-hydroxydeoxyguanosine (8-OHdG: a mutagen formed by the effect of •OH at the C8 position of deoxyguanosine base) in colonic mucosa in UC patients compared to normal mucosa in healthy controls. Furthermore, 8-OHdG concentrations were higher in UC patients with dysplasia, with longer disease duration, and with clinical and histological activity, and were lower in the rectum, suggesting that the 5-aminosalicylate enemas used by most of the study patients might have had an antioxidant effect (D'Inca et al., 2004). Other evidence supporting the contribution of oxidative stress to colorectal carcinogenesis came from the study by Hussain et al. examining the mutation spectrum of *p53* tumour suppressor gene at codons 247 and 248. They found in more than 50% of colonic mucosal specimens from UC patients, a higher frequency of G to A transitions at the CpG site of codon 248 and C to T transitions at the third base of codon 247 (Hussain et al., 2000). In addition, these abnormalities were only detected in inflamed mucosa (Hussain et al., 2000). Finally, alterations of *p53* were associated with increased iNOS activity suggesting that oxidative stress plays a role in colorectal carcinogenesis (Oshitani et al., 1993). An exhaustive overview on this specific topic has been recently published (Roessner et al., 2008).

Numerous reports have suggested that oxidative stress may play a role in colon carcinogenesis. In colon cancer cell lines, ROS such as •O_2^-, •OH, hypochlorite anion, and, in particular H_2O_2 induce frameshift mutations and inactivate the DNA mismatch repair system (Gasche et al., 2001; Chang et al., 2002). Concerning this point, several studies indicate that mesalazine is able to inhibit ROS production and/or their deleterious effects (Allgayer et al., 1992; Allgayer, 2003).

3.3.2 5-aminosalicylates and cyclooxygenase-2 inhibition

As stated in Section 2.2.6 COX-2 represents an important target in colorectal cancer in general, and CAC in particular. Due to its structural similarity with other COX inhibitors and to the over-expression of COX-2 in inflamed UC colonic mucosa, it has been suggested that 5-ASA chemoprotective properties against CAC were linked to its capacity to inhibit COX-2 activity. However, experimental data remain controversial. In an experimental study published by Stolfi et al., 5-ASA effectively inhibited colon cancer cell line HCT-115 (which expresses constitutively COX-2) proliferation and, in addition, down-regulated COX-2 mRNA and protein expression, and finally decreased prostaglandin E2 production (Stolfi et al., 2008). However, addition of exogenous prostaglandin E2 to cell culture does not reverse 5-ASA's inhibitory effect on HCT-115 proliferation. Furthermore, Stolfi et al. showed that 5-ASA inhibits proliferation in DLD-1 human colon cancer cell line (which does neither express COX-1, nor COX-2), a result we reproduced recently (unpublished data) (Stolfi et al., 2008). Therefore, inhibition of colon carcinogenesis by 5-ASA appears partially independent of its effects on COX-2.

3.3.3 Peroxisome proliferator-activated receptor-γ activation

Peroxisome proliferator-activated receptor-γ is a nuclear receptor highly expressed in the colonic mucosa. Several studies have demonstrated that its activation both decreased tumour cells proliferation and increased pro-apoptotic activities (Matthiessen et al., 2005; Shimada et al., 2002;), inhibited aberrant crypt foci formation (Tanaka et al., 2001), and reduced colorectal cancer development (Osawa et al., 2003), presumably through an interaction with the Wnt/β-catenin pathway (Jansson et al., 2005; Lu et al., 2005). Rousseaux et al. have demonstrated that 5-ASA acts like a PPAR-γ ligand (Rousseaux et al., 2005). Performing both *in vitro* and *in vivo* animal experiments, they showed that 5-ASA increased PPAR-γ expression, thereby reducing inflammation in experimental colitis in mice (Rousseaux et al., 2005). Additionally, Schwab et al. showed that the anti-proliferative and pro-apoptotic properties of 5-ASA were, at least partly, mediated by PPAR-γ-dependent mechanisms (Schwab et al., 2008). Finally, in immunodeficient SCID mice engrafted with human colorectal cancer cells, locally administered mesalazine significantly inhibited xenografts' growth, an effect blocked by concomitant administration of the PPAR-γ-selective antagonist GW9662 (Desreumaux & Ghosh, 2006).

3.3.4 5-aminosalicylic acid and nuclear factor NF-kappa B

The clinical efficacy of 5-ASA as a chemopreventive drug against CAC may probably also be the result of its inhibition of the pro-inflammatory and pro-oncogenic nuclear factor kappa B (NF-κB). Nuclear factor-κB is a transcription factor controlling the expression of numerous genes implicated both in inflammatory and immune response, and additionally in initiation, development and propagation of colorectal cancer in UC patients. Although few data are available, the key role of NF-κB both in regulating inflammatory/immune response in IBD patients, and its implication in colorectal carcinogenesis, pointed researchers interest towards its role in CAC. In particular, the close link between TNF-α (clearly recognized as a pro-carcinogen in CAC) and NF-κB, suggested that NF-κB probably contributes to CAC onset and development. Until now, this has only been shown in an animal study (Onizawa et al., 2009) and suspected from the results published by Popivanova et al. in 2008 (Popivanova et al., 2008;).

3.3.5 Effects on the Wnt/β-catenin and the epidermal growth factor receptor pathways

Recent studies have hypothesized that 5-ASA may also exert its chemopreventive properties directly, and not only through its actions on mucosal inflammation. Mesalamine has been reported to decrease the activity of the wingless and integration site growth factor (Wnt)/β-catenin pathway [which is constitutively activated in up to 80% of sporadic colorectal cancers due to somatic mutation of the *Apc* tumour suppressor gene, although lesser in CAC (Viennot et al., 2009; Laurent et al., 2011)], by inhibiting protein phosphatase A2 (which results in a enhancement of β-catenin phosphorylation, and induces activation of carcinogenetic genes such as *cyclin D1*, *c-met* and *c-myc*) (Bos et al., 2006).

5-aminosalicylic acid has also been reported to inhibit epidermal growth factor receptor (EGFR) pathway. This pathway has been shown to be highly activated in colorectal cancer, and is one of the targets of currently used biotherapies in sporadic colorectal cancer (cetuximab, Erbitux®). In CAC, over-expression of EGFR is frequent (Svrcek et al., 2007), and *in vitro* human colon cancer cell lines exposure to 5-ASA markedly decreased EGFR signaling, at least in part by enhancing the activity of phosphatase SH-PTP2, one of the phosphatases inhibiting EGFR phosphorylation, an essential event for its pro-carcinogenetic effects (Moghal et al., 1999; Monteleone et al., 2006).

4. Conclusion and current clinical recommendations

Colitis-associated cancer prevention in UC (and colonic CD) remains a controversial subject. Following initial data reporting an important increase in colorectal cancer in UC patients, more recent studies performed not only in reference centres but also considering the general UC patients population, reported a CAC risk probably lower than the risk reported in earlier work. In addition, despite numerous (but also often contradictory experimental data on 5-ASA effects on colorectal cancer initiation, development and progression) suggesting a protective role of 5-ASA against CAC in UC patients, most of the data are retrospective, some data are contradictory, and a clear conclusion could not been drawn. In addition, it seems unlikely that a prospective, large population-based study to evaluate 5-ASA chemopreventive properties against CAC would be performed, due to its costs, duration, and number of patients needed to participate.

As a conclusion, clinicians should therefore be very cautious but also consider each UC (or colonic CD) patient as a particular case. Nevertheless, in our opinion and despite several uncertainties, the best remains to follow practical guidelines recommended by numerous gastroenterological scientific societies. These guidelines usually propose a systematic chemopreventive use of 5-ASA (usually around 1.8 to 2 g/day) in addition to systematic colonoscopic dysplasia and CAC screening including chromoendoscopy using either indigo carmine or methylene blue.

5. References

Agoff, S.N.; Brentnall, T.A.; Crispin, D.A.; Taylor, S.N.; Raaka, S.; Haggitt, R.C.; Reed, M.W.; Afonina, I.A.; Rabinovitch, P.S.; Stevens, A.C.; Feng, Z. & Bronner, M.P. (2000). The role of cyclooxygenase 2 in ulcerative colitis-associated neoplasia. *The American Journal of Pathology*, 157, 3, Septembre 2000, 737-745, ISSN: 0002-9440.

Allgayer, H. (2003). Review article: mechanisms of action of mesalazine in preventing colorectal carcinoma in inflammatory bowel disease. *Alimentary Pharmacology and Therapeutics*, 18 (Suppl. 2), September 2003, 10-14, ISSN: 0269-2813.

Allgayer, H.; Höfer, P.; Schmidt, M.; Böhne, P.; Kruis, W. & Gugler, R. (1992). Superoxide, hydroxyl and fatty acid radical scavenging by aminosalicylates. Direct evaluation with electron spin resonance spectroscopy. *Biochemical Pharmacology*, 43, 2, January 1992, 259-262, ISSN: 0006-2952.

Askling, J.; Dickman, P.W.; Karlén, P.; Brostrom, O.; Lapidus, A., Löfberg, R. & Ekbom A. (2001a). Family history as a risk factor for colorectal cancer in inflammatory bowel disease. *Gastroenterology*, 120, 6, May 2001, 1356-1362, ISSN: 0016-5085.

Askling, J.; Dickman, P.W.; Karlén, P.; Brostrom, O.; Lapidus; A., Löfberg, R. & Ekbom A. (2001b). Colorectal cancer rates among first-degree relatives of patients with inflammatory bowel disease: a population-based cohort study. *Lancet*, 357, 9252, January 2001, 262-266, ISSN: 0140-6736.

Azadkahn, A.K.; Truelove, S.C. & Aronson, J.K. (1982). The disposition and metabolism of sulphasalasine (salicylazosulphapyridine) in man. *British Journal of Clinical Pharmacology*, 16, 4, April 1982, 523-528, ISSN: 0306-5251.

Bernstein, C.N.; Nugent, Z. & Blanchard, J.F. (2011). 5-aminosalicylate is not chemoprophylactic for colorectal cancer in IBD: a population-based study. *The American Journal of Gastroenterology*, 106, 4, April 2011, 731-736, ISSN: 0002-9266.

Bernstein, C.N.; Blanchard, J.F.; Kliewer, E. & Wajda, A. (2001). Cancer risk in patients with inflammatory bowel disease: a population-based study. *Cancer*, 91, 4, February 2001, 854-862, ISSN: 0008-543X.

Biasco, G.; Zannoni, U.; Paganelli, G.M.; Santucci, R.; Gionchetti, P. ; Rivolta, G.; Miniero, R.; Pironi, L.; Calabrese, C.; Di Febo, G. & Miglioli, M. (1997). Folic acid supplementation and cell kinetics of rectal mucosa in patients with ulcerative colitis. *Cancer Epidemiology Biomarkers & Prevention*, 6, 6, June 1997, 469-471, ISSN: 1055-9965.

Boland, C.R.; Luciani, M.G.; Gasche, C. & Goel, A. (2005). Infection, inflammation, and gastrointestinal cancer. *Gut*, 54, 9, September 2005, 1321-1231, ISSN: 0017-5749.

Bos, C.L.; Diks, S.H.; Hardwick, J.C.; Walburg, K.V.; Peppelenbosch, M.P. & Richel, D.J. (2006). Protein phosphatase 2A is required for mesalazine-dependent inhibition of Wnt/β-catenin pathway activity. *Carcinogenesis*, 27, 12, December 2006, 2371-2382, ISSN: 0143-3334.

Broomé, U.; Löfberg, R.; Veress, B. & Eriksson L.S. (1995). Primary sclerosing cholangitis and ulcerative colitis. Evidence for increased neoplastic potential. *Hepatology*, 22, 5, November 1995, 1404-1408, ISSN: 0270-9139.

Cao, Y.; Pearman, A.T.; Zimmerman, G.A.; McIntyre, T.M. & Prescott, M. (2000). Intracellular unesterified arachidonic acid signals apoptosis. *Proceedings of the National Academy of Sciences of the United States of America*, 97, 21, October 2000, 11280-11285, ISSN: 0027-8424.

Chang, C.L.; Marra, G.; Chauhan, D.P.; Ha, H.T.; Chang, D.K.; Ricciardiello, L.; Randolph, A.; Carethers, J.M. & Boland, C.R. (2002). Oxidative stress inactivates the human DNA mismatch repair system. *American Journal of Physiology. Cell Physiology*, 283, 1, July 2002, C148-C154, ISSN: 0363-6143.

Chourasia, M.K. & Jain, S.K. (2003). Pharmaceutical approaches to colon targeted drug delivery systems. *Journal of Pharmacy & Pharmaceutical Sciences*, 6, 1, January-April 2003, 33-66, ISSN: 1482-1826.

Cosnes, J.; Gower-Rousseau, C.; Seksik, P. & Cortot, A. (2011). Epidemiology and natural history of inflammatory bowel diseases. *Gastroenterology*, 140, 6, May 2011, 1785-1794, ISSN: 0016-5085.

D'Inca, R.; Cardin, R.; Benazzato, L.; Angriman, I.; Martines, D. & Sturniolo, G.C. (2004). Oxidative DNA damage in the mucosa of ulcerative colitis increases with disease duration and dysplasia. *Inflammatory Bowel Disease*, 10, 1, January 2004, 23-27, ISSN: 1078-0998.

Desreumaux, P. & Ghosh, S. (2006). Review article: mode of action and delivery of 5-aminosalicylic acid - new evidence. *Alimentary Pharmacology and Therapeutics*, 24 Suppl 1, September 2006, 2-9, ISSN: 0269-2813.

Eaden, J.; Abrams, K.; Ekbom, A.; Jackson, E. & Mayberry, J. (2000). Colorectal cancer prevention in ulcerative colitis: a case-control study. *Alimentary Pharmacology and Therapeutics*, 14, 2, February 2000, 145-153, ISSN: 1078-0998.

Eaden, J.; Abrams, K.R. & Mayberry, J.J. (2001). The risk of colorectal cancer in ulcerative colitis: a meta-analysis. *Gut*, 48, 4, April 2001, 526-535, ISSN: 0017-5749.

Eaton, J.E.; Silveira, M.G.; Pardi, D.S.; Sinakos, E.; Kowdley, K.V.; Luketic, V.A.; Harrison, M.E.; McCashland, T.; Befeler, A.S.; Harnois, D.; Jorgensen, R.; Petz, J. & Lindor, K.D. (2011). High-dose ursodeoxycholic acid is associated with the development of colorectal neoplasia in patients with ulcerative colitis and primary sclerosing cholangitis. *The American Journal of Gastroenterology*, May 2011 (in press), ISSN: 0002-9266.

Ekbom, A.; Helmick, C.; Zack, M. & Adami, H.O. (1990). Ulcerative colitis and colorectal cancer. A population-based study. *The New England Journal of Medicine*, 323, 18, November 1990, 1228-1233, ISSN: 0028-4793.

Garrity-Park, M.; Loftus, E.V. Jr.; Sandborn, W.J. & Smyrk, T.C. (2011). Myeloperoxydase immunohistochemitry as a measure of disease activity in ulcerative colitis: association with ulcerative colitis-colorectal cancer, tumor necrosis factor polymorphism and RUNX3 methylation. *Inflammatory Bowel Disease*, March 2011 (in press), ISSN: 1078-0998.

Gasche, C.; Chang, C.L.; Rhees, J.; Goel, A. & Boland, C.R. (2001). Oxidative stress increases frameshift mutations in human colorectal cancer cells. *Cancer Research*, 61, 20, October 2001, 7444-7448, ISSN: 0008-5472.

Gerrits, M.M.; Chen, M.; Theeuwes, M.; van Dekken, H.; Sikkema, M.; Steverberd, E.W.; Lingsma, H.F.; Siersema, P.D.; Xia, B.; Kusters, J.G.; van der Woude, C.J. & Kuipers, E.J. (2011). Biomarker-based prediction or inflammatory bowel disease-related colorectal cancer: a case-control study. *Cellular Oncology (Dordrecht)*, 34, 2, April 2011, 107-117, ISSN: 2211-3436.

Giovannucci, E.; Stampfer, M.J.; Colditz, G.A.; Hunter, D.J.; Fuchs, C.; Rosner, B.A.; Speizer, F.E. & Willett, W.C. (1998). Multivitamin use, folate, and colon cancer in women in the Nurses' Health Study. *Annals of Internal Medicine*, 129, 7, October 1998, 517-524, ISSN: 0003-4819.

Giovannucci, E.; Stampfer, M.J.; Colditz, G.A.; Rimm, E.B.; Trichopoulos, D.; Rosner, B.A.; Speizer, F.E. & Willett, W.C. (1993). Folate, methionine, and alcohol intake and risk of colorectal adenoma. *Journal of the National Cancer Institute*, 85, 11, June 1993, 875-884, ISSN: 0027-8874.

Gupta, R.B.; Harpaz, N.; Itzkowitz, S.; Hossain, S.; Matula, S.; Kornbluth, A.; Bodian, C. & Ullman, T. (2007). Histologic inflammation is a risk factor for progression to colorectal neoplasia in ulcerative colitis: a cohort study. *Gastroenterology*, 133, 4, October 2007, 1099-1105, ISSN: 0016-5085.

Harnois, D.M.; Angulo, P.; Jorgensen, R.A. ; Larusso, N.F. & Lindor, K.D. (2001). High-dose ursodeoxycholic acid as a therapy for patients with primary sclerosing cholangitis. *The American Journal of Gastroenterology*, 96, 5, May 2001, 1558-1562, ISSN: 0002-9266.

Heuschen, U.A.; Hinz, U.; Allemeyer, E.H.; Stern, J.; Lucas, M.; Autschbach, F.; Herfarth, C. & Heuschen, G. (2001). Backwash ileitis is strongly associated with colorectal cancer in patients with ulcerative colitis. *Gastroenterology*, 120, 4, March 2001, 841-847, ISSN: 0016-5085.

Hofseth, L.J.; Saito, S.; Hussain, S.P.; Espey, M.G.; Miranda, K.M.; Araki, Y.; Jhappan, C.; Higashimoto, Y.; He, P.; Linke, S.P.; Quezado, M.M.; Zurer, I.; Rotter, V.; Wink, D.A.; Appella, E. & Harris, C.C. (2003). Nitric oxide-induced cellular stress and p53 activation in chronic inflammation. *Proceedings of the National Academy of Sciences of the United States of America*, 100, 1, January 2003, 143-148, ISSN: 0027-8424.

Hudson, J.D.; Shoaibi, M.A.; Maestro, R.; Carnero, A.; Hannon, G.J. & Beach, D.H. (1999). A proinflammatory cytokine inhibits p53 tumor suppressor activity. *The Journal of Experimental Medicine*, 190, 10, November 1999, 1375-1382, ISSN: 0022-1007.

Hussain, S.P.; Amstad, P.; Raja, K.; Ambs, S.; Nagashima, M.; Bennett, W.P.; Shields, P.G.; Ham, A.J.; Swenberg, J.A.; Marrogi, A.J. & Harris, C.C. (2000). Increased p53 mutation load in noncancerous colon tissue from ulcerative colitis: a cancer-prone chronic inflammatory disease. *Cancer Research*, 60, 13, July 2000, 3333-3337, ISSN: 0008-5472.

Hussain, S.P.; Hofseth, L.J. & Harris, C.C. (2003). Radical causes of cancer. *Nature Reviews Cancer*, 3, 4, April 2003, 276-285, ISSN: 1474-175X.

Jansson, E.A.; Are, A.; Greicius, G.; Kuo, I.C.; Kelly, D.; Arulampalam, V. & Pettersson, S. (2005). The Wnt/beta-catenin signaling pathway targets PPARgamma activity in colon cancer cells. *Proceedings of the National Academy of Sciences of the United States of America*, 102, 5, February 2005, 1460-1465, ISSN: 0027-8424.

Kim, Y.I.; Pogribny, I.P.; Basnakian, A.G.; Miller, J.W.; Selhub, J.; James, S.J. & Mason, J.B. (1997). Folate deficiency in rats induces DNA strand breaks and hypomethylation within the p53 tumor suppressor gene. *The American Journal of Clinical Nutrition*, 65, 1, January 1997, 46-52, ISSN: 0002-9165.

Kimura, H.; Hokari, R.; Miura, S.; Shigematsu, T.; Hirokawa, M.; Akiba, Y.; Kurose, I.; Higuchi, H.; Fujimori, H.; Tsuzuki, Y.; Serizawa, H. & Ishii, H. (1998). Induced expression of an inducible isoform of nitric oxide synthase and the formation of peroxynitrite in colonic mucosa of patients with active ulcerative colitis. *Gut*, 42, 2, February 1998, 180-187, ISSN: 0017-5749.

Kulaylat, M.N. & Dayton, M.T. (2010). Ulcerative colitis and cancer. *Journal of Surgical Oncology*, 15, 8, June 2010, 706-712, ISSN: 0022-4790.

Lashner, B.A. (1993). Red blood cell folate is associated with the development of dysplasia and cancer in ulcerative colitis. *Journal of Cancer Research and Clinical Oncology*, 119, 9, September 1993, 549-554, ISSN: 0171-5216.

Lashner, B.A.; Heudenreich, P.A.; Su, G.L.; Kane, S.V. & Hanauer, S.B. (1989) Effect of folate supplementation on the incidence of dysplasia and cancer in chronic ulcerative colitis. *Gastroenterology*, 97, 2, August 1989, 255-259, ISSN: 0016-5085.

Lashner, B.A.; Provencher, K.S.; Seidner, D.L.; Knesebeck, A. & Brzezinski A. (1997). The effect of folic acid supplementation on the risk for cancer or dysplasia in ulcerative colitis. *Gastroenterology*, 112, 1, January 1997, 29-32, ISSN: 0016-5085.

Laurent, C.; Svrcek, M.; Flejou, J.F.; Chenard, M.P.; Duclos, B.; Freund, J.N. & Reimund, J.M. (2011). Immunohistochemical expression of CDX2, *ß*-catenin and TP53 in inflammatory bowel disease-associated colorectal cancer. *Inflammatory Bowel Disease*, 17, 1, January 2011, 232-240, ISSN: 1078-0998.

Lichtenstein, G.R. & Rutgeerts, P. (2010). Importance of mucosal healing in ulcerative colitis. *Inflammatory Bowel Disease*, 16, 2, February 2010, 338-346, ISSN: 1078-0998.

Loftus, E.V. Jr.; Aguilar, H.I.; Sandborn, W.J.; Tremaine, W.J.; Krom, R.A.; Zinsmeister, A.R.; Graziadai, I.W. & Wiesner, R.H. (1998). Risk of colorectal neoplasia in patients with primary sclerosing cholangitis and ulcerative colitis following orthotopic liver transplantation. *Hepatology*, 27, 3, March 1998, 685-690, ISSN: 0270-9139.

Lu, D.; Cottam, H.B.; Corr, M. & Carson, D.A. (2005). Repression of beta-catenin function in malignant cells by nonsteroidal anti-inflammatory drugs. *Proceedings of the National Academy of Sciences of the United States of America*, 102, 51, December 2005, 18567-18571, ISSN: 0027-8424.

Lutgens, M.W.; van der Heijden, G.J.; Vleggaar, F.D. & Oldenburg, B. (2008) A comprehensive meta-analysis of the risk of colorectal carcinoma in ulcerative colitis and Crohn's disease. *Gut*, 57 (Suppl II), A131, ISSN: 0017-5749.

Lutgens, M.W.M.D.; Vleggaar, F.P.; Schipper, M.E.I.; Stokkers, P.C.F.; van der Woude, C.J.; Hommes, D.W.; de Jong, D.J.; Dijkstra, G.; van Bodegraven, A.A.; Oldenburg, B & Samsom, M. (2008). High frequency of early colorectal cancer in inflammatory bowel disease. *Gut*, 57, 9, September 2008, 1246-1251, ISSN: 0017-5749.

Mardini, H.A.; Lindsay, D.C.; Deighton, C.M. & Record, C.O. (1987). Effect of polymer coating on faecal recovery of ingested 5-aminosalicylic acid in patients with ulcerative colitis. *Gut*, 28, 9, September 1987, 1084-1089, ISSN: 0017-5749.

Matthissen, M.W.; Pedersen, G.; Albrektsen, T.; Adamsen, S.; Fleckner, J. & Brynskov, J. (2005). Peroxisome proliferator-activated receptor expression and activation in normal colonic epithelial cells and tubular adenomas. *Scandinavian Journal of Gastroenterology*, 40, 2, February 2005, 198-205, ISSN: 0036-5521.

Moghal, N. & Sternberg, P.W. (1999). Multiple positive and negative regulators of signaling by the EGF-receptor. *Current Opinion in Cell Biology*, 11, 2, April 1999, 190-196, ISSN: 0955-0674.

Monteleone, G.; Franchi, L.; Fina, D.; Carusao, R.; Vavassori, P.; Monteleone, I.; Calabrese, E.; Naccari, G.C.; Bellinvia, S.; Testi, R. & Pallone, F. (2006). Silencing of SH-PTP2 defines a crucial role in the inactivation of epidermal growth factor receptor by 5-aminosalicylic acid in colon cancer cells. *Cell Death and Differentiation*, 13, 2, February 2006, 202-211, ISSN: 1350-9047.

Moody, G.A.; Jayanthi, V.; Probert, C.S.; Mac Kay, H. & Mayberry, J.F. (1996). Long-term therapy with sulphasalazine protects against colorectal cancer in ulcerative colitis: a retrospective study of colorectal cancer risk and compliance with treatment in Leicestershire. *European Journal of Gastroenterology and Hepatology*, 8, 12, December 1996, 1179-1183, ISSN: 0954-691X.

Nuako, K.W.; Ahlquist, D.A.; Mahoney, D.W.; Schaid, D.J.; Siems, D.M. & Lindor, N.M. (1998). Familial predisposition for colorectal cancer in ulcerative colitis: a case-control study. *Gastroenterology*, 115, 5, November 1998, 1079-1083, ISSN: 0016-5085.

Onizawa, M.; Nagaishi, T.; Kanai, T.; Nagano, K.; Oshima, S.; Nemoto, Y.; Yoshioka, A.; Totsuka, T.; Okamoto, R.; Nakamura, T.; Sakamoto, N.; Tsuchiya, K.; Aoki, K.; Ohya, K.; Yagita, H. & Watanabe, M. (2009). Signaling pathway via TNF-alpha/NF-kappaB in intestinal epithelial cells may be directly involved in colitis-associated carcinogenesis. *American Journal of Physiology. Gastrointestinal and Liver Physiology*, 296, 4, April 2009, G850-859, ISSN: 0193-1857.

Osawa, E.; Nakajima, A.; Wada, K.; Ishimine, S.; Fujisawa, N.; Kawamori, T.; Matsuhashi, N.; Kadowaki, T.; Ochiai, M.; Sekihara, H. & Nakagama, H. (2003). Peroxisome proliferator-activated receptor gamma ligands suppress colon carcinogenesis induced by azoxymethane in mice. *Gastroenterology*, 124, 2, February 2002, 361-367, ISSN: 0016-5085.

Oshitani, N.; Kitano, A.; Okabe, H.; Nakamura, S.; Matsumoto, T. & Kobayashi, K. (1993). Location of superoxide anion generation in human colonic mucosa obtained by biopsy. *Gut*, 35, 7, July 1993, 284-285, ISSN: 0017-5749.

Pardi, D.S.; Loftus, E.V. Jr.; Kremers, W.K.; Keach, J. & Lindor, K.D. (2003). Ursodeoxycholic acid as a chemopreventive agent in patients with ulcerative colitis and primary sclerosing cholangitis. *Gastroenterology*, 124, 4, April 2003, 889-893, ISSN: 0016-5085.

Phelip, J.M.; Ducros, V.; Faucheron, J.L.; Flourié, B. & Roblin, X. (2008). Association of hyperhomocysteinemia and folate deficiency with colon tumors in patients with inflammatory bowel disease. *Inflammatory Bowel Disease*, 14, 2, February 2008, 242-248, ISSN: 1078-0998.

Pinczowski, D.; Ekbom, A.; Baron, J.; Yuen, J. & Adami, H.O. (1994). Risk factors for colorectal cancer in patients with ulcerative colitis: a case-control study. *Gastroenterology*, 107, 1, July 1994, 117-120, ISSN: 0016-5085.

Popivanova, B.K.; Kitamura, K.; Wu, Y. ; Kondo, K. ; Kagava, T.; Kaneko, S.; Oshima, M.; Fujii, C. & Mukaida, M. (2008). Blocking TNF-α in mice reduces colorectal carcinogenesis associated with chronic colitis. *The Journal of Clinical Investigation*, 118, 2, February 2008, 560-570, ISSN: 0021-9738.

Rachmilewitz, D.; Stamler, J.S.; Bachwich, D.; Karmeli, F.; Ackerman, Z. & Podolsky, D.K. (1995). Enhanced colonic nitric oxide generation and nitric oxide synthase activity in ulcerative colitis and Crohn's disease. *Gut*, 36, 5, May 1995, 718-723, ISSN: 0017-5749.

Ransohoff, D.F. (1988). Colon cancer in ulcerative colitis. *Gastroenterology*, 94, 4, April 1988, 1089-1091, ISSN: 0016-5085.

Rijk, M.C.; van Schaik, A. & van Tongeren, J.H. (1988). Disposition of 5-aminosalicylic acid by 5-aminosalicylic acid-delivering compounds. *Scandinavian Journal of Gastroenterology*, 23, 1, January 1988, 107-112, ISSN: 0036-5521.

Roessner, A.; Kuester, D.; Malfertheiner, P. & Schneider-Stock, R. (2008). Oxidative stress in ulcerative colitis-associated carcinogenesis. *Pathology, Research and Practice*, 204, 7, June 2008, 511-524, ISSN: 0344-0338.

Rousseaux, C.; Lefebvre, B.; Dubuquoy, L.; Lefebvre, P.; Romano, O.; Auwerx, J.; Metzger, D.; Wahli, W.; Desvergne, B.; Naccari, G.C.; Chavatte, P.; Farce, A.; Bulois, P.; Cortot, A.; Colombel, J.F. & Desreumaux, P. (2005). Intestinal anti-inflammatory effect of 5-aminosalicylic acid is dependent on peroxisome proliferator-activated receptor-gamma. *The Journal of Experimental Medicine*, 201, 8, April 2005, 1205-1215, ISSN: 0022-1007.

Rutter, M.D.; Saunders, B.P.; Wilkinson, K.H., Rumbles, S.; Schofield, G.; Kamm, M.; Williams, C.B.; Price, A.B.; Talbot, I.C. & Forbes, A. (2004a). Cancer surveillance in longstanding ulcerative colitis: endoscopic appearances help predict cancer risk. *Gut*, 53, 12, December 2004, 1813-1816, ISSN: 0017-5749.

Rutter, M.; Saunders, B; Wilkinson, K.; Rumbles, S.; Shofield, G.; Kamm, M.; Williams, C.; Price, A.; Talbot, I. & Forbes, A. (2004b). Severity of inflammation is a risk factor for colorectal neoplasia in ulcerative colitis. *Gastroenterology*, 126, 2, February 2004, 451-459, ISSN: 0016-5085.

Rutter, M.D.; Saunders, P.P.; Wilkinson, K.H.; Rumbles, S.; Schofield, G.; Kamm, M.; Williams, C.B.; Price, A.B.; Talbot, I.C. & Forbes, A. (2006). Thirty years analysis of colonoscopic surveillance program for neoplasia in ulcerative colitis. *Gastroenterology*, 130, 4, April 2006, 1030-1038, ISSN: 0016-5085.

Sandborn, W.J. & Hanauer, S.B. (2003). Systematic review: the pharmacokinetic profiles of oral mesalazine formulations and mesalazine pro-drugs used in the management of ulcerative colitis. *Alimentary Pharmacology and Therapeutics*, 17, 1, January 2003, 29-42, ISSN: 1078-0998.

Shimada, T.; Kojima, K.; Yoshiura, K.; Hiraishi, H. & Terano, A. (2002). Characteristics of the peroxisome proliferator receptor gamma (PPARgamma) ligand induced apoptosis in colon cancer cells. *Gut*, 50, 5, May 2002, 658-664, ISSN: 0017-5749.

Sjöqvist, U.; Tribukait, B.; Ost, A.; Einarsson, C.; Oxelmark, L. & Löfberg, L. (2004). Ursodeoxycholic acid treatment in IBD patients with colorectal dysplasia and/or DNA-aneuploidy: a prospective, double-blind, randomized controlled pilot study. *Anticancer Research*, 24, 5B, September-October 2004, 3121-3127, ISSN: 0250-7005.

Sokol, H.; Cosnes, J.; Chazouillieres, O.; Beaugerie, L.; Tiret, E.; Poupon, R. & Seksik P. (2008). Disease activity and cancer risk in inflammatory bowel disease associated with primary sclerosing cholangitis. *World Journal of Gastroenterology*, 14, 22, June 2008, 3497-3503, ISSN 1007-9327.

Stolfi, C.; Fina, D.; Caruso, R.; Caprioli, F.; Sarra, M.; Fantini, M.C.; Rizzo, A.; Pallone, F. & Monteleone, G. (2008). Cyclooxygenase-dependent and –independent inhibition of proliferation of colon cancer cells by 5-aminosalicylic acid. *Biochemical Pharmacology*, 75, 3, February 2008, 668-676, ISSN: 0006-2952.

Svrcek, M; Cosnes, J.; Tiret, E.; Bennis, M.; Park, Y. & Flejou, J.F. (2007). Expression of epidermal growth factor receptor (EGFR) is frequent in inflammatory bowel disease (IBD)-associated intestinal cancer. *Virchows Archives*, 450, 2, February 2007, 243-244, ISSN: 0945-6317.

Tanaka, T.; Kohno, H.; Yoshitani, S.; Takashima, S.; Okumura, A.; Murakami, A. & Hosokawa, M. (2001). Ligands for peroxisome proliferator-activated receptors alpha and gamma inhibit chemically induced colitis and formation of aberrant crypt foci in rats. *Cancer Research*, 61, 6, March 2001, 2424-2428, ISSN: 0008-5472.

Terdiman, J.P.; Steinbuch, M.; Blumentals, W.A.; Ullman, T.A. & Rubin, T.D. (2007). 5-aminosalicylic acid therapy and the risk of colorectal cancer among patients with inflammatory bowel diseases. *Inflammatory Bowel Disease*, 13, 367-371, ISSN: 1078-0998.

Torres, J.; de Chambrun, G.P.; Itzkowitz, S.; Sachar, D.B. & Colombel, J.F. (2011). Review article: colorectal neoplasia in patients with primary sclerosing cholangitis and inflammatory bowel disease. *Alimentary Pharmacology and Therapeutics*, June 2011 (in press), ISSN: 0269-2813.

Van Hogezand, R.A.; van Hees, P.A.; van Gorp, J.P.; van Lier, H.J.; Bakker, J.H.; Wesseling, P.; van Haelst, U.J. & van Tongeren, J.H. (1988). Double-blind comparison of 5-aminosalicylic acid and acetyl-5-aminosalicylic acid suppositories in patients with idiopathic proctitis. *Alimentary Pharmacology and Therapeutics*, 2, 1, February 1988, 33-40, ISSN: 1078-0998.

van Staa, T.P.; Card, T.; Logan, R.F. & Leufkens, H.G.M. (2005). 5-Aminosalicylate use and colorectal cancer risk in inflammatory bowel disease: a large epidemiological study. *Gut*, 54, 11, November 2005, 1573-1578, ISSN: 0017-5749.

Velayos, F.S.; Loftus, E.V. Jr.; Jess, T.; Harmsen, W.S.; Bida, J.; Zinsmeister, A.R.; Tremaine, W.J. & Sandborn, W.J. (2006). Predictive and protective factors associated with colorectal cancer in ulcerative colitis: a case-control study. *Gastroenterology*, 130, 7, June 2006, 1941-1949, ISSN: 0016-5085.

Velayos, F.S.; Terdiman, J.P. & Walsh, J.M. (2005). Effect of 5-aminosalicylate use on colorectal cancer and dysplasia risk: a systematic review and metaanalysis of observational studies. *The American Journal of Gastroenterology*, 100, 6, June 2005, 1354-1356, ISSN: 0002-9266.

Viennot, S.; Deleporte, A.; Moussata, D.; Nancey, S.; Flourié, B. & Reimund, J.M. (2009). Colon cancer in inflammatory bowel disease: recent trends, questions and answers. *Gastroentérologie Clinique et Biologique*, 33 Suppl 3, June 2009, S190-201, ISSN: 0399-8320.

Vree, T.B.; Dammers, E.; Exler, P.S.; Sorgel, F.; Bondesen, S. & Maes, R.A. (2000). Liver and gut mucosa acetylation of mesalazine in healthy volunteers. *International Journal of Clinical Pharmacology and Therapeutics*, 38, 11, November 2000, 514-522, ISSN: 0946-1965.

Winther, K.V.; Jess, T.; Langholz, E.; Munkholm, P. & Binder, V. (2004). Long-term risk of cancer in ulcerative colitis: a population-based cohort study from Copenhagen County. *Clinical Gastroenterology and Hepatology*, 2, 12, December 2004, 1088-1095, ISSN: 1542-3565.

Wolf, J.A.; Rybicki, L.A. & Lashner, B.A. (2005). The impact of ursodeoxycholic acid on cancer , dysplasia and mortality in ulcerative colitis patients with primary scleosing cholangitis. *Alimentary Pharmacology and Therapeutics*, 22, 9, November 2005, 783-788, ISSN: 1078-0998.

Yakut, M.; Ustün, Y.; Kabaçam, G. & Soykan, I. (2010). Serim vitamin B12 and folate status in patients with inflammatory bowel disease. *European Journal of Internal Medicine*, 21, 4, August 2010, ISSN: 0953-6205.

9

Ulcerative Colitis

Yousef Ajlouni[1] and Mustafa M. Shennak[2]
[1]*IBD, Consultant Gastroenterologist, Internist, King Hussein Medical Center*
[2]*GI and Liver Division, Faculty of Medicine, University of Jordan and Hospital*
Jordan

1. Introduction

Ulcerative colitis (UC) is a chronic inflammatory disease that primarily affects the colonic mucosa; it is most commonly diagnosed in patients aged 15-35 years, although the condition can affect patients of any age and of either sex. It's exact etiologie remain uncertain. The annual incidence of ulcerative colitis in western countries is estimated to be 6-8 cases per 100,000 individuals, with the prevalence reaching 70-150 cases per 100,000 individuals. The disease course is generally relapsing-remitting, with patients experiencing few or no gastrointestinal symptoms between symptomatic relapses.

As medical options increase, decisions about the sequence and timing of therapy and surgery in particular become more difficult. Consequently a therapeutic strategy is necessary, keeping an eye on the direction of travel to avoid going round in circles from one incompletely effective therapy to another. Patients live with a considerable symptom burden despite medical treatment in the hope that a cure for ulcerative colitis will emerge. This article reviews the new advances in ulcerative colitis, epidemiology, pathogenesis, diagnosis, new therapeutic goals, as well as therapy that occurred in the past year.

2. Epidemiology

The prevalence of ulcerative colitis (UC) rapidly increased in western countries in the second half of the twentieth century and is becoming more common in the rest of the world as different countries adopt a Western lifestyle.[(1)] There are many similarities between Asian and Western populations, even significant differences do exist. These differences in genetic and environmental influences represent an important opportunity to understand the influences that lead to the development UC. [(2)] UC tends to be a disease of young adulthood.[(3)] There are slightly more women affected than men. Cigarette smoking protective in ulcerative colitis, an effect that has yet to be satisfactorily explained. It is well known that smoking reduces the severity of disease in ulcerative colitis, reducing the number of hospitalizations and need for steroids or surgery. By contrast, smoking increases the severity of Crohn's disease, increasing the number of exacerbations and the need for steroids.[(4)] Additionally, early appendectomy (before age 20) has resulted in a lower risk of ulcerative colitis.[(5,6)] Accurate descriptive epidemiology is needed now more than ever, so that it can be applied to the various populations with inflammatory bowel disease (IBD) such that further genetic and clinical studies can be conducted.

3. Genetics in ulcerative colitis

It is well known that IBD is a disease that has appeared over the last century and that its incidence varies markedly with geographic location, urbanization, and industrial development. Such data clearly highlight the presumptive importance of environmental factors in modulating disease evolution in IBD. However, a variety of other epidemiologic data also highlight the intimate role played by genetic factors in IBD pathogenesis. For instance, marked ethnic and racial differences in disease prevalence have been noted, particularly in Ashkenazi Jews. Furthermore, twin studies have demonstrated a much higher rate of disease concordance in monozygotic compared with dizygotic twins, particularly in Crohn's disease. However, it should also be highlighted that over 60% of monozygotic twins are not concordant for IBD. Thus, genetic susceptibility alone, while important, is clearly not sufficient for the development of disease.

The greatest identifiable risk factor for the development of IBD is having a first-degree family member affected by the disease. Affected first-degree relatives are more frequently identified in patients with Crohn's disease (9% to 15%) than in those with ulcerative colitis (6% to 9%), and appear to be more common in patients with earlier disease onset and in those of Jewish descent. Siblings of an affected individual are at highest risk. The risk of disease in the offspring of patients is very difficult to calculate accurately due to the paucity of data. Offspring of couples who are both affected by IBD (either Crohn's disease, ulcerative colitis, or "mixed" [ie, 1 parent with Crohn's disease and the other with ulcerative colitis]) appear to have about a 30% chance of developing disease by 30 years of age. If only a single parent has IBD, then the risk appears to be much less: approximately 9% if the parent has Crohn's disease, and about 6% if the parent has ulcerative colitis.

The substantial heterogeneity seen in IBD suggests that it does not encompass only 2, but many inflammatory disorders. Various epidemiologic data support this concept. Multiply-affected families show surprising concordance for disease phenotype, including age of onset, disease location, and extra-intestinal manifestations. Longitudinal studies examining changes in Crohn's disease phenotype over time demonstrate the stability of disease location, but the progression of disease behavior following diagnosis. The current genetic model for IBD attempts to encompass these observations. It is generally believed that there may be a number of "susceptibility genes" that confer a general predisposition to IBD. Other "modifier genes," although they don't initiate disease, then act to influence specific phenotypic characteristics such as disease behavior, complications, and treatment response, among others. Both "susceptibility" and "modification" may be further influenced by interaction with environmental factors.

4. Mechanisms of disease and pathogenesis

Chronic intestinal inflammation in UC results from the interactions of genetic, immunologic, microbial and environmental factors.(7) It is proposed that IBD results from the failure to appropriately downregulate nonspecific inflammation initiated by an environmental trigger, such as an acute, self-limited infection or NSAID use. (8) Normal hosts quickly clear infections of invasive enteric bacteria, downregulate innate immune responses and heal the injured mucosa without stimulating effector T-cell responses. (9) By contrast, genetically susceptible hosts who are unable to clear an invading pathogen and/or generate tolerogenic immune response to commensal microbial agents—by mounting appropriate innate immunity, downregulating immune responses or healing the mucosal barrier—subsequently activate pathogenic T-cell responses to commensal bacteria and proceed to chronic, relapsing intestinal inflammation. Resistance to T-cell apoptosis, lack of response to downregulatory signals and continuous exposure to luminal antigens and adjuvants help sustain this inflammatory response.(10)

Many environmental factors can influence mucosal immune responses and enteric bacteria composition, including diet, smoking, stress, altered microenvironment and NSAID exposure. (11) Although It postulated that self-limited, nonspecific infections can initiate the onset of chronic inflammation and reactivate quiescent disease, it is possible that a persistent pathogen could cause disease in individuals unable to clear infections, or that the commensal bacteria of some patients could acquire virulence factors (e.g. toxins, adherence and/or invasion properties) that might cause chronic intestinal inflammation.(12)

5. Diagnosis of ulcerative colitis

Endoscopy; Colonoscopy is more sensitive than radiographic studies in detecting early changes associated with UC, and represents the primary modality to obtain tissue for histologic evaluation. Clinicians should be cognizant that even if the colonic mucosa appears macroscopically normal, there may be histologic changes diagnostic of UC. Therefore, it is of paramount importance that biopsies be procured, even from tissue that appears endoscopically normal. Histology represents the most sensitive measure of disease extent and activity. In 10% of all patients, colonoscopy with biopsy is unable to differentiate between Crohn's colitis and ulcerative colitis. (13)

In early-stage edema, confluent erythema with rectal involvement is typical. As the disease progresses, granularity and contact bleeding is appreciated endoscopically. With progression of disease to the late stages, discrete ulcerations with pus/exudate and loss of haustral folds is characteristic. The presence of aphthoid ulcerations is not seen in patients with ulcerative colitis. Chronic inflammation frequently leads to diffuse mucosal atrophy, leaving behind hypertrophic areas of swollen, edematous tissue and areas of granulation that assume a polypoid configuration. These areas, known as pseudopolyps, have no malignant potential and occur in both ulcerative colitis and Crohn's disease. (14) Histologically, ulcerative colitis has alterations of crypt architecture including crypt architectural distortion. Paneth cells are commonly found in normal individuals, proximal to the hepatic flexure; however, in patients with ulcerative colitis, it is not uncommon to discern their presence distal to the hepatic flexure suggestive of prior crypt destruction and subsequent regeneration. It is most common to find these features distally. It is also common to find basal plasma cells and many basal lymphoid cells, indicating the presence of chronicity. (19) Basal plasma cells are, however, not specific for ulcerative colitis and may be seen in other chronic disorders, such as collagenous colitis and Crohn's disease and, rarely, in infectious colitis. Other minor features of ulcerative colitis include hyperplasia of argentaffin cells, mucosal vascular congestion with edema, and focal hemorrhage. Depletion of goblet cell mucin is a characteristic and consistent finding in acute ulcerative colitis, and except where dysplasia is present, is another reliable indicator of disease activity. (15)

Radiographic Studies; Radiographic imaging for evaluation of patients with ulcerative colitis also remains a standard and helps to differentiate ulcerative colitis from Crohn's disease. The presence of mucosal granularity is the earliest radiographically detectable evidence of disease in ulcerative colitis. The granular pattern is thought to result from abnormalities associated with edema and hyperemia. [16] Early ulcer formation in ulcerative colitis appears as fine speckled barium collections superimposed on a granular-appearing mucosa. Other associated findings may be present, including haustral fold thickening, colonic shortening, polyps and pseudopolyps, strictures, dysplasia, colorectal cancer, and toxic dilation for various disease stages. [17]

Serologic Testing; Combined serologic testing has also been proposed to help differentiate between ulcerative colitis and Crohn's disease in cases of indeterminate colitis. At this time, there is insufficient evidence to demonstrate that perinuclear anti-neutrophilic cytoplasmic antibody (pANCA) and anti-Saccharomyces cerevisiae antibody (ASCA) testing alone is completely reliable in reaching a definitive diagnosis.[18] The presence of ANCA, pANCA, ASCA, anti-OmpC (outer membrane porin from Escherichia coli), and anti-CBir1 (anti-CBir1 flagellin) markers appears to be associated with ulcerative colitis and Crohn's disease.[19,20] More markers and combined serologic testing represent a promising step forward for diagnosis.

6. Backwash Ileitis in ulcerative colitis

Involvement of the distal ileum in ulcerative colitis (UC) is termed backwash ileitis (BWI). Most authors agree that BWI has a similar morphologic pattern of mucosal inflammation and injury to UC and does not have the features typical of CD. [21] Features that favor a diagnosis of CD rather than chronic UC with BWI, are an extensive length of involved small bowel, involvement of the jejunum, proximally located regions of active ileitis separated by skip regions of uninvolved cecum or distal ileum, greater inflammatory activity and mucosal injury in the ileum than the cecum, transmural ileal inflammation with granulomas and neural hyperplasia, and mucous gland (so-called pyloric gland) metaplasia of the ileal mucosa. [22] In endoscopic biopsy specimens, features that suggest a diagnosis of CD include mucous gland metaplasia or the constellation of focal lamina propria edema with crypt disarray and no to mild active inflammation that involves a small region of a tissue fragment surrounded by normal small bowel mucosa. Mild BWI consists of active inflammation and edema that is located predominantly in villus tips without significant lamina propria focal edema or crypt disarray. In BWI, mild ileal mucosal injury is found in association with moderate or markedly active cecal colitis. Focal ileal erosions with mild active inflammation seen in association with mildly active cecal colitis should be considered CD. [23]

7. Indeterminate colitis

Although some patients who are initially labelled as having indeterminate colitis eventually have classic features of ulcerative colitis or Crohn's disease, others who remain indeterminate may have a unique phenotype. If a unique phenotype exists, novel diagnostic tests are needed to positively identify this group, instead of relying on current tests that can only exclude ulcerative colitis and Crohn's disease. Until indeterminate colitis becomes a diagnosis based on positive test results, data regarding the epidemiology, response to therapy and cancer risk will likely remain difficult to interpret.[24,25] At present time serological tests can not diagnose or predict the course of indeterminate colitis. The serological tests would not be diagnostic for indeterminate colitis until there exists at least one test that positively identifies the subgroup of indeterminate colitis. [26]

8. Treatment of ulcerative colitis

Clinical trials on ulcerative colitis have all used different endpoints to define response and remission. Some outcomes that matter to patients, such as hospitalization, time off work, surgery and mortality, are difficult to measure, but are only now being captured in large trials. Other outcomes (steroid-free remission, speed of response, time to relapse) also matter to patients, are readily understood, easily measured and more informative than composite indices. Surrogate markers for determining improved outcomes, such as fewer hospital visits, or surgery, include mucosal healing.

9. 5-Aminosalicylic Acid (5-ASA)

When free 5-ASA is administered orally, it is nearly completely systemically absorbed from the proximal small intestine and then extensively metabolized to N-acetyl-5-ASA in intestinal epithelial cells and the liver; it is then excreted in the urine. [27] 5-ASA has been shown to have a topical mechanism of action in the treatment of ulcerative colitis.[28] Therefore, strategies to "protect" orally administered 5-ASA from absorption until it reaches the colon have been developed. These strategies include the use of prodrugs; delayed-release formulations; controlled-release formulations; and, more recently, sophisticated formulations that combine both delayed-release and sustained-release mechanisms.

Prodrug Formulations; The first strategy employed to protect 5-ASA until it reaches the colon was to design prodrugs that release active drug in the colon by the bacterial enzyme azo reductase. Three such drugs were developed: sulfasalazine, olsalazine, and balsalazide. The oldest of these agents, sulfasalazine, consists of 5-ASA linked to sulfapyridine by an azo bond. Olsalazine comprises 2 molecules of 5-ASA linked by an azo bond as a dimer, and balsalazide consists of 5-ASA linked by an azo bond to 4-amino-benzoyl-beta-alanine. Sulfasalazine is formulated as a 500-mg tablet containing 200 mg of 5-ASA. Sulfasalazine is administered orally 4 times daily to minimize side effects associated with the sulfapyridine moiety. Olsalazine is formulated as a 250-mg capsule and is administered orally twice daily. Balsalazide is formulated as a 750-mg tablet that contains 262 mg of 5-ASA. Balsalazide is administered orally 3 times daily. A capsule formulation of balsalazide is currently under development. [29]

Delayed-Release Formulations; The second strategy employed to protect 5-ASA until it reaches the colon was to coat the drug with polymers that release at pH 6 or pH 7, thus delaying release of active drug until it reaches the small bowel or the cecum. Four such oral drugs were developed: Asacol (Ohio), Salofalk (Germany), Mesasal (Canada), and Claversal (Germany). Asacol is a delayed-release tablet formulation of 5-ASA that is coated with a polymer called Eudragit-S, which releases drug in the terminal ileum and colon at pH ≥ 7.0. Salofalk, Mesasal, and Claversal are delayed-release tablet formulations that are coated with a polymer called Eudragit-L, which releases drug in the distal jejunum and proximal ileum. Asacol is formulated as a 400-mg tablet and as an investigational 800-mg tablet (currently available only in Canada); it is administered orally 2-3 times daily. Salofalk, Mesasal, and Claversal are formulated as 250- and 500-mg tablets and are administered orally 3-4 times daily. [30]

Controlled-Release Formulations; The third strategy employed to protect 5-ASA until it reaches the colon was to formulate the 5-ASA as ethylcellulose-coated microgranules that gradually release beginning in the duodenum and continuing throughout the jejunum, the ileum, and the colon to the rectum. (31) Only 1 controlled-release drug was developed: Pentasa (Pennsylvania). After the ethylcellulose-coated microgranules release the drug throughout the small intestine and colon.[(32) Pentasa is formulated as 250-mg and 500-mg tablets, 250-mg and 500-mg capsules, and 1000-mg sachets; this agent is administered orally 1 g once or twice daily for induction of remission and treatment of mild-to-moderate active ulcerative colitis.

Delayed- and Sustained-Release Formulations; The fourth strategy employed to protect 5-ASA until it reaches the colon was the use of a sophisticated formulation that coats pellets or matrices containing 5-ASA with polymers that release at pH 6 or pH 7, thus delaying release of pellets or matrices until they reach the small bowel or the cecum. The pellets or matrices contain 5-ASA that gradually releases, beginning in the distal small bowel and continuing throughout the colon to the rectum. Two such drugs have been developed: mesalamine pellets (Salofalk GranuStix; Germany) and mesalamine with MMX technology (Lialda in the United States and as Mezavant in Europe).

Mesalamine pellets have an outer coating of the Eudragit-L polymer and an additional retarding polymer in the pellet core. The entire mesalamine pellet dose passes unaltered to the distal jejunum and proximal ileum. After the Eudragit-L polymer disintegrates at pH 6.0 in the distal jejunum and proximal ileum and the 5-ASA is then released from the pellet core. (33) Mesalamine pellets are formulated as 500-mg sachets and are administered orally 1-3 times daily.

MMX technology has a pH-sensitive film which delays the release of 5-ASA until the tablet reaches the terminal ileum. Intestinal fluids are thought to interact with hydrophilic excipients causing the tablet to form a viscous gel, which slows diffusion of 5-ASA into the colonic lumen. It is supposed that other lipophilic excipients reduce the rate of dissolution and extend the process of delivery of 5-ASA. It is clear that it works, for both inducing and maintaining remission in single or twice daily doses. (34-36)

Once-daily mesalamine

Once-daily oral formulations of 5-aminosalicylic acid (5-ASA) are likely to be preferred if they offer comparable efficacy and improved adherence. This premise appears correct with Pentasa showed a better remission rate at 1 year in the single daily dose group. Questionnaires confirmed significantly greater compliance and acceptability in the once-daily group. Same results with mesalamine MMX and Salofalk (37,38) the effect is likely to be generic rather than compound specific.

High-dose 5-aminosalicylic acid

The benefit of mesalamine 4.8 over 2.4 g/day is limited to symptom improvement rather than remission in mild or moderately active colitis, as confirmed in the large ASCEND I trial and a systematic review. (39,40)

Induction and maintenance of remission with 5-aminosalicylic acid therapy

The efficacy of oral and rectal formulations of 5-aminosalicylate acid (5-ASA) has been demonstrated in clinical trials as both induction and maintenance agents for mildly to moderately active ulcerative colitis. Two large meta-analyses showed that 5-ASAs were significantly more effective than placebo for induction of remission, and within the limits of this analysis, there was no significant difference between the efficacy of sulfasalazine and the other 5-ASA therapies. (41)

At present, there are no published maintenance-of-remission studies involving mesalamine pellets or MMX mesalamine in patients with active ulcerative colitis.
As with other chronic diseases requiring maintenance therapy, compliance with the prescribed medical regimen is a challenge. Although compliance in clinical trials, which involve a highly selected and motivated patient group, is greater than 80%, much lower rates were seen in community-based, "real-world" studies (40% to 60%).(42) Noncompliance results in an increased risk for disease relapse, a diminished quality of life, and a possible increase in the risk for colorectal cancer. (43) Therefore, successful management of patients with ulcerative colitis requires treatment strategies that encourage and confirm compliance with the prescribed therapeutic plan.

10. Combination oral and topical 5-ASA therapy

A fundamental principle of 5-ASA therapy is delivery of the drug to the site of disease. Several studies, including a meta-analysis, confirmed the efficacy of 5-ASA in an enema formulation in both inducing and maintaining remission in left-sided ulcerative colitis (defined as distal to the splenic flexure). (44,45) The addition of topical 5-ASA to oral therapy increases mucosal levels of mesalamine by 3-fold in the descending colon and over 20-fold in the rectum.(51) Moreover, it has been demonstrated repeatedly that the combination of 5-ASA in oral and enema formulations is superior to either therapy alone in inducing and maintaining remission of extensive colitis. (46)

11. Corticosteroids

Systemic corticosteroids are often given to ulcerative colitis patients with moderately to severely active disease. Over 5 years study, those patients who had achieved complete response with steroid treatment had less need for immunosuppression, fewer hospitalizations, and a longer time interval to relapse in comparison with the group not received steroids. However, colectomy rates were similar among all patient groups. Therefore, the study authors suggested that more aggressive therapy, probably with immunosuppressants, is required for patients who do not completely respond to their first corticosteroid course. (47)
The impact of prednisone on bone density, independent of disease activity, has been the subject of debate, as clinicians have reported osteoporosis in corticosteroid-naive UC patients, and found normal bone densities in some patients on long-term steroids.
The most serious complication associated with corticosteroid therapy in UC is avascular necrosis (osteonecrosis). A search of a large database identified 94 patients with IBD and avascular necrosis; these subjects were matched to IBD controls without avascular necrosis. Important to note was that 6 patients with avascular necrosis had never been exposed to corticosteroids. Likely risk factors for avascular necrosis included systemic steroid exposure, IBD severity, parenteral nutrition, estrogen exposure, and cigarette smoking in ulcerative colitis patients. Although some of these risk factors are modifiable, above all, corticosteroid therapy must be minimized in IBD patients. (48,49)
Dexamethasone encapsulated into the patient's own erythrocytes and infused back into the patient may offer a way to deliver adequate steroid therapy to tissues while minimizing the adverse effects often associated with steroid use. Autologous erythrocytes can be used as drug carriers, owing to the capability of their membrane to be opened and resealed in

appropriate conditions. An ideal drug to be encapsulated into erythrocytes is dexamethasone 21-phosphate (Dex 21-P), a biologically inactive compound. In this randomized clinical trial involving 40 patients with mildly to moderately active ulcerative colitis, subjects received either dexamethasone encapsulated into erythrocytes at entry and at day 14; prednisolone 0.5 mg/kg with tapering; or sham infusions of dexamethasone encapsulated into erythrocytes. At 8 weeks, remission was achieved in 85% of patients who received the erythrocyte-mediated delivery of dexamethasone, in 80% of prednisolone-treated patients, and in 20% of sham-treated patients ($P < .01$). No patient treated with encapsulated dexamethasone experienced steroid-related side effects, as compared with 80% of the prednisolone-treated group. The study authors concluded that very low doses of dexamethasone delivered via encapsulated erythrocytes may be as effective as prednisolone but without the steroid-related side effects. [50,51]

Steroid resistance remains a major clinical challenge, but emerging knowledge of the pathogenesis of IBD is enabling the development of new agents to overcome this resistance. Many difficult questions remain to be answered, such as whether steroid resistance is an inherent property of an individual or if it is acquired. The demonstration of steroid resistance in the lymphocytes of healthy individuals would suggest that it is an inherent property of an individual that is only of relevance in the presence of inflammatory disease.[52] However, the observation that some individuals become less responsive to steroids over time makes this hypothesis more difficult to support. The clonal nature of lymphocyte proliferation raises the possibility that steroid treatment gradually depletes activated steroid-sensitive lymphocytes leaving behind a highly steroid-resistant population over time. May be, combination treatment with existing treatments, such as is employed in the treatment of TB or even malignancy will offer the answer to preventing the development of steroid-resistant lymphocyte clones. Steroid-resistant UC remains a difficult condition to treat. We must consider when designing future trials whether response to treatment is an adequate end point. Patients need to be in steroid-free remission, and this is what we should aspire to achieve. [53]

12. Azathioprine/6-Mercaptopurine

Thiopurines are widely used in the treatment of inflammatory bowel disease (IBD). However, in clinical practice, azathioprine (AZA) or mercaptopurine (MP) are not effective in one-third of patients and up to one-fifth of patients discontinues thiopurine therapy because of adverse events. [54] Dosing recommendations for the thiopurine analogs have traditionally been based on the patient's weight and the impact on hematologic and hepatic parameters. More recently, measurement of the levels of the 2 primary metabolites, 6-thioguanine (6-TGN; thought to be a marker of drug efficacy), and 6-methylmercaptopurine (6-MMP; associated with hepatotoxicity in some instances), as well as the activity of the thiopurine methyltransferase (TPMT) enzyme, has been purported to provide a more accurate prediction of patient response to therapy and of appropriate dosing. [55]

In patients refractory to thiopurines who have high TPMT activity and preferentially metabolize the agents to produce the 6-MMP metabolite instead of the 6-TGN metabolite. The addition of low-dose allopurinol (100 mg or less daily) along with a greatly reduced dose of the purine analog (often 25-50 mg) not only resulted in treatment success, but also in a reversal of the 6-TGN:6-MMP nucleotide ratio to favor production of the 6-TGN nucleotide. The 6-mercaptopurine dose ranged from 0.35 mg/kg to 0.61 mg/kg, although the study authors suggested lowering the dose to 25 mg daily for 4 weeks prior to initiating the allopurinol. Due to the risk for serious hematologic consequences, further research recommended be done prior to the adoption of this combination of therapies in clinical practice. (56)

Intolerance to 6-mercaptopurine does not necessarily mean that the same patient will be unable to be treated with azathioprine, although severe hematologic reactions and pancreatitis resulting from treatment with one of the agents usually precludes challenge with the other. A previous study suggested that patients with an intolerance to azathioprine could subsequently receive 6-mercaptopurine. (57) A practical option for patients who cannot tolerate thiopurines (both azathioprine and 6-mercaptopurine) is to try mycophenolate mofetil. In a case series of 70 patients, 24% achieved steroid-free remission for almost 3 years. (58)

13. Calcineurin inhibitors (Cyclosporine/Tacrolimus)

Clinical improvement usually occur within 1-4 weeks of treatment with calcineurin inhibitors and duration of therapy is 3-6 months. (59)

Cyclosporine has demonstrated efficacy in the treatment of severe steroid-refractory ulcerative colitis, but questions persist as to the long-term outcomes of those patients treated with the "salvage" agent. In a study of 75 patients, 79% avoided colectomy during their hospitalization; 56% were well at 6 months; and 45% were still well at a mean of 14.7 years later. Higher rates were seen among the 69 patients in the latter subset, with 80% initially avoiding colectomy, 73% well at 6 months, and 54% still well at a mean of 8.6 years later. (60-62)

Tacrolimus showed better results than cyclosporine as it has powerful immunosuppressant, 10 to 20 times greater than cyclosporine and it has consistent absorption even in the presence of gastrointestinal disease. Its intravenous dose 0.01-0.02 mg/kg/day and 0.1-0.2mg/kg/day orally. (63)

Prophylaxis against Pneumocystis carinii pneumonia is strongly recommended when using the calcineurin inhibitors. (64)

14. Anti-tumour necrosis factor therapy for ulcerative colitis

Infliximab therapy for ulcerative colitis showed modest steroid-free remission rate (21% at 6 months in the combined active ulcerative colitis trials ACT 1 and ACT 2). Nevertheless, subsequent analysis showed an associated reduction in colectomy,(65) but whether this benefit is maintained remains unclear. Outside of clinical trial settings, outpatient case series have reported colectomy rates of up to 50% after a median follow up of 13 months, (66) but lower rates in less refractory patients. Older patients and those who are perinuclear antineutrophil cytoplasmic antibody (p-ANCA) positive may respond less well.(67) A single series of 10 patients with ulcerative colitis who had lost response to infliximab were given adalimumab (160/80) in a 4-week open-label trial. Four patients improved, six did not respond, and of these, two went onto colectomy. (68) Phase III studies of adalimumab for ulcerative colitis are in progress. Infliximab for acute severe colitis is best considered separately, as is the question of whether to continue immunomodulators. The "real-world" experience with infliximab in ulcerative colitis seems to recapitulate efficacy results seen in the large clinical trials. (69)

15. Long-lasting clinical remission in patients with ulcerative colitis

The induction of an effective and long-lasting clinical remission, including tissue mucosal healing, is of the utmost importance in reducing the need for surgery and in lessening the incidence of dysplasia and cancer. Maintenance therapy should begin only after a patient has achieved a favorable clinical response to induction therapy. (70)
The US FDA has set the stage in adopting stringent criteria for clinical remission, including tissue healing with symptomatic improvement, for future clinical trials investigating the efficacy of medical therapies in patients with ulcerative colitis. This renewed standardization of controlled clinical trials will lead to the development of more effective therapies that improve patient outcome while potentially avoiding complications of long-standing ulcerative colitis. (71)

16. Acute severe ulcerative colitis

Intravenous corticosteroids remain the mainstay for acute severe colitis. In case of steroid refractory severe ulcerative colitis, the choice for rescue therapy in 2008 is between infliximab and calcineurin inhibitors (cyclosporine A or tacrolimus).(72) Controlled trials are needed, because case series report 20-75% coming to colectomy after infliximab for intravenous-steroid resistant ulcerative colitis.(73) Safety is a key factor, especially if surgery becomes necessary. While it is generally accepted that elective surgery in the presence of infliximab is safe, the same may not apply to emergency colectomy for acute severe colitis. Combination therapy in an attempt to avoid colectomy cannot be recommended. (74) The message should be to use objective indices that predict outcome at an early stage (on the third day of intravenous steroid treatment). A new index for patients with acute severe colitis has been developed and validated which depend on C-reactive protein and stool frequency. (75)

17. Surgery for ulcerative

Colectomy is an integral component of an overall therapeutic strategy. Patients with an ileal pouch anal anastomosis (IPAA) have a quality of life similar to patients with ulcerative colitis in remission or mild disease, although it depends on the measure used. (76) Complications of IPAA have been reviewed, but a common dilemma is the impact of pelvic surgery on fecundity and pregnancy on pouch function. Infertility rate was 12% before and 26% after IPAA among 945 patients in seven studies. No significant difference was seen in pouch function after vaginal delivery, but elective caesarean section for patients with a pouch tends to be favoured after discussion with the obstetrician and patient. (77)

18. Pouchitis

Pouchitis, a non-specific, idiopathic inflammation of the ileal reservoir, has become the most frequent long-term complication following pouch surgery for UC. The reported incidence of pouchitis is largely variable because of differences in nature and duration of the follow-up and, particularly, because a myriad of diagnostic criteria have been used to define this syndrome. Most patients who develop acute pouchitis do so within the first year, but some may suffer their first attack some years following surgery. (78)

Metronidazole appears to be an effective therapy for active chronic pouchitis. Bismuth carbomer foam enemas may not be an effective therapy for chronic active pouchitis. Oral probiotic therapy with VSL - 3 appears to be an effective therapy for maintaining remission in patients with chronic pouchitis in remission. There is no evidence of a difference in the maintenance of symptomatic remission in patients with chronic pouchitis treated with glutamine versus butyrate suppositories, and it is unknown whether glutamine and butyrate are equally effective or ineffective. Additional randomized, double - blind, placebo - controlled, dose - ranging clinical trials are needed to determine the efficacy of empiric medical therapies currently being used in patients with pouchitis. (79-81)

19. Novel therapies

Although conventional therapy accounts for the management of at least 90% of patients with ulcerative colitis, it is often new treatment that attracts attention. Therapeutic targets other than tumour necrosis factor (TNF) are sorely needed, since conventional therapy, however well used, is reaching its limits.(82)

Visilizumab; This anti-CD3 monoclonal antibody binding to activated T cells to induce apoptosis showed real promise as rescue therapy for intravenous steroid-resistant ulcerative colitis. The phase 1 dose-ranging study has been reported, but sadly the phase III study was suspended in 2007 when interim analysis showed no benefit.(83)

Phosphodiesterase 4 Inhibitor; Phosphodiesterase 4 is a key enzyme in cell homeostasis and inflammation, and its inhibition has been useful in rheumatoid arthritis and other diseases. A phase II study of tetomilast (OPC-6535) in 186 patients with active ulcerative colitis showed potential benefit in those with more active disease, but did not reach significance for remission or overall response.(84)

Phosphatidylcholine; Insufficient phosphatidylcholine in colonic mucus fits with current concepts of a primary defect in barrier function. Significantly more patients given phosphatidylcholine 2 g/day were able to stop steroids compared with placebo.(85)

Other Agents; Interferon-β still seeks a role for treating ulcerative colitis, although a case report describes the onset of the condition during treatment with interferon-β for multiple sclerosis. A similar disparity applies to rituximab, an anti-CD20-antibody that might inhibit B-cell-mediated destruction of epithelial cells. It is undergoing pilot studies in ulcerative colitis, but a case report describes disease exacerbation. Abatacept prevents T-cell activation by inhibiting costimulation through CD28 and worked in two animal models of colitis; it is undergoing clinical trials at present. (86)

20. IV Iron therapy for anaemia in ulcerative colitis

In most studies testing oral iron, 100–200 mg of ferrous salts (fumarate or sulphate) were administered. As only small amounts of iron are absorbed (10–30 mg) the majority of ingested iron passes along within the bowel content. (87) At sites of ulcers, the iron-rich luminal matter may increase the formation of hydroxyl radicals (by catalysing the Fenton reaction: $Fe^{2+} + H_2O_2 \rightarrow Fe^{3+} + OH^{\bullet} + OH^{-}$). The hydroxyl radical is the primary oxidizing species; it can be used to oxidize and break apart organic molecules and thereby may enhance tissue damage and disease activity of the underlying IBD. As this hypothesis is difficult to test in patients, it has been subject of several studies using animal model of IBD. (88) Many publications that tested the effect of iron on intestinal disease activity, oxidative stress or the degree of mucosal inflammation in rodent models of IBD. Although the experimental setting, the iron dose and the readout are quite diverse, these studies unanimously support the hypothesis of iron-induced hydroxyl radical generation in the inflamed tissue leading to worsening of intestinal inflammation and increased colon carcinogenesis. (89)

From eight studies that tested oral iron in IBD, intolerance was a common finding leading to discontinuation in up to 21%. Two studies using ferric iron reported fewer side effects despite good effectiveness. Some case–control studies saw similar intolerance to non-IBD patients in others the frequency and spectrum of side effects (increase in diarrhoea vs. constipation) was considerably different. A 15-year-old girl developed typical symptoms of UC after treatment of anaemia with ferrous sulphate. Recently, some worsening of proctosigmoiditis was demonstrated by rigid sigmoidoscoy. (90)

Intravenous iron therapy for IBD-associated anaemia has been suggested in the 1970s, but clinical trials have not been performed until the early 1990s. Studies during the last 10 years showed that IV iron polymaltose or iron sucrose appear effective and safe. Iron sucrose may be administered undiluted as a 100 mg slow intravenous injection over 2 to 5 minutes or as an infusion of 100 mg, diluted in a maximum of 100 mL of 0.9% NaCl over a period of at least 15 minutes per session for a total cumulative dose of 1000 mg within the 14 day period. There is limited experience with administration of an infusion of 500 mg iron sucrose diluted in a maximum of 250 mL of 0.9% NaCl, over a period of 3.5 to 4 hours on day 1 and day 14. Hypotension may occurred in up to 10% of patients treated.

Patients receiving regular parenteral iron therapy require monitoring of hematologic parameters and iron indices (Hb, Hct, transferrin saturation, and ferritin).

Sufficient IV iron should be administered to maintain transferrin saturation between 20% and 50%. Iron therapy should be withheld in patients with transferrin saturation ≥50%. Since transferrin saturation values increase rapidly after IV administration of iron sucrose, serum iron values may be reliably obtained 48 hours after IV iron sucrose dosing. (91,92)

21. Colorectal cancer in ulcerative colitis

There is no doubt that patients with ulcerative colitis have an increased risk for colorectal cancer, and that colorectal cancer remains an important cause of death in IBD patients. It is interesting to note that worldwide, ulcerative colitis related colorectal cancer rates seem to be diminishing, possibly due to the benefits of cancer surveillance programs, chemopreventive efforts, or to a changing risk-factor profile. Cancer surveillance colonoscopy programs have been in place for IBD patients for at least 30 years. Perhaps the efforts of gastroenterologists have been successful in decreasing cancer rates over that time period. It is encouraging to see that many patients with advanced neoplasia (high-grade dysplasia or cancer) have had earlier examinations where low-grade dysplasia was detected. Inflammation appears to be an important biological risk factor for the development of CRC. Clinically, duration and anatomic extent of colonic inflammation are the most important risk factors for CRC in chronic ulcerative colitis. Chronic inflammation increases oxidative stress; promotes repeated cycles of injury, regeneration, and repair; and accelerates the accumulation of oncogenic mutations. Over time, accumulation of these mutations may result in dysplasia, an unequivocal neoplastic change in the colon. With additional key mutations, dysplasia can transform into invasive colorectal cancer.(93) Other established risk factors include primary sclerosing cholangitis (PSC) (increases the relative risk of CRC 4.8-

fold compared with just chronic ulcerative colitis alone) and a family history of CRC (increases the risk of CRC 2.5-9.2 fold compared with chronic ulcerative colitis alone). (94) Other risk factors such as backwash ileitis and young age at diagnosis (in some studies) have been described; however, the clinical role of these factors remains to be determined. (95) Smoking reduces the risk of CRC in chronic ulcerative colitis by 50%, but increases the risk of CRC in Crohn's disease 4-fold. (96) Pseudopolyps also increase the risk of CRC in chronic ulcerative colitis, by 2.5-fold, perhaps either as a historical marker of more severe inflammation or because pseudopolyps may obscure the sensitivity of surveillance colonoscopy. (97)

The ultimate protective factor against the development of CRC in chronic ulcerative colitis is proctocolectomy for all patients, beginning 8-10 years after the onset of disease. The currently recommended strategy for preventing CRC in this setting is to perform regular surveillance colonoscopy in all patients beginning at 8-10 years after the onset of disease, with proctocolectomy reserved for those patients with histologic evidence of dysplasia on mucosal biopsies. A colectomy at the time of low-grade dysplasia detection would have prevented advanced neoplasia from developing. (98)

22. Chemoprevention

5-ASA agents; have been suggested to have chemopreventive properties because of their structural and partial functional relationship with aspirin. A 2005 meta-analysis of 9 observational studies identified a significant risk reduction associated with 5-ASA therapy, with the OR for dysplasia and colorectal cancer combined (ie, combined endpoint) at 51% in patients with ulcerative colitis. Although the existing evidence for the protective association between 5-ASA use and colorectal cancer or dysplasia is promising but inconclusive, the potential benefit is based on good clinical rationale, and given the excellent safety profile of this class of drugs, will likely encourage compliance with long-term prescribed therapy. (99)

Steroids, aspirin, NSAIDs. There are several studies that suggest steroids, aspirin, and NSAIDs may reduce the risk of CRC in chronic ulcerative colitis. Although the long-term use of these therapies is not routinely encouraged in this patient population, these data are helpful in suggesting that a common anti-inflammatory or anticancer mechanism shared with 5-ASA may be important. (100)

Immunomodulators; data regarding the effects of these agents on CRC risk are mixed. The reason for these observed differences may relate to differences in the molecular properties of immunomodulators compared with other anti-inflammatory therapies, differences in the reduction in inflammation or mucosal healing achieved with each medication, or differences in the neoplasia risk of the underlying population taking each medication. (101)

Ursodeoxycholic acid. The strongest for chemoprevention is for ursodeoxycholic acid in PSC-chronic ulcerative colitis patients reducing the risk of CRC by 80%. Ursodeoxycholic acid is an antioxidant that reduces the colonic concentration of the secondary bile acid deoxycholic acid, a carcinogen. (102)

Folate. In the setting of sporadic CRC, low folate levels have been associated with an increased risk of developing colorectal adenomas and carcinomas. Patients with IBD are at risk for low folate levels due to reduced intestinal absorption because of competitive inhibition from sulfasalazine use and because of folate loss due to active disease. Several case-control studies show a nonstatistical trend that patients with chronic ulcerative colitis who consume folate tend to have a reduced risk of CRC. Despite lack of definitive clinical evidence, many experts recommend folate supplementation in patients with long-standing chronic ulcerative colitis, on the basis of biological rationale and safety. (103,104)

5-ASA Formulation	Clinical Response	Induction Remission	Maintenance Remission	Mucosal Healing
Delayed and sustained release	+	+	+	+
Delayed release	+	-	+	-
Olsalazine	-	-	+	-
Balsalazide	+	-	-	-

Table 1. Proven efficacy of 5-ASA therapy in patients with ulcerative colitis

23. Pregnancy with ulcerative colitis

Fertility is affected in postsurgical ulcerative colitis. There are no increases in adverse outcomes with quiescent ulcerative colitis. Active disease at conception increases the risk for adverse outcomes. The majority of medications for ulcerative colitis are safe in pregnancy and breastfeeding as shown in table 2 and table 3. (105-109)

Category B Medications	Category C, D Medications	Contraindicated
Oral, topical mesalamine	Corticosteroids	Methotrexate
Sulfasalazine, olsalazine, balsalazide	Azathioprine	Thalidomide
Infliximab	6- mercaptopurine	
Ciprofloxacin, metronidazole (after first trimester)	Cyclosporine	
Loperamide	Diphenoxylate + atropine	

Table 2. Safety of IBD Medications During Pregnancy

Safe to Use When Indicated	Limited No Data	Contraindicated
Oral, topical mesalamine	Infliximab	Methotrexate
Sulfasalazine, olsalazine, balsalazide	Azathioprine	Thalidomide
Low doses of steroids (< 20 mg)	6- mercaptopurine	Cyclosporine

Table 3. Safety of IBD Medications During Breastfeeding

The indications for surgery during pregnancy are identical to those for nonpregnant patients, including obstruction, perforation, abscess, and hemorrhage. Although the obstetric indications for caesarean section do not differ in women with IBD, women with IBD undergo elective caesarean sections more frequently than do women in the normal population. (110)

24. Quality of living for patients with ulcerative colitis

Ulcerative colitis negatively affects physical and psychosocial well-being. Quality of Living is diminished in many patients with ulcerative colitis; strategies for improvement of Quality of Living must therefore be included in any therapeutic plan and there must be a multifaceted approach to improve Quality of Living. (111)
Disease activity seems to be the principal factor affecting Quality of Living. Identifying other potential factors that have a negative impact on Quality of Living is vital in order to achieve therapeutic success. Although drug therapy for ulcerative colitis is effective in achieving and maintaining remission, medication nonadherence remains a considerable obstacle, especially in quiescent disease. Patient-physician communication is crucial for successful management of patients with ulcerative colitis. Ultimately, choosing a therapy that is convenient, effective, and safe will help improve adherence, maintain remission, and potentially decrease the need for surgery or development of colorectal cancer. (112,113)

25. References

[1] Binder V. Clinical epidemiology - how important now? Gut. 2005;54:574-575.
[2] Loftus EV. Clinical epidemiology of inflammatory bowel disease: incidence, prevalence and environmental influences. Gastroenterology. 2004;126:1504-1517.
[3] Hanauer SB. Inflammatory bowel disease: epidemiology, pathogenesis and therapeutic opportunities. Inflamm Bowel Dis. 2006;12:S3-9.
[4] Birrenbach T, Bocker U. Inflammatory bowel disease and smoking. A review of the epidemiology, pathophysiology and therapeutic implications Inflamm Bowel Dis. 2004;10:848-859.
[5] Anderson RE, Olaison G, Tysk C, Ekbom A. Appendectomy and protection against ulcerative colitis. N Engl J Med. 2001;344:808-814.
[6] Gasche C, Grundtner P. Genotypes and phenotypes in Crohn's disease: Do they help in clinical management? Gut. 2005;54:162-167.
[7] Newman B and Siminovitch KA. Recent advances in the genetics of inflammatory bowel disease. Curr Opin Gastroenterol 2005. 21: 401–407
[8] Barnich N et al. GRIM-19 interacts with nucleotide oligomerization domain 2 and serves as downstream effector of anti-bacterial function in intestinal epithelial cells. J Biol Chem 2005. 280: 19021–19026
[9] Kobayashi KS et al. Nod2-dependent regulation of innate and adaptive immunity in the intestinal tract. Science 2005. 307: 731–734
[10] Noble CL et al. The contribution of OCTN1/2 variants within the IBD5 locus to disease susceptibility and severity in Crohn's disease. Gastroenterology 2005. 129: 1854–1864
[11] Stoll M et al. Genetic variation in DLG5 is associated with inflammatory bowel disease. Nat Genet 2005. 36: 476–480.
[12] Ho GT et al. Allelic variations of the multidrug resistance gene determine susceptibility and disease behavior in ulcerative colitis. Gastroenterology 2005. 128: 288–296.
[13] Farrell RJ, Peppercorn MA. Endoscopy in inflammatory bowel disease. In: Sartor RB, Sandborn WJ, eds. Kirsner's Inflammatory Bowel Disease. 6th ed. Philadelphia: WB Saunders; 2004:380-398.

[14] Lois A, Waldleigh F, Neri B. Development of a hybrid algorithm based on learning classifiers that improves diagnosis of inflammatory bowel disease and differentiation between Crohn's and ulcerative colitis in a multi-marker system. Gastroenterology. 2006;130:Abstract M 1198.
[15] Krok K, Lichtenstein GR. Inflammatory bowel disease. In: Ginsberg GG, Kochman ML, Norton I, Gostout CJ. Clinical Gastrointestinal Endoscopy. Philadelphia: Elsevier-Saunders; 2005:311-332.
[16] Lo SK, Mehdizadeh S. Therapeutic uses of double-balloon enteroscopy. Gastrointest Endosc Clin N Am. 2006;16:363-376.
[17] Lashner BA. Sensitivity-specificity trade-off for capsule endoscopy in IBD: Is it worth it? Am J Gastroenterol. 2006;101:965-966.
[18] Dubinsky MC, Ofman JJ, Urman M, Targan SR, Seidman EG. Clinical utility of serodiagnostic testing in suspected pediatric inflammatory bowel disease. Am J Gastroenterol. 2001;96:758-765.
[19] Targan SR, Landers CJ, Yang H, et al. Antibodies to CBir1 flagellin define a unique response that is associated independently with complicated Crohn's disease. Gastroenterology. 2005;128:2020-2028.
[20] Peeters M, Joossens S, Vermeire S, Viietinck R, Bossuyt X, Rutgeerts P. Diagnostic value of anti-Saccharomyces Cervesiae and antineutrophil cytoplasmic autoantibodies in inflammatory bowel disease. Am J Gastroenterol. 2001;96:730-734.
[21] Matsui T, Yao T, Sakurai T, et al. Clinical features and pattern of indeterminate colitis: Crohn's disease with ulcerative colitis-like clinical presentation. J Gastroenterol. 2003;38:647-655.
[22] Abdelrazeq AS, Wilson TR, Leitch DL, et al. Ileitis in ulcerative colitis: is it a backwash? Dis Colon Rectum. 2005;48:1542-1549.
[23] Odze RD, Greenson JK. Inflammatory diseases of the large intestine. In: Odze RD, Goldblum JR, Crawford JM, eds. Surgical Pathology of the GI Tract, Liver, Biliary Tract, and Pancreas. Philadelphia, PA: Saunders; 2004:213-246.
[24] Silverberg MS, Satsangi J, Ahmad T, et al. Toward an integrated clinical, molecular and serological classification of inflammatory bowel disease: Report of a Working Party of the 2005 Montreal World Congress of Gastroenterology. Can J Gastroenterol 2005; 19 (Suppl. A): 5–36.
[25] Satsangi J, Silverberg MS, Vermeire S, Colombel JF. The Montreal classification of inflammatory bowel disease: controversies, consensus, and implications. Gut 2006; 55: 749–53.
[26] Carvalho RS, Abadom V, Dilworth HP, Thompson R, Oliva-Hemker M, Cuffari C. Indeterminate colitis: a significant subgroup of pediatric IBD. Inflamm Bowel Dis 2006; 12: 258–62.
[27] Sandborn WJ, Hanauer SB. Systematic review: the pharmacokinetic profiles of oral mesalazine formulations and mesalazine pro-drugs used in the management of ulcerative colitis. Aliment Pharmacol Ther. 2003;17:29-42.
[28] Prescribing information for Pentasa (mesalamine). Wayne, Pa: Shire USA Inc. Package Insert 2005.
[29] Hanauer SB, Sandborn WJ, Kornbluth A, et al. Delayed-release oral mesalamine at 4.8 g/day (800 mg tablet) for the treatment of moderately active ulcerative colitis: The ASCEND II trial. Am J Gastroenterol. 2005;100:2478-2485.

[30] Marakhouski Y, Fixa B, Holoman J, et al; The International Salofalk Study Group. A double-blind dose-escalating trial comparing novel mesalazine pellets with mesalazine tablets in active ulcerative colitis.[erratum appears in Aliment Pharmacol Ther. 2005;21(6):793]. Aliment Pharmacol Ther. 2005;21:133-140.
[31] Rubin DT, LoSavio A, Yadron N, Huo D, Hanauer SB. Aminosalicylate therapy in the prevention of dysplasia and colorectal cancer in ulcerative colitis. Clin Gastroenterol Hepatol. 2006;4:1346-1350.
[32] Kane SV, Cohen RD, Aikens JE, Hanauer SB. Prevalence of nonadherence with maintenance mesalamine in quiescent ulcerative colitis. Am J Gastroenterol. 2001;96:2929-2933.
[33] Kane S, Huo D, Magnanti K. A pilot feasibility study of once daily dosing versus conventional dosing mesalamine for maintenance of ulcerative colitis. Clin Gastroenterol Hepatol. 2003;1:170-173.
[34] Sandborn WJ. Treatment of ulcerative colitis with mesalamine: advances in drug formulation, efficacy expectations and dose response, compliance, and chemoprevention. Rev Gastroenterol Disord. 2006;6:97-105.
[35] Kamm MA, Sandborn WJ, Gassull M, et al. Once-daily high concentration MMX mesalamine in active ulcerative colitis. Gastroenterology. 2007;132:66-75.
[36] Lichtenstein GR, Kamm MA, Boddu P, et al. Effect of once- or twice-daily MMX mesalamine (SPD476) for the induction of remission of mild to moderately active ulcerative colitis. Clin Gastroenterol Hepatol. 2007;5:95-102.
[37] Ghosh S, Mitchell R. Results of the European Federation of Crohn's and Colitis Associations (EFCCA) patient survey: prevalence and impact on quality of life. J Crohn's Colitis (in press).
[38] Dignass A, Vermeire S, Adamek H, et al. Improved remission rates from once- versus twice-daily mesalazine (Pentasa®) granules for the maintenance of remission in ulcerative colitis: results from a multinational randomised controlled trial [abstract]. Gut 2007; 56 (Suppl III):A46.
[39] Kamm MA, Sandborn WJ, Gassull M, et al. Once-daily, high-concentration MMX mesalamine in active ulcerative colitis. Gastroenterology 2007; 132:66-75.
[40] Lichtenstein G, Kamm M, Boddu P, et al. Effect of once- or twice-daily MMX mesalamine (SPD476) for the induction of remission of mild to moderately active ulcerative colitis. Clin Gastroenterol Hepatol 2007; 5:95-102.
[41] Sandborn WJ, Kamm MA, Lichtenstein GR, et al. MMX Multi Matrix System mesalazine for the induction of remission in patients with mild-to-moderate ulcerative colitis: a combined analysis of two randomized, double-blind, placebo-controlled trials. Aliment Pharmacol Ther 2007; 26:205-215.
[42] Kamm MA, Lichtenstein GR, Sandborn WJ, et al. Randomised trial of once- or twice-daily MMX™ mesalazine for maintenance of remission in ulcerative colitis. Gut 2008; 13 February [Epub ahead of print].
[43] Kruis W, Gorelov A, Kiudelis G, et al. Once daily dosing of 3 g mesalamine (Salofalk granules) is therapeutic equivalent to a three-times daily dosing of 1 g mesalamine for the treatment of active ulcerative colitis [abstract]. Gastroenterology 2007; 132 (Suppl 4):A-130.
[44] Hanauer SB, Sandborn WJ, Dallaire C, et al. Delayed-release oral mesalamine 4.8 g/day (800 mg tablets) compared to 2.4 g/day (400 mg tablets) for the treatment of mildly

to moderately active ulcerative colitis: the ASCEND I trial. Can J Gastroenterol 2007; 21:827-834.
[45] Safdi AV, Cohen RD. Review article: increasing the dose of oral mesalazine therapy for active ulcerative colitis does not improve remission rates. Aliment Pharmacol Ther 2007; 26:1179-1186.
[46] Eliakim R, Tulassay Z, Kupcinskas L, et al. Clinical trial: randomized-controlled clinical study comparing the efficacy and safety of a low-volume vs. a high-volume mesalazine foam in active distal ulcerative colitis. Aliment Pharmacol Ther 2007; 26:1237-1249.
[47] Kornbluth A, Sachar DB. Ulcerative practice guidelines in adults (update): American College of Gastroenterology Practice Parameters Committee. Am J Gastroenterol 2004;99:1371–85.
[48] Lichtenstein GR, Abreu MT, Cohen T, et al. For the American Gastroenterological Association. American Gastroenterological Association Institute technical review on corticosteroids, immunomodulators, and infliximab in inflammatory bowel disease. Gastroenterology 2006;130:940–87.
[49] Faubion WA, Loftus EV, Harmsen WS, et al. The natural history of corticosteroid therapy for inflammatory bowel disease: A population-based study. Gastroenterology 2001;121:255–60.
[50] Yang YX, Lichtenstein GR. Corticosteroids in Crohn's disease. Am J Gastroenterol 2002;97:803–23.
[51] D'Ascenzo M, Antonelli A, Chiarantini L, et al. Red blood cells as a glucocorticoids delivery system. In: Sprandel U, Way JL, eds. Erythrocytes as drug carriers in medicine. New York, NY: Plenum Press, 1997:81–8.
[52] Rossi L, Serafini S, Generini L, et al. Erythrocyte-mediated delivery of dexamethasone in patients with chronic obstructive pulmonary disease. Biotechnol Appl Biochem 2001;33:85–9.
[53] Rossi L, Castro M, D'Orio F, et al. Low doses of dexamethasone constantly delivered by autologous erythrocytes slow progression of lung disease in cystic fibrosis patients. Blood Cells Mol Dis 2004;33:57–63.
[54] Timmer A, McDonald JW, Macdonald JK. Azathioprine and 6-mercaptopurine for maintenance of remission in ulcerative colitis. Cochrane Database Syst Rev 2007; (1):CD000478.
[55] Chande N, MacDonald JK, McDonald JW. Methotrexate for induction of remission in ulcerative colitis. Cochrane Database Syst Rev 2007; (4):CD006618.
[56] Yip JS, Woodward M, Abreu MT, Sparrow MP. How are azathioprine and 6-mercaptopurine dosed by gastroenterologists? Results of a survey of clinical practice. Inflamm Bowel Dis 2008; 14:514-518.
[57] Sparrow MP, Hande SA, Friedman S, et al. Effect of allopurinol on clinical outcomes in inflammatory bowel disease nonresponders to azathioprine or 6-mercaptopurine. Clin Gastroenterol Hepatol 2007; 5:209-214.
[58] Palaniappan S, Ford AC, Greer D, et al. Mycophenolate mofetil therapy for refractory inflammatory bowel disease. Inflamm Bowel Dis 2007; 13:1488-1492.
[59] Loftus CG, Egan LJ, Sandborn WJ. Cyclosporine, tacrolimus, and mycophenolate mofetil in the treatment of inflammatory bowel disease. Gastroenterol Clin North Am 2004; 33: 141-69.

[60] Sandborn W. A critical review of cyclosporine therapy in inflammatory bowel disease. Inflamm Bowel Dis 1995; 1: 48-63.
[61] Sandborn WJ, Present DH, Isaacs KL, et al. Tacrolimus for the treatment of fistulas in patients with Crohn's disease: a randomized, placebo-controlled trial. Gastroenterology 2003; 125: 380-8.
[62] Ierardi E, Principi M, Francavilla R, et al. Oral tacrolimus long-term therapy in patients with Crohn's disease and steroid resistance. Aliment Pharmacol Ther 2001; 15: 371-7.
[63] Gonzalez Lama Y, Abreu LE, Vera MI, et al. Long-term oral tacrolimus therapy in refractory to infliximab fistulizing Crohn's disease. Inflamm Bowel Dis 2005; 111: 8-15.
[64] Baumgart DC, Wiedenmann B, Dignass AU. Rescue therapy with tacrolimus is effective in patients with severe and refractory inflammatory bowel disease. Aliment Pharmacol Ther 2003; 17: 1273-81.
[65] Sandborn WJ, Rutgeerts P, Feagan BG, et al. Infliximab reduces colectomy in patients with moderate-to-severe ulcerative colitis: colectomy analysis from ACT1 and ACT 2 [abstract]. Gut 2007; 56(Suppl III):A26.
[66] Jakobovits SL, Jewell DP, Travis SP. Infliximab for the treatment of ulcerative colitis: outcomes in Oxford from 2000 to 2006. Aliment Pharmacol Ther 2007; 25:1055-1060.
[67] Ferrante M, Vermeire S, Katsanos KH, et al. Predictors of early response to infliximab in patients with ulcerative colitis. Inflamm Bowel Dis 2007; 13:123-128.
[68] Peyrin-Biroulet L, Laclotte C, Roblin X, Bigard MA. Adalimumab induction therapy for ulcerative colitis with intolerance or lost response to infliximab: an open-label study. World J Gastroenterol 2007; 13:2328-2332.
[69] Regueiro M, Curtis J, Plevy S. Infliximab for hospitalized patients with severe ulcerative colitis. J Clin Gastroenterol 2006; 40:476-481.
[70] Cuffari C, Bayless TM, Hanauer SB, Lichtenstein G, Present DH. Optimizing therapy in patients with pancolitis. IBD. 2005;11:937-946.
[71] Hanauer S. Medical therapy for ulcerative colitis. In: Sartor R, Sandborn W, eds. Kirsner's Inflammatory Bowel Diseases. Sixth ed. Philadelphia, Pa: WB Saunders; 2004:503-530.
[72] Su C, Lewis JD, Goldberg B, et al. A meta-analysis of the placebo rates of remission and response in clinical trials of active ulcerative colitis. Gastroenterology 2007; 132:516-526.
[73] D'Haens G, Sandborn WJ, Feagan BG, et al. A review of activity indices and efficacy end points for clinical trials of medical therapy in adults with ulcerative colitis. Gastroenterology 2007; 132:763-786.
[74] Jess T, Riis L, Vind I, et al. Changes in clinical characteristics, course, and prognosis of inflammatory bowel disease during the last 5 decades: a population-based study from Copenhagen, Denmark. Inflamm Bowel Dis 2007; 13:481-489.
[75] Hoie O, Wolters FL, Riis L, et al. Low colectomy rates in ulcerative colitis in an unselected European cohort followed for 10 years. Gastroenterology 2007; 132:507-515.
[76] Roberts SE, Williams JG, Yeates D, Goldacre MJ. Mortality in patients with and without colectomy admitted to hospital for ulcerative colitis and Crohn's disease: record linkage studies. BMJ 2007; 335:1033.

[77] Society for Surgery of the Alimentary Tract. SSAT patient care guidelines: management of ulcerative colitis. J Gastrointest Surg 2007; 11:1203-1206.
[78] Stack WA, Long RG, Hawkey CJ. Short- and long-term outcome of patients treated with cyclosporin for severe acute ulcerative colitis. Aliment Pharmacol Ther 1998;12:973–8.
[79] Leijonmarck CE, Brostrom O, Monsen U, et al. Surgical treatment of ulcerative colitis in Stockholm County, 1955 to 1984. Dis Colon Rectum 1989;32:918–26.
[80] Stahlberg D, Gullberg K, Liljeqvist L, et al. Pouchitis following pelvic pouch operation for ulcerative colitis. Incidence, cumulative risk, and risk factors. Dis Colon Rectum 1996;39:1012–18.
[81] Korsgen S, Keighley MR. Causes of failure and life expectancy of the ileoanal pouch. Int J Colorectal Dis 1997;12:4–8.
[82] Musch E, Andus T, Malek M, et al. Successful treatment of steroid refractory active ulcerative colitis with natural interferon-beta: an open long-term trial. Z Gastroenterol 2007; 45:1235-1240.
[83] Plevy S, Salzberg B, Van Assche G, et al. A phase I study of visilizumab, a humanized anti-CD3 monoclonal antibody, in severe steroid-refractory ulcerative colitis. Gastroenterology 2007; 133:1414-1422.
[84] Schreiber S, Keshavarzian A, Isaacs KL, et al. A randomized, placebo-controlled, phase II study of tetomilast in active ulcerative colitis. Gastroenterology 2007; 132:76-86.
[85] Stremmel W, Ehehalt R, Autschbach F, Karner M. Phosphatidylcholine for steroid-refractory chronic ulcerative colitis: a randomized trial. Ann Intern Med 2007; 147:603-610.
[86] Yang X, Stetsko D, Xie J, et al. Targeting T-cell costimulation with abatacept is effective in TNBS-induced colitis [abstract]. Gastroenterology 2007; 132:A153.
[87] Carrier JC, Aghdassi E, Jeejeebhoy K, Allard JP. Exacerbation of dextran sulfate sodium-induced colitis by dietary iron supplementation: role of NF-kappaB. Int J Colorectal Dis 2006; 21: 381–7.
[88] Erichsen K, Milde AM, Arslan G, et al. Low-dose oral ferrous fumarate aggravated intestinal inflammation in rats with DSS-induced colitis. Inflamm Bowel Dis 2005; 11: 744–8.
[89] Seril DN, Liao J, Yang CS, Yang GY. Systemic iron supplementation replenishes iron stores without enhancing colon carcinogenesis in murine models of ulcerative colitis: comparison with iron-enriched diet. Dig Dis Sci 2005; 50: 696–707.
[90] de Silva AD, Tsironi E, Feakins RM, Rampton DS. Efficacy and tolerability of oral iron therapy in inflammatory bowel disease: a prospective, comparative trial. Aliment Pharmacol Ther 2005; 22: 1097–105
[91] Schroder O, Mickisch O, Seidler U, et al. Intravenous iron sucrose vs. oral iron supplementation for the treatment of iron deficiency anemia in patients with inflammatory bowel disease–a randomized, controlled, open-label, multicenter study. Am J Gastroenterol 2005; 100: 2503–9.
[92] Erichsen K, Ulvik RJ, Nysaeter G, et al. Oral ferrous fumarate or intravenous iron sucrose for patients with inflammatory bowel disease. Scand J Gastroenterol 2005; 40: 1058–65.
[93] Eaden JA, Abrams KR, Mayberry JF. The risk of colorectal cancer in ulcerative colitis: a meta-analysis. Gut. 2001;48:526-535.

[94] Ekbom A, Helmick C, Zack M, Adami HO. Ulcerative colitis and colorectal cancer. A population-based study. N Engl J Med. 1990;323:1228-1233.
[95] Winther KV, Jess T, Langholz E, Munkholm P, Binder V. Long-term risk of cancer in ulcerative colitis: a population-based cohort study from Copenhagen County. Clin Gastroenterol Hepatol. 2004;2:1088-1095.
[96] Jess T, Loftus EV Jr, Velayos FS, et al. Risk of intestinal cancer in inflammatory bowel disease: a population-based study from Olmsted County, Minnesota. Gastroenterology. 2006;130:1039-1046.
[97] Munkholm P, Loftus EV, Reinacher-Schick A, et al. Prevention of colorectal cancer in inflammatory bowel disease: value of screening and 5-aminosalicylates. Digestion. 2006;73:11-19.
[98] Delaunoit T, Limburg PJ, Goldberg RM, Lymp JF, Loftus EV Jr. Colorectal cancer prognosis among patients with inflammatory bowel disease. Clin Gastroenterol Hepatol. 2006;4:335-342.
[99] van Staa,TP, Card T, Logan RF, Leufkens HG. 5-Aminosalicylate use and colorectal cancer risk in inflammatory bowel disease: a large epidemiological study. Gut. 2005;54:1573-1578.
[100] Bernstein CN, Blanchard JF, Metge C, Yogendran M. Does the use of 5-aminosalicylates in inflammatory bowel disease prevent the development of colorectal cancer? Am J Gastroenterol. 2003;98:2784-2788.
[101] Matula S Croog V, Itzkowitz S, et al. Chemoprevention of colorectal neoplasia in ulcerative colitis: the effect of 6-mercaptopurine. Clin Gastroenterol Hepatol. 2005;3:1015-1021.
[102] Tung BY, Emond MJ, Haggitt RC, et al. Ursodiol use is associated with lower prevalence of colonic neoplasia in patients with ulcerative colitis and primary sclerosing cholangitis. Ann Intern Med. 2001;134:89-95.
[103] Lashner BA, Heidenreich PA, Su GL, Kane SV, Hanauer SB. Effect of folate supplementation on the incidence of dysplasia and cancer in chronic ulcerative colitis. A case-control study. Gastroenterology. 1989;97:255-259.
[104] Lashner BA, Provencher KS, Seidner DL, Knesebeck A, Brzezinski A. The effect of folic acid supplementation on the risk for cancer or dysplasia in ulcerative colitis. Gastroenterology. 1997;112:29-32.
[105] Korelitz BI. Inflammatory bowel disease and pregnancy. In Pregnancy and Gastro-intestinal disorders. Gastroenterol Clin North Am. 1998;27:213-224.
[106] Baird DD, Narendranathan M, Sandler RS. Increased risk of preterm birth for women with inflammatory bowel disease. Gastroenterology. 1990;9:987-994.
[107] Mayberry JF, Weterman IT. European survey of fertility and pregnancy in women with Crohn's disease: A case control study by European collaborative group. Gut. 1986;27:821-825.
[108] Olsen KO, Berndtsson I, Oresland T, et al. Ulcerative colitis: Female fecundity before diagnosis, during disease, and after surgery compared with a population sample. Gastroenterology. 2002;122:15-19.
[109] Johnson P, Richard C, Ravid A, et al. Female fertility after ileal pouch-anal anastomosis for ulcerative colitis. Dis Colon Rectum. 2004;47:1119-1126.
[110] Nielsen OH, Andreasson B, Bondensen S, et al. Pregnancy in ulcerative colitis. Scand J Gastroenterol. 1983;18:735-742.

[111] Irvine EJ. Quality of life of patients with ulcerative colitis: past, present, and future. Inflamm Bowel Dis. 2008;14:554-565.
[112] Langhorst J, Mueller T, Luedtke R, et al. Effects of a comprehensive lifestyle modification program on quality-of-life in patients with ulcerative colitis: a twelve-month follow-up. Scand J Gastroenterol. 2007;42:734-745.
[113] Larsson K, Loof L, Ronnblom A, Nordin K. Quality of life for patients with exacerbation in inflammatory bowel disease and how they cope with disease activity. J Psychosom Res. 2008;64:139-148.

10

Current and Novel Treatments for Ulcerative Colitis

Cuong D. Tran, Rosa Katsikeros and Suzanne M. Abimosleh
Gastroenterology Unit, Women's and Children's Health Network, North Adelaide
Discipline of Physiology, School of Medical Sciences, University of Adelaide
Australia

1. Introduction

Ulcerative colitis and Crohn's disease are defined by a common term of inflammatory bowel disease. These chronic diseases result in significant morbidity and mortality. While there are no cures for these diseases, the last two decades have been a period of major advancement in our understanding of the biology of intestinal inflammation. This can be attributed to a steadily increasing number of experimental animal models with some clinical manifestation similar to those observed in human inflammatory bowel disease. These experimental animal models have also contributed greatly to our current understanding of the immunological, pathological and physiological features of chronic intestinal inflammation. However, specific causes of ulcerative colitis and Crohn's disease remain unknown. Conventional treatments for the disease include corticosteroids and immunosuppressives, however treatments in many patients are not entirely effective with many therapies associated with significant adverse effects. Thus, treatments that are effective and have little or no side effects remain an unmet need. There are numerous emerging therapeutic strategies which may be useful in the alleviation of chronic intestinal inflammation and this chapter will focus on novel therapies that may be effective for ulcerative colitis in the future.

2. Etiology of ulcerative colitis

While the precise etiology of inflammatory bowel disease is unknown, genetic susceptibility, environmental factors, impaired barrier function, imbalances or disruption to the commensal host microflora and an abnormal intestinal immune response are thought to play an important role in its manifestation.

2.1 The immune response

It is clear that not one single component of inflammatory bowel disease pathogenesis can trigger and maintain the disease. Understanding mucosal immunity in Crohn's disease and ulcerative colitis is fundamental in unraveling the complex mechanisms of chronic gut inflammation which can then provide some insight into the treatment of inflammatory bowel disease. The immune response is divided into two components, innate immunity and adaptive immunity.

2.2 Innate immunity

In the normal intestine, macrophages are conditioned by the mucosal microenvironment to express a non-inflammatory phenotype which is translated by a down-regulated expression of innate immunity receptors and constrained production of pro-inflammatory cytokines (1). In contrast, in inflammatory bowel disease-affected intestinal tissue, macrophages newly recruited from the peripheral blood still express monoctyic CD14 markers but are primed for the production of various pro-inflammatory cytokines such as interleukin (IL)1α, IL1β, and tumour necrosis factor (TNF)α (2-3). It has been reported that in Crohn's disease these $CD14^+$ pro-inflammatory macrophages are increased and subsequently result in more IL23 and TNFα production compared to controls and ulcerative colitis and contribute to the production of interferon (IFN)γ by T cells (4).
Intestinal dendritic cells (DC) are antigen-presenting cells involved in the initiation and regulation of local innate immune response but also play a role in adaptive immunity (5). Similar to macrophages, their function is dependent on the mucosal microenvironment and function to provide protection and defense, induce tolerance or mediate inflammation (6). It has been shown that in inflammatory bowel disease, intestinal DC is activated, increasing the expression of microbial receptors and production of pro-inflammatory cytokines like IL12 and IL6 (7).

2.3 Adaptive immunity

B cell immunity

There is limited focus given to B cell immunity in inflammatory bowel disease even though in active inflammatory bowel disease there is antibody production and secretion of immunoglobulin (Ig)M, IgG and IgA, by both peripheral blood and mucosal mononuclear cells (8). The patterns of antibody class production differ in ulcerative colitis and Crohn's disease; in ulcerative colitis there is a disproportional increase in IgG1 secretion, whereas in Crohn's disease IgG1, IgG2 and IgG3 are increased compared to control cells (9).

T cell immunity

There has been a considerable increase in our understanding of adaptive immunity since the identification of $CD4^+$ T helper 1 (Th1) and T helper 2 (Th2) subsets in mice (10) and humans (11). The T cell immunity field is still evolving and in addition to IFNγ-producing Th1 cells and IL4, IL5 and IL13-producing Th2 cells, new Th subsets have been identified including IL17 producing Th17 cells (12) and dual IFNγ- and IL17-producing Th17 cells (13). More recently, two new subsets of $CD4^+$ effector Th cells have been described, Th9 and Th22, however, their function are not clearly understood (14). Furthermore, Cosmi et al. (15) reported that Th cells can produce both IL17 and IL4 which is a dual Th17 and Th2-mediated immune response.
In addition to Th cells, another major subset is made up of T regulatory (Treg) cells whose function is to monitor the immune response and prevent an excessive and potentially harmful immune response (16-17). It has been speculated that Th17 and Treg cells share common pathways, suggesting developmental and functional links between Treg and Th17 cells (18-19). Regulatory T cells are accepted to be key players in the maintenance of tolerance and prevention of autoimmunity (20). Of particular interest are the $CD4^+$ CD25bright $Foxp3^+$ Regulatory T cell (Treg), where mutations of the transcription factor Foxp3, crucial in the development and function of Tregs, manifest in multiple autoimmune

diseases in both mice and humans (21). In both cases a severe early onset of inflammatory bowel disease is observed as part of the pathology. A deficiency of number and/or function of Tregs are also seen in other autoimmune diseases including multiple sclerosis and systemic lupus, and the transfer of Tregs has been shown to treat experimental murine colitis and type 1 diabetes.

The Th17 effector cell is a relatively new effector cell lineage distinct from the Th1/Th2 dichotomy, and is driven by the transcription factor retinoic acid-related orphan receptor-γt, (RORγt). Th17 cells secrete predominately IL17 and potentially provide critical protection against fungi and extra cellular bacteria which are not covered by Th1/Th2 immunity (22). There is good evidence that Crohn's disease has a dominant Th1 component as shown by an elevated production of IFNγ and IL12 by lamina propria mononuclear cells (23-24). As well there is an increased production of IL-17 by Th17 cells and dual IFNγ- and IL17-producing mucosal Th cells (13, 25). In contrast, ulcerative colitis is considered an atypical Th2 response based on studies demonstrating increased IL5 and IL13 production of Th cells and also IL13 by natural killer (NK) T cells in the inflamed mucosa (26). The increased production of IL13 has been shown to induce cytotoxicity and apoptosis and impair mucosal barrier function (27), which may be a contributor to the overall pathogenesis of ulcerative colitis.

3. Characteristics of ulcerative colitis

The remainder of the chapter will focus on animal models of ulcerative colitis and novel therapeutic approaches in treating this condition. The clinical symptoms of ulcerative colitis consist of severe abdominal pain and increased frequency of bloody diarrhoea. Unlike Crohn's disease, ulcerative colitis is characterized by inflammation contained to the large intestine, which affects only the mucosal layer and is superficial in comparison to the inflammation seen in Crohn's disease. Inflammation commonly extends proximally from the rectum, and extensive superficial ulceration is typical (28). Inflammation is accompanied by ulceration, edema, and hemorrhage along the length of the colon. Complications of ulcerative colitis differ from Crohn's disease, with increased risk of perforation, toxic megacolon and a higher incidence of bowel cancer. Histopathological features include the presence of neutrophil infiltrates which form crypt abscesses (29).

4. Animal models of experimental ulcerative colitis

Even with a wealth of information on the etiology of ulcerative colitis there is still no cure. As a consequence numerous animal models of ulcerative colitis have been established to elucidate the potential mechanism of ulcerative colitis and to develop therapeutic strategies within the preclinical phase.

5. Chemical-induced colitis

5.1 Dextran Sulphate Sodium(DSS)-induced colitis

Features of DSS-induced colitis

The DSS model of experimental colitis (30) is one of the most popular and widely utilized and characterized animal models of ulcerative colitis. DSS is a synthetic sulphated polysaccharide composed of dextran and sulphated anhydroglucose unit (31).

Supplementing the drinking water of rodents with low molecular weight DSS (54,000 mol. wt.) results in histopathological and symptomatic features resembling ulcerative colitis (31-32). Histologically, DSS-induced colitis resembles the damage manifested in human ulcerative colitis patients with an inflammatory response consistent with human inflammatory bowel disease (33). DSS administration also produces visual signs of disease activity including rectal bleeding, weight loss and diarrhea (32), all common features of ulcerative colitis.

The DSS-induced ulcerative colitis model has been well characterized morphologically and biochemically (34-35). After a four-day treatment with 3% DSS in the drinking water, mice show signs of acute colitis including weight loss, bloody stools, and diarrhoea (34). Histologically, DSS produces submucosal erosions, ulceration, inflammatory cell infiltration and crypt abscesses as well as epithelioglandular hyperplasia (35). The luminal bacteria in the colon induce the production of the inflammatory cytokines, IL6 and TNFα, which cause colitis. The damage induced by DSS has been reported to affect the distal colon and caecum preferentially, with lesser damage evident in the proximal colon (32). This model is particularly useful to study the contribution of the innate immune mechanism towards colitis as well as for the study of epithelial repair mechanisms.

Mechanism of action

The mouse model of colitis induced by DSS histologically resembles human ulcerative colitis, and although the exact mechanism of DSS-induced mucosal injury is not fully understood, a topical toxic effect of DSS on the colonic epithelial cells has been proposed (36). This results in loss of barrier function which would likely result in an increased uptake of luminal antigens (bacteria and bacterial products) as well as activation of lamina propria immune cells and the inflammatory response (37). It has been reported that DSS-induced colitis alters the tight junction complex resulting in the loss of barrier function thereby facilitating the development of the inflammatory infiltrate and development of intestinal inflammation (38).

Chronic model of DSS-induced colitis

DSS is commonly administered in a dose range of 3-10% for 7-10 days to induce an acute inflammation depending on the susceptibility of the species or the molecular weight of DSS (39). The DSS-induced acute colitis model may be extrapolated to a chronic colitis model by simply prolonging the administration of DSS. It has been suggested that to induce chronicity, DSS is normally administered in three to five cycles with a 1- to 2-week rest between cycles (40-41). This is useful in understanding disease progression as well as pathological inflammatory changes observed in ulcerative colitis. Interestingly, in inbred rats administered 5% DSS for 215 days, intestinal tumors (adenomas, adenocarcinomas as well as papillomas) were seen (42) predominantly in the colon and caecum.

5.2 2, 4, 6-Trinitrobenzene sulfonic acid (TNBS)-induced colitis

Features of TNBS-induced colitis

Another model that has been used widely is the well characterized haptene reagent TNBS-induced colitis. This model of chronic colitis also resembles human ulcerative colitis in its various histological features including infiltration of colonic mucosa by neutrophils and macrophages. There is also increased production of inflammatory mediators including Th1 profile of cytokines (IFNγ, TNFα and IL12) resulting in substantial inflammation and tissue injury (43). Studies (44-45) have indicated that the TNBS-induced colitis model is useful for testing therapeutic strategies for humans. More specifically, when TNBS is introduced into the colon of susceptible mice it induces a T cell-mediated immune response within the colonic mucosa, leading to dense infiltration of T cells and marcophages throughout the entire wall of the large bowel (46). In addition, this histopathologic characteristic is accompanied by clinical features of progressive weight loss, bloody diarrhoea, rectal prolaspe and large bowel wall thickening (47). The TNBS-induced colitis model has been very useful in studying many important aspects of gut inflammation, including cytokine secretion patterns, mechanisms of oral tolerance, cell adhesion and immunotherapy.

Induction of TNBS colitis

In 2001, Scheiffele and Fuss (48) described the induction of TNBS colitis in mice. Colitis is induced by the administration of TNBS through a trocar needle using a rubber catheter inserted via the anus (49). Scheiffele and Fuss (48) recommended using 0.5 to 4.0 mg TNBS in 45% to 50% ethanol intra-rectally. Inherent in this model and other similar models is the need for ethanol at high concentrations as a vehicle for intra-colonic administration of the hapten. It seems that ethanol is a prerequisite since it acts as a barrier breaker, and allows TNBS to enter the mucosa to induce colitis (50). Ethanol by itself causes severe inflammation in the intestinal mucosa therefore it is difficult to distinguish between the ethanol-induced inflammation and hapten-induced inflammation (51). There are no standard practices for this model subsequently a critical appraisal of the various studies using TNBS colitis and a recommendation for future use of this model has been extensively reviewed by te Velde et al. (52). Intra-rectal administration of TNBS results in ulceration and thickening of the bowel wall which may persist for at least 8 weeks (53). Furthermore, granulomas and Langhans-type giant cells were also observed at the site of ulceration and inflammation. The inflammation was characterized by high myeloperoxidase and decreased glutathione levels (53).

Mechanism of action

TNBS dissolved in ethanol is required to break the mucosal barrier. TNBS can bind covalently to the E-amino group of lysine and modify cell surface proteins. Colitis may develop when pre-sensitized T lymphocytes lyse hapten-modified autologous cells (54-55). T-lymphocytes will lyse hapten-modified autologous cells only if the animal has been pre-sensitized, whereas macrophages will destroy TNBS-modified autologous cells in the absence of pre-sensitization (56). In addition, TNBS may be metabolized to yield O_2^- and H_2O_2 from the interaction between ascorbate and TNBS (57) indicating that TNBS-induced colitis may partly be mediated by cytotoxic reactive oxygen species generated by the oxidative metabolism of TNBS.

A variety of inflammatory mediators may be involved in TNBS-induced colitis. The predominant arachidonate metabolites found in TNBS colitis are leukotriene B4 (LTB4) and the monhydroxyl fatty acids 5-HETE, 12-HETE and 15-HETE (58). The synthesis of LTB4 increased within 4 h and peaked 24-72 h after the administration of TNBS and this increase is correlated with colonic myeloperoxidase activity (59). Furthermore, it has been shown that a significant level of luminal eicosanoids such as prostaglandin E2 (PGE2), 6-keto $PGF_1\alpha$, TXB2 and LTB4 were increased 3 days after intracolonic instillation of TNBS (59) suggesting that eicosanoids play an important role in the pathogenesis of TNBS-induced colitis. Another potential mechanism of TNBS-induced colitis may be the increased level of platelet-activating factor (PAF). High PAF production was not seen during the time of maximal neutrophil infiltration (1-4 days after TNBS) but was seen 1-3 weeks after the induction of colitis (60). This finding suggests that PAF is unlikely to play an important role in the acute inflammatory response but may be important in the prolongation of the inflammation in this model.

Types of TNBS-induced colitis models

The TNBS-induced colitis model may be used in 3 different scenarios, (i) in acute TNBS-induced colitis in which the primary phase of the induction of Th1 response, a nonspecific inflammatory response, is analyzed (ii) established TNBS-induced colitis in which the local delayed-type hypersensitivity response is mimicked and a specific response can be analyzed and (iii) chronic TNBS-induced colitis in which repeated local induction of DTH response will lead to fibrotic lesions and a Crohn's disease-like cytokine profile (52). These forms are not well described and documented in current practices therefore it is essential to predefine the objective for using this type of experimental colitis to better understand the pathophysiology of the chosen type of colitis.

5.3 Dinitrobenzene sulfonic acid (DNBS) model of colitis

Features of DNBS-induced colitis

DNBS is another hapten which can be used to induce colonic inflammation. DNBS is less hazardous than TNBS and can be used safely in a well-ventilated room with personnel wearing protective gloves, clothing and goggles. The DNBS model produces acute and chronic inflammation and ulceration in the colon similar to TNBS (61). The feature of colitis in this model is similar to that of the TNBS model with bloody diarrhea and significant loss of body weight evident. Four days after DNBS administration, colon damage was characterized by areas of mucosal necrosis and neutrophil infiltration and the colon appeared flaccid and filled with liquid stool. The macroscopic inspection of caecum, colon and rectum showed presence of mucosal congestion, erosion, and hemorrhagic ulcerations (62). The histopathological features included a transmural necrosis and oedema and diffuse leukocyte cellular infiltrate in the submucosa.
In comparison, rats treated with DNBS have no granulomas whereas about half of the TNBS rats have granulomas (53). In the rat, DNBS causes an overproduction of nitric oxide (NO) due to induction of inducible nitric oxide synthase (iNOS), which contributes to the inflammatory process (63-64). As in the TNBS model, DNBS induces a strong inflammatory response and a significant increase in myeloperoxidase (MPO) activity compared to controls (60). Since TNBS is no longer available in the United States, DNBS can be an alternative compound for inducing experimental models of ulcerative colitis.

Induction of TNBS colitis

Colitis was induced by using a technique of acid-induced colon inflammation as described by Morris et al., (53). In fasted rats lightly anaesthetized with isoflurane, a 3.5 F catheter was inserted into the colon via the anus until the splenicflexure was reached (approximately 8 cm from the anus). 2,4-dinitrobenzenesulphonic acid (DNBS; 25 mg/rat), dissolved in 50% ethanol (total volume, 0.8 ml) was administered as an enema. While other investigator have modified the method that was first described (53), where colitis was induced in lightly anesthetized mice by an intra-rectal injection of 3 mg of DNBS in 100 μl of 50% ethanol, delivered 3 cm into the colon via a polyethylene catheter (65).

Mechanism of action

DNBS and TNBS both bind to proteins, but TNBS has an additional active nitro group and binds more readily at lower concentrations. However, DNBS is more selective and binds only to the ε-amino group of lysine (61).

5.4 Oxazolone-induced colitis

Features of oxazolone-induced colitis

A number of experimental models of colitis have been proposed. However, there are limited colitis models that have a Th2 profile. The oxazolone-induced colitis model is Th2-mediated and has important implications for investigating the pathogenesis and treatment of ulcerative colitis (66-67). The administration of low intrarectal doses of a inducing agent (oxazolone) in ethanol to BALB/c mice every 7 days for 10 weeks showed that in the first 3 weeks of this treatment, the mice lost about 10-15% of their starting weight and exhibited ruffled coats, hunched posture, and restricted movement. During this period 10-15% of animals died. Over the next 3 weeks the surviving mice regained weight and no longer exhibited obvious signs of chronic illness. Repetitive administration of intra-rectal ethanol alone led to a weight loss of up to 5% in the early phase of the disease (68).

Induction of oxazolone colitis

The oxazolone-induced colitis model is established by painting the skin with 0.2 ml 3% oxazolone in 100% ethanol on days 0 and 1 followed by intrarectal administration of 0.15 ml 1% oxazolone in 50% ethanol on day 7 (66). However, another study (51) used carmellose sodium/peanut oil as a non-irritating vehicle in place of ethanol and found that the oxazolone-induced colitis model was still a reproducible animal model of human colonic inflammation. The oxazolone challenge resulted in rapid development of inflammation characterized by diarrhoea, mild ulcerations, hyperemia, infiltration of inflammatory cells, epithelial damage and submucosal edema.

More recently, oxazolone-induced colitis has been established as a chronic model via repeated intrarectal administration of oxazolone in ethanol. This allows the model to be used to define specific features of the inflammatory milieu that favors tumor development (69). Chronic oxazolone-induced colitis begins as severe inflammation with corresponding weight loss, which transforms into chronic inflammation and partial weight recovery. The inflammation is marked by the rapid increase in the production of IL13 in the lamina propria and the appearance of NK T cells, which are both immunologic features of acute oxazolone-induced colitis (69). The authors also concluded that the chronic oxazolone-induced colitis model supports epithelial tumour development induced by administration of a carcinogenic agent, azoxymethane.

Mechanism of action

Similar to the TNBS-induced colitis model, oxazolone, a hapten, induces delayed-type hypersensitivity and contact hypersensitivity reactions to subsequently induce inflammation. Oxazolone-induced colitis has been suggested to be dependent on the presence of IL13 producing invariant NK T cells (70). Thus the oxazolone-induced colitis model is one of the few models suitable for the study of the Th2 dependent immune response in intestinal inflammation.

5.5 Carrageenin-induced colitis

Carrageenan is a high molecular weight sulfated polygalactan, derived from several species of red seaweeds (*Rhodophyceae*) including *Gigartina, Chondrus,* and *Eucheuma* (71). The most common forms of carrageenan are lambda (λ), kappa (κ), and iota (ι) (71). Carrageenans are used by the food industry to improve the texture of food products by thickening, stabilizing, or emulsifying dairy products, salad dressings, infant formulas, processed meat, soy milk, and other food products (72-73). Its use has increased markedly during the last half century, and is known to induce inflammation in rheumatological models and in intestinal models of colitis (71).

Features of carrageenan-induced colitis

Early work in animal models has demonstrated that carrageenan may cause gastrointestinal pathology, including ulcerations and tumours of the gastrointestinal tract (71-72). In guinea pigs deprived of ascorbic acid, the oral administration of degraded *E. spinosum* carrageenan induced mild to moderate colitis, while E. cottonii carrageenan consistently induced severe colitis. The severe colitis induced by *E. cottonii* in scorbutic animals markedly affected the mid and distal colon and showed histological changes similar to human ulcerative colitis (74). Delivery of 10% carrageen (degraded carrageenan) for 10 days in the drinking water of CF1 mice induced bloody diarrhoea and pericryptal inflammation, and produced marked dilatation of the cecum and ascending colon (75). Histologically, the mucosa was characterized by distorted crypt architecture, inflammatory infiltration of the lamina propria, and ulceration, conditions which were more pronounced in the proximal colon but were also present in the distal colon.

Induction of carrageenan colitis

Carrageenan causes a reproducible inflammatory reaction and remains a standard chemical for examining acute inflammation and effects of anti-inflammatory drugs. With or without sensitizing the animals with carrageenan, colitis is induced by supplementing the drinking water of 2-10% degraded carrageenan (74-75).

Mechanism of action

Carrageenan has been widely used to induce inflammation in experimental models of colitis in animal models (72-73), that resemble human ulcerative colitis. NFκB is a key determinant of the intestinal epithelial inflammatory cascade and occupies a central role in the transcriptional activation of pro-inflammatory genes (76). Furthermore, Borthakur et al. (71) suggested that activation of NFκB in the intestinal cells following carrageenan exposure is largely attributable to an increase in Bcl10. Bcl10 resides in the cytoplasm which relays receptor mediated signals to activate NFκB (77).

6. Genetic-induced colitis

More recently, various experimental animal model of colitis, especially transgenic mice models with spontaneous colitis (78-79) have been reported and demonstrated that T cells are necessary for involvement and initiation of intestinal inflammation. New genetically engineered animals with spontaneous colitis, such as IL2 and IL10 knockout mice models, are promising tools for further understanding of the etiology of intestinal inflammation.

6.1 IL2 knockout mice

When reared and maintained under conventional specific pathogen-free conditions, IL2 deficient ($IL2^{-/-}$) mice spontaneously develop disorders of the hemopoietic and immune system characterized by anemia, lymphocytic hyperplasia, progressive loss of B cells, and disturbances in bone marrow hemopoietic cells. Animals that survive more than 8-9 weeks of age also develop a chronic, non-granulomatous inflammation of the colonic and caecal submucosa and mucosa. (80).

Features of IL2 deficiency-induced colitis

The histopathology of colitis observed in $IL2^{-/-}$ mice seems to vary depending on the method of induction and the location of animal housing. The original paper (80) described the features of spontaneously developing colitis in $IL2^{-/-}$ mice which included ulceration, crypt abscesses, destruction of the mucosal layer with epithelial dysplasia, but also mononuclear cell infiltration of the mucosa and submucosa. However, the histopathology of immunization-induced colitis and spontaneously-developing colitis in mice reared at the NIH animal facility, seem to resemble human Crohn's disease (transmural inflammation, lymphoid hyperplasia) (81). These findings suggest that the histopathological characteristics in these animals may not only be dependent on genetic but also on environmental factors.

Mechanism of action

$IL2^{-/-}$ mice reared and maintained under gnotobiotic conditions do not develop intestinal lesions (82). Furthermore, colitis that develops in $IL2^{-/-}$ mice under conventional conditions suggests a direct result of an abnormal immune response in the colonic mucosa to intestinal bacterial flora. It is not known specifically how the absence of IL2 accounts for colitis in $IL2^{-/-}$ mice and the role this cytokine plays in homeostatic regulation of mucosal immunity. However, Baumgart et al. (83) suggests that IL2 is required for the generation and the function of a regulatory population of mucosal T cells or is directly involved in preventing the development of inflammatory responses to enteric antigens.

6.2 IL10 knockout mice

Only a small number of spontaneous models of chronic colitis have been employed by researchers to yield detailed information on the penetrance, severity and reproducibility of the gut inflammation (84). The most widely used of the gene-targeted models of spontaneous colitis is the IL10 deficient ($IL10^{-/-}$) mouse model. The $IL10^{-/-}$ model is a well established Th1-mediated model of transmural colitis (85). $IL10^{-/-}$ mice were generated by disrupting the IL10 gene in embryonic stem cells and although the mice were considered to have normal lymphocyte development and antibody response, growth retardation and anemia were observed (86).

Features of IL-10 deficiency-induced colitis

Mice with targeted disruption of the IL10 gene develop spontaneous pancolitis and caecal inflammation by 2-4 months of age (85). Histopathological examination of the colons obtained from mice with active disease show many of the same characteristics as those observed in human inflammatory bowel disease. The initial changes in intestinal inflammation consisted of small, focal infiltrates of inflammatory cells in the lamina propria with minimal or no epithelial hyperplasia (85, 87). Inflammatory infiltrates consisted of a mixture of lymphocytes, plasma cells, and macrophages with smaller numbers of neutrophils and eosinophils. $IL10^{-/-}$ mice also develop ulcers and crypt abscesses, exhibit epithelial hyperplasia, mucin production is reduced, an increased numbers of mitotic figures were observed and increased expression of major histocompatibility complex class II molecule were also observed in the intestinal epithelial cells (85-87). As mice become older, inflammation involved the submucosa or less frequently became transmural (87).

Mechanism of action

It has been demonstrated that there is a lower number of caecal bacteria observed before colitis (7 weeks of age) in $IL10^{-/-}$ compared to C57Bl/6J mice. This suggests differences in intestinal bacteria that might be associated with the genotype which could contribute to the development of colitis in this mouse model (88).

6.3 $CD45RB^{Hi}$ T cell transfer model of colitis

$CD4^+$ T cells can be separated on the basis of their CD45RB expression into populations expressing high ($CD4^+$ $CD45RB^{Hi}$) or low ($CD4^+$ $CD45RB^{Lo}$) levels of this antigen (89). $CD4^+$ $CD45RB^{Hi}$ T cells isolated via fluorescence activated cell sorting from spleens of donor mice transferred to immuno-deficient SCID or $RAG1/2^{-/-}$ recipient mice cause a wasting syndrome with transmural intestinal inflammation primarily in the colon starting 5-10 weeks after cell transfer (90-91).

Features of $CD45RB^{Hi}$ T cell transfer model of colitis

Initial lesions consisted of minimal multifocal or diffuse inflammatory cell infiltrates in the lamina propria.In mice with more severe colitis, changes were diffuse and sometimes transmural (90). Inflammatory infiltrates consisted of macrophages and lymphocytes, accompanied by smaller numbers of neutrophils and eosinophils (90-91). Occasional multinucleated giant cells and ulcers were observed, whereas crypt abscesses were sparse (90-91). Epithelial changes included hyperplasia with lengthening and branching of glands, mucin depletion, increased numbers of mitotic figures, and enhanced levels of major histocompatibility complex class II molecule expression on intestinal epithelial cells (90).

Mechanism of action

Recipient mice repopulated with the $CD^+CD45RB^{Lo}$ T cell subset or both populations ($CD^+CD45RB^{Hi}$ and $CD^+CD45RB^{Lo}$ T cell subsets) do not develop colitis. $CD25^+FoxP3^+$ cells within the $CD^+CD45RB^{Lo}$ population account for the prevention of colitis since depletion of $CD25^+$ cells from $CD45RB^{Lo}$ cells abrogates their colitis prevention potential (92). Treg cells which produce IL-10 due to co-culture with IL-10, prevent the onset of gut inflammation and antigen-specific immune responses when transferred together with pathogenic $CD4^{+-}$ $CD45RB^{Hi}$ T cells. Furthermore, SCID mice administered both $CD45RB^{Hi}$ T cells and Treg cells together with anti-IL10 receptor antibodies develop colitis (93). These results suggest that the progeny of $CD45RB^{Hi}$ T cells mount a pathogenic Th1-like response in the colon of these immuno-deficient mice.

6.4 Which colitis model to use?

As increasingly more sophisticated experimental colitis models are being described and characterized, researchers have the potential to exploit the unique potential of each model to ask specific questions. No single experimental model of colitis recapitulates all of the pathogenic and clinical features of human ulcerative colitis, however each animal model has contributed to our understanding of the mechanisms underlying initiation and perpetuation of chronic intestinal inflammation.

7. Current treatments for ulcerative colitis

At present, conventional therapies or pharmaceutical treatments have remained the mainstay of treatment for most patients suffering from ulcerative colitis. However, these treatments are variably effective with significant adverse effects and approximately 25 to 40% of patients will eventually require colectomy (94). The aim of these treatments is to induce and maintain the patient in remission. First line therapy for mild to moderate ulcerative colitis comprise of anti-inflammatory drugs containing 5-aminosalycylic acid (5-ASA), such as oral and rectal mesalamine. Sulfasalazine, the archetype for this class of medications, is cleaved upon reaching the colon releasing mesalamine. Second generation 5-ASA medications include olsalazine and balsalazide (95). Approximately 60 and 80% of patients are adequately treated with these medications and the remainder who exhibit severe ulcerative colitis are treated with a combination of corticosteriods (prednisolone). Immunosuppressives or immunomodulators such as a azathioprine and mercaptopurine that treat severe inflammatory bowel disease and/or administered to patients who have inadequate response to corticosteroids can be beneficial but there is little information about their effectiveness in treating ulcerative colitis and are also associated with risks of infection and malignancy (96). Up to 20% of inflammatory bowel disease sufferers discontinue immunosuppressant therapy because of side effects (97). Biologic drugs that interfere with the inflammatory response such as the anti-TNFα agent infliximab can be effective in inducing remission for ulcerative colitis patients that are refractory to initial treatments.

It has been demonstrated that colonic bacteria may initiate inflammation of inflammatory bowel disease (97-98) and a combination therapy with antibiotics has been shown to offer significant benefit in ulcerative colitis (99-100). Most clinicians use antibiotics as an adjuvant therapy for severe ulcerative colitis despite relatively few trials conducted on their use. Although recent advances have been made in understanding the etiology and pathophysiological mechanisms underlying the pathogenesis of ulcerative colitis, the problem still remains for patients refractory to conventional treatments or not responding and being able to maintain remission effectively with maintenance treatments (101).

Currently, there is no cure for ulcerative colitis and there is increasing evidence that alternative therapies (102-103) may provide some insights into developing a potential successful treatment. The remainder of this chapter will focus on the potential therapeutic interventions which target various aspects of the etiology of ulcerative colitis including the use of pre- and probiotics to manipulate the gut microflora and molecules that mediate the action of inflammatory cells (104). Biological therapies for ulcerative colitis will not be covered in this chapter as this area is reviewed by Rutgeerts et al. (105).

8. Novel therapies for ulcerative colitis

8.1 n-3 fatty acids

Over the years, dietary n-3 fatty acids have gained a reputation in preventing and treating several disorders including cardiovascular diseases, rheumatoid arthritis and Alzheimer's disease by way of anti-inflammatory, antithrombotic, antiarrythmic, hypolipidemic and vasodilatory activities (101, 106-111). It has been shown in human and animal studies that these n-3 fatty acids have potent immunomodulatory and anti-inflammatory effects by inhibiting the production of inflammatory mediators, eicosanoids, PGE2 and LTB4 and cytokines, TNFα and IL1β (112). It stands to reason that supplemental n-3 fatty acids might therefore be beneficial in treating or preventing relapse in chronic inflammatory diseases such as ulcerative colitis (113).

Animal studies

There have been numerous studies utilising experimentally induced colitis animal models to define the role of dietary n-3 fatty acids in disease prevention and progression. In a severe combined immunodeficient (SCID) mouse model of colitis, Whiting et al. (114) found that dietary n-3 fatty acids reduced clinical colitis and colonic immunopathology by decreasing the synthesis of proinflammatory cytokines, reducing myeloid cell recruitment and activation, and enhancing epithelial barrier function and mucosal wound healing mechanisms. Li et al. (115) demonstrated within the TNBS rat colitis model that rats pretreated with n-3 fatty acids showed significant attenuation of colonic injury and protection. Compromised epithelial barrier in ulcerative colitis by chronic immune cell activation might be explained by the altered expression and distribution of tight junction proteins in tight junction membrane microdomains of the intestinal mucosa, and n-3 fatty acids have been shown to positively affect this altered expression and distribution (115). Many studies have shown adiponectin, a protein hormone produced and secreted primarily by adipocytes and more recently by colonic myofibroblasts to play a beneficial role in ulcerative colitis due to it's anti-inflammatory effect (116-118). Interestingly, Matsunaga et al. (119) who found a decrease in adiponectin expression in DSS-induced colitic mice also found a further decrease in adiponectin expression in colitic mice fed with n-3 fatty acids, which could have contributed to the observed exacerbated colitis for this group. This is in contrast to the beneficial effects other studies have shown regarding dietary n-3 fatty acids and colitis.

Human studies

Fish oil is the best source of n-3 fatty acids. Although numerous studies have focused on oral supplementation in patients with inflammatory bowel disease which ultimately results in the incorporation of n-3 fatty acids into the gut mucosal tissue thereby modifying inflammatory mediators (120-121), the evidence of clinical benefits remains unclear due to conflicting results. A systematic review of the effects of fish oil in human ulcerative colitis by MacLean et al. (113) found significant improvements in clinical scores in three studies at one or more time points relative to the comparative study arm. Studies that were restricted to patients with ulcerative colitis (122-123) reported a statistical improvement in the endoscopic score with fish oil relative to comparative treatment. Together with studies that observed induction of remission (122, 124), prevention of relapse (124-128) and the requirement for immunosuppressive agents (122, 124, 129). MacLean et al. (113) deduced that there were insufficient data to draw any conclusions. However, the observed efficacy of fish oil delivered by enteric coated capsule on reducing steroid requirements did warrant more attention (113).

Another systematic review and meta-analyses by Turner et al. (101) looked at the efficacy and safety of n-3 fatty acid or fish oil therapy in maintaining remission in inflammatory bowel disease. Of the nine studies eligible for inclusion, only three involved ulcerative colitis. There was no difference in the relapse rate between the n-3 fatty acid therapy (fish oil) and control groups. Pooled analysis showed an increase in diarrhea and symptoms of the upper gastrointestinal tract in the n-3 fatty acid group (fish oil) suggesting troublesome side effects. In short, there was insufficient data to recommend the use of n-3 fatty acids for the maintenance of remission of ulcerative colitis. Given the biologic rationale and the benefit of n-3 fatty acid therapy derived from tissue samples and animal models, it is difficult to explain the lack of clinical benefit in inflammatory bowel disease, although it has been suggested that the dosing regimen may be inadequate or the formulation not optimal (101). Enterically coated n-3 fatty acid that has a timed release of 60 minutes upon ingestion was found to be more beneficial with the lowest adverse events compared with other timed release points and triglyceride compounds (130). In conclusion, further studies are warranted to address appropriate dosing and delivery systems of fish oil for the treatment of ulcerative colitis.

8.2 Plant derived therapies

Other novel therapies that possess anti-oxidant, anti-inflammatory and immuno-modulatory properties have been investigated in experimentally-induced animal colitis models and to some extent in human trials for the treatment of ulcerative colitis. Persistent ulcerative colitis is associated with a 10-fold increased risk of colorectal cancer (131) and therefore limiting chronic colonic inflammation will appear to reduce this risk.

Resveratrol

Resveratrol is a natural polyphenol found in fruits and vegetables and abundantly in grapes and red wine. Sanchez-Fidalgo et al. (132) investigated the protective/preventive effects of dietary resveratrol in the DSS-induced colitis mouse model. There were significant attenuations of clinical signs of colitis such as loss of body weight, diarrhea and rectal bleeding. All mice fed the resveratrol diet survived and finished the treatment while mice fed the standard diet showed a 40% mortality rate. Resveratrol caused significant reductions in TNFα and IL1β and an increase in IL10, an anti-inflammatory cytokine. Expression of prostaglandin E synthase-1 (PGES-1), cyclooxygenase (COX-2) and iNOS, proteins involved in the inflammatory response, were also reduced. Cui et al. (133) investigated the protective/preventive effects as well as the chemopreventive properties of dietary resveratrol in the chronic DSS-induced colitis mouse model. Resveratrol was shown to ameliorate colitis in a dose dependant manner and reduce the tumour incidence by 60%. The number of tumours per animal was also reduced. Resveratrol is tolerated at high doses and a diet rich in this polyphenol could represent a novel approach to treating ulcerative colitis and preventing colon cancer associated with ulcerative colitis.

Andrographis paniculata

Andrographis paniculata, a member of the plant family Acanthaceae, is used extensively in Asian countries, Sweden and Chile for the treatment of various inflammatory and infectious diseases. HMPL-004, an aqueous ethanol herbal extract of Andrographis paniculata has been shown to inhibit TNFα and IL1β and prevent colitis in animal models. A pilot human clinical trial conducted by Tang et al. (134) investigated the efficacy and safety of HMPL-004 in patients with mild to moderate ulcerative colitis. In comparison to a parallel group treated with the standard first line therapy, mesalazine, there were no significant differences observed for clinical remission and disease activity. 13% of patients treated with HMPL-004 and 27% treated with mesalazine had at least one adverse event although the majority of events were not strongly linked to the study medications. In conclusion, HMPL-004 could be an efficacious alternative to mesalazine for the treatment of ulcerative colitis.

Black raspberries

As well as exhibiting ability to limit the inflammatory response in cell culture (135-137), black raspberries (BRB) have the highest concentration of antioxidant polyphenols compared to other dark berries (138-139). These antioxidants (anthocyanins and ellagic acid) have been shown to scavenge free radicals, increase expression of detoxification enzymes and increase the capacity of the cell to absorb radicals (140-143). A study conducted by Montrose et al. (144), the first to utilise a DSS-induced mouse model of ulcerative colitis to explore the effects of freeze-dried BRB on disease severity, demonstrated the high anti-inflammatory potency of BRB. Dietary BRB markedly reduced colonic injury to the epithelium and tissue levels of TNFα and IL1β were suppressed. Biomarkers of oxidative stress remained unaffected by BRB treatment, however the findings still demonstrated potent anti-inflammatory properties which support a possible therapeutic role for the treatment of ulcerative colitis.

American ginseng

American ginseng (AG), a natural herb, has been shown to improve mental performance and end points associated with conditions such as cardiovascular disease, cancer and diabetes (145-147). In a study by Jin et al. (148), AG extract was mixed in with the chow of DSS-induced colitic mice and given before and after the onset of colitis. Results showed prevention and treatment of colitis with AG along with the downregulation of iNOS and COX-2 and p53 (induced by inflammatory stress). In part, leukocyte activation in colitis causes mucosal and DNA damage which was shown to be inhibited by AG *in vitro* and *in vivo*. A dysfunctional intestinal immune system is a major mechanism by which chronic inflammation occurs in ulcerative colitis and defects in apoptosis of mucosal inflammatory cells is critical in the pathogenesis of ulcerative colitis. Another study conducted by Jin et al. (149), showed that AG extract can drive apoptosis of inflammatory cells through the p53 mechanism *in vitro* which is consistent with dietary AG protecting against DSS-induced colitis in the mouse model.

Ginkgo biloba

Ginkgo biloba extract (EGB) is derived from the green leaves of the Gingko biloba tree and has been used extensively in conditions associated with inflammatory mediators such as acute pancreatitis, central neural system disorders, heart and intestine injury/reperfusion injury (150-152). Zhou et al. (153) investigated the mechanism by which EGB ameliorates inflammation in TNBS-induced colitic rats and its effects on the production of inflammatory mediators. Four weeks of EGB therapy provided protection in ulcerative colitis possibly by radical scavenging and down regulating some of the inflammatory mediators including TNFα, NFκBp65 and IL6. All inflammatory mediators in this study were affected by EGB in a dose dependant manner resulting in the improvement of ulcerative colitis. Another study by Kotakadi et al (154) showed that EGBs have anti-inflammatory properties *in vitro* and prevent and treat colitis in the DSS-induced mouse model. The mechanism underlying the treatment of ulcerative colitis is in part due to the ability of EGB to drive $CD4^+$ effector T cell apoptosis which is fundamental in regulating many chronic inflammatory and autoimmune diseases (155-156).

8.3 Other potential therapies

Crocetin

Crocetin, a carotenoid compound derived from *Crocus sativus L* (saffron) has been used to treat different diseases (157). In the TNBS-induced colitis mouse model, it was revealed that treatment with 50 mg/kg/day intragastrically for 8 days significantly ameliorated diarrhea, inflammation and colonic tissue injury (158). The mechanisms by which crocetin exerted these beneficial effects is through the reduction of neutrophil infiltration and MDA in the inflamed colon. Increased production of NO by iNOS and activation of NFκB, known to play a central role in the early steps of inflammation were also reduced. With further investigation, crocetin could prove to be an alternative therapy or perhaps be used alongside conventional therapies.

Pomegranate

Punica granatum or the pomegranate is used in traditional medicine in China, India, Europe and South Africa. Studies have shown that pomegranate has protective properties against liver fibrosis and ultraviolet-induced pigmentation (159-160). Furthermore, it has antibacterial, anti-inflammatory, anti-diabetic effects and is cardio-protective (161-163). Singh et al. (164) explored the effect of Punica granatum extract and its component, ellagic acid, in the DSS-induced colitis mouse model and found significant attenuation of colonic inflammation. Mast cell degranulation, which releases various inflammatory mediators, including histamine, has been implicated in the pathogenesis of ulcerative colitis and the use of mast cell stabilizers have been documented to attenuate the severity of ulcerative colitis in humans (165). Singh et al (164) found that Punica granatum extract and its ellagic acid component had anti-ulcerative effects comparable to sodium cromoglycate (mast cell stabilser) and sulphasalazine (standard first line treatment for ulcerative colitis).

Helminths

Immune-mediated diseases such as inflammatory bowel disease are becoming more prevalent in highly developed and industrialized countries (166). It is suggested that the adoption of hygienic lifestyles in these countries have contributed to a decline in helminths or parasitic worm infections (166). Epidemiological studies (167-169) have suggested that helminths may provide protection against some immune-mediated diseases and the eradication may in fact promote these diseases. Animal studies have shown helminth protection by promoting regulatory immune responses. In a DNBS-induced mouse colitis model Melon et al. (170) showed that mice infected with the tapeworm, *Hymenolepis diminuta*, increased the production of IL4 and IL10 that protected them from colitis, in contrast to steroid treatment (dexamethasone) which offered little benefit. Khan et al. (171) also showed protection with the nematode, *Trichinella spiralis*, in the TNBS- induced colitis mouse model. However, it was found that helminth infection enhanced disease severity in the oxazolone induced colitis mouse model (172). In a human randomized crossover trial conducted by Summers et al (173), a significant percentage of patients with ulcerative colitis receiving the porcine whipworm, *Trichuris suis*, improved when compared to placebo. As well, the treatment seemed to be safe with no reported side effects. In conclusion, there is potential value for helminth therapy for specific inflammatory bowel disease patients however further studies are needed to fully understand the mechanisms underlying the pathophysiology of ulcerative colitis and the type of helminth therapy required to avoid the possibility of disease aggravation.

8.4 Prebiotics

There is a diverse and large population of micro-organisms naturally living on the mucosal surfaces or in the lumen of the human intestine. The number of resident bacteria increases along the small bowel, with the colon being the most heavily populated region of intestine. The microbiota refers to the particular ecological niche of a host individual in which the community of living micro-organisms is assembled (174). A healthy or balanced microbiota has been considered to be predominantly saccharolytic and comprises of significant numbers of lactobacilli and bifidobacteria (175). A prebiotic can be defined as a non-digestible food ingredient that exerts a beneficial effect on the host through the selective stimulation and metabolism in the intestine, thereby improving host health (176). Inulin and oligofructose are prebiotic carbohydrates that resist digestion by intestinal and pancreatic enzymes in the human gastrointestinal tract and are fermented by bacteria living in the intestinal ecosystem. Prebiotics increase saccharolytic activity within the gut and selectively promote the growth of bifidobacteria when administered in significant amounts (177-178).

Animal models

Videla et al. (179) investigated the effectiveness of inulin, which stimulates intracolonic generation of butyrate and growth of lactic acid bacteria, in the protection against colitis. In a rat model of DSS-induced colitis, oral inulin treatment significantly reduced colonic tissue MPO activity and mucosal release of inflammatory mediators (179). Histologically, oral inulin treatment reduced the extent of damaged mucosa, decreased the severity of crypt disruption and lowered histological damage severity scores compared with controls. Inulin induced an acidic environment from the caecum to the left colon and increased counts of Lactobacilli (179).

Fructooligosaccharides (FOS) increase the growth of lactic acid bacteria and promote butyrate and lactate production, therefore possessing beneficial properties for intestinal inflammation (180). Intracolonic TNBS-induced colitic rats treated with intragastric infusions of FOS resulted in a reduction of pH and inflammation assessed by MPO activity. Furthermore, FOS treatment increased lactate and butyrate concentrations including lactic acid bacteria counts in the caecum (180).

Madsen et al. (181) investigated the role of colonic aerobic luminal bacteria and lactobacillus species in IL10 gene-deficient mice that spontaneously develop colitis. These knockout mice have a decreased level of lactobacillus species in the colon and an increase in adherent and translocated bacteria in the neonatal period. Normalising Lactobacillus levels via oral lactulose therapy reduced colonic mucosal bacteria and prevented colitis (181). Similarly, lactulose treatment has demonstrated protective effects against DSS- and TNBS-models of colitis (182-183). Rumi et al. (182) demonstrated that lactulose therapy ameliorated DSS-induced colitis in a dose-dependent manner and significantly reduced the severity of colonic lesions and decreased MPO activity. Furthermore, Camuesco et al. (183) indicated that lactulose treatment in TNBS-induced colitis exerted a preventive anti-inflammatory effect as evidenced by a significant reduction of MPO activity, a decrease of colonic TNFα and leukotriene B4 production and an inhibition of colonic inducible nitric oxygen synthase expression, which is a result of the inflammatory process (183). Furthermore, this effect was associated with increased levels of lactobacilli and bifidoacteria species in colonic content when compared with untreated colitic rats (183). Overall, the experimental evidence provides significant indications of the anti-inflammatory and beneficial properties of prebiotics in settings of ulcerative colitis.

Clinical studies

Recently, Casellas et al. (184) tested the effect of oligofructose-enriched inulin, which promote the selective growth of saccharolytic bacteria with low inflammatory potential, in patients with active ulcerative colitis. Eligible patients in the randomized, placebo-controlled double blinded pilot trial had been previously in remission with mesalazine as maintenance therapy or no drug, and presented with a relapse of mild to moderate activity (184). Nineteen subjects were treated with mesalazine and randomly allocated to receive either oligofructose-enriched inulin or placebo for two weeks. Patients treated with oligofructose-enriched inulin displayed a reduction of faecal calprotectin, a protein found in granulocytes that resist metabolic degradation (184).

8.5 Probiotics

Probiotics are defined as living, non-pathogenic bacteria which are able to exert beneficial therapeutic or physiologic activities when administered in sufficient numbers (185). Bacteria can be derived from various sources such as cultured food and the normal human microbiota. Lactobacillus or bifidobacterium genera are the most common strains of probiotic bacteria and have also been identified from enterococcus, streptococcus, and lactococcus species, while certain non-pathogenic Escherichia strains are also classified as probiotics (186). Furthermore, genetic engineering of probiotic strains can ensure the release of bioactive compounds16. The beneficial effects of probiotics are highly species and strain specific and therefore the mechanism of action is not well understood. Common mechanisms of action identified in probiotics include improvement of epithelial barrier function, inhibition of pathogenic enteric bacteria and manipulation of host immunoregulation (185).

In vitro models

The effects of probiotics have been investigated using recent comprehensive cell culture experiments which are model systems of inflammation and infection similar to ulcerative colitis. Schlee et al. (187) investigated the ability and mechanism by which different probiotic lactobacillus strains, including *L. Acidophilus PZ1138, L. Fermentum PZ-1138, E. coli Nissle 1917* and VSL#3 (a combination of 8 bacterial strains), stabilize gut barrier function via induction of the anti-microbial peptide human beta defensin-2 (hBD2) gene. The expression of hBD2 gene by probiotic bacteria was both time- and dosage-dependent, and the promoter activation by probiotics was completely inhibited via deletion of NFκB and activator protein-1 (AP1) binding sites on the hBD-2 promoter (187). Furthermore, hBD-2 induction was also hindered by the inhibition of mitogen-activated protein kinase (MAPK). Overall, Schlee et al. (187) demonstrated that lactobacilli and the VSL#3 bacterial combination strengthened intestinal barrier functions via the up-regulation of hBD-2 through induction of MAPKs and pro-inflammatory pathways including NFκB and AP1. In support of the finding of Schlee et al. (187), *E. coli Nissle 1917* was further demonstrated to strengthen intestinal barrier function using a polarized T84 epithelial monolayer model to monitor barrier disruption by E.coli infection (188). Co-incubation of the enteropathogenic *E. coli* strain with *E. coli Nissle 1917* or addition of *E. coli Nissle 1917* following infection abolished barrier disruption and restored barrier integrity (188). DNA-microarray analysis of T84 cells incubated with the enteropathogenic *E. coli* identified altered expression of over 300 genes, including the distribution of zonla occludens-2 (ZO-2) protein and of distinct protein kinase C isotypes, all of which are involved in the maintenance of epithelial tight junctions (188).

Furthermore, *E. coli Nissle 1917* has been shown to exert anti-inflammatory effects on human colonic epithelial cells *in vitro* (189). Enzyme-linked immunosorbent assays and real-time quantitative PCR demonstrated that *E. coli Nissle 1917* treatment in vitro suppressed TNFα-induced IL8 transcription and production and inhibited IL8 promoter activity. These properties, in conjunction with the hBD2 results from Schlee et al (187) and T84 epithelial monolayer model results from Zyrek et al. (188) contribute to the reported efficacy in the treatment of inflammatory bowel diseases. Due to the unfortunate idiopathic nature of IBD, pre-treatment with probiotics may be more beneficial for either genetically susceptible individuals or to help IBD sufferers maintain remission.

Animal models

Several murine models of intestinal damage have been utilised to assess the efficacy of probiotics *in vivo* (190-192). Ukena et al. (191) orally administered the probiotic *E. coli Nissle 1917* to BALB/c mice with acute dextran sulphate sodium (DSS)-induced colitis. The probiotic treatment resulted in an upregulation of the tight junction molecule ZO-1 in intestinal epithelial cells at both mRNA and protein levels and reduced intestinal barrier permeability (191). Additionally, infiltration of the colon with leukocytes was ameliorated in E.coli Nissle 1917 inoculated mice (191). Furthermore, Grabig et al (193) demonstrated that *E. coli Nissle 1917* treatment in a wildtype DSS-induced colitis mouse model significantly reduced pro-inflammatory cytokine expression, myeloperoxidase (found in the intracellular granules of neutrophils) activity and disease activity. The inability of *E. coli Nissle 1917* to exert its beneficial effect in the absence of toll-like receptor (TLR)-2 and TLR4 signaling using TLR2 and TLR4 knockout mice indicates that the amelioration of experimentally-indiced colitis in mice was elicited via TLR2- and TLR4-dependent pathways (193). This finding highlights the fact that *E. coli Nissle 1917* may improve the ability of TLRs, which are key components of the innate immune system that trigger antimicrobial host defence responses, to recognise microbial pathogens, improving the host immune response.

Lee et al. (194) demonstrated that oral *L. plantarum HY115* treatment to mice with DSS-induced colitis inhibited colon shortening and MPO production. Furthermore, *L. plantarum HY115* repressed the mRNA expressions of IL1β, TNFα and IFNγ, including colonic IL1 beta and IL6 protein expression and reduced the degradation activities of chondroitin sulphate and hyaluronic acid of intestinal bacteria (194). Similarly, Schultz et al. (195) immune-mediated colitic (induced by IL10 deficiency) mice treated with L. plantarum had decreased levels of mucosal IL12, IFNγ and immunoglobulin G2a (195).

A study by Peran et al. (196) assessed the intestinal anti-inflammatory effects of probiotics with immunomodulatory properties in the TNBS rat model of colitis. *L. casei, L. acidophilus* and bifidobacterium lactis elicited intestinal anti-inflammatory effects, evidenced macroscopically by a decreased colonic weight/length ratio and biochemically, all probiotics restored colonic glutathione levels, depleted due to oxidative stress (196). Interestingly, each probiotic displayed a unique anti-inflammatory profile; bifidobacterium lactis reduced colonic TNFα production, L. casei decreased colonic COX-2 expression and L. acidophilus reduced leukotrine B4 production and MPO activity (196). These findings indicate that probiotics exert their beneficial effects via different mechanisms. Menard et al. (197) inoculated gnotobiotic mice with bifidobacterium longum NCC2705 and nine bifidobacterium strains isolated from infants' faecal flora to investigate the effect of these probiotics on the Th1/Th2 balance. Immunomodulatory responses including induction of the Th1 and Th2 cytokines, increased ileal IL10, IL4, TNFα and IFNγ secretions and TGFβ1 gene expressions, were observed from only specific strains (197). It was concluded that bifidobacterium's capacity to stimulate immunity is species specific however its influence on the orientation of the immune system is strain specific.

Clinical trials

To date, probiotics have been investigated in several clinical trials as treatments for ulcerative colitis, with conflicting results. However, there have been relatively few large, placebo-controlled, randomised and double-blinded clinical studies to test the efficacy of probiotics in humans (198). Tsuda et al. (199) evaluated the efficacy of the probiotics combination therapy BIO-THREE, comprising of Streptococcus faecalis T-110, Clostridium butyricum TO-A and Bacillus mesentericus TO-A, in patients with mild to moderate distal ulcerative colitis. Patients ingested nine BIO-THREE tablets per day for four weeks. Clinical symptoms and endoscopic findings were evaluated as ulcerative colitis disease activity index and faecal samples were collected to assess the microflora, pre- and post-treatment (199). Remission was observed in nine patients (45%), response in two patients (10%), no response in eight patients (40%) and worsening in one patient (5%) (199). Interestingly, terminal restriction fragment length polymorphism (T-RFLP) analysis indicated that the principal alteration in microflora was an increase in bifidobacteria (199); an unusual finding as no bifidobacteria was administered in the probiotic supplement.

8.6 Zinc

Zinc is ubiquitous in biologic systems and has abundant and varied functions. The zinc atom has the ability to participate in readily exchangeable ligand binding in addition to assuming a number of coordination geometries to provide functional needs to other ligands (200). Zinc has numerous central roles in DNA and RNA metabolism (201). Zinc metalloenzymes and zinc-dependent enzymes have been identified and are involved in nucleic acid metabolism and cellular proliferation, differentiation and growth (202). Zinc also plays a regulatory role in apoptosis (203), with cytoprotective functions that suppress major pathways, leading to programmed cell death.

Animal studies

Zinc administration has been shown to suppress the development of DSS-induced colitis in mice as indicated by decreased clinical disease activity index and histological severity scores (204-206). Ohkawara et al. (205) demonstrated that polaprezinc (N-(3-Aminopropionyl)-L-histidinato zinc), an anti-ulcer drug, suppresses DSS-induced colitis in mice, partly through inhibition of production of pro-inflammatory cytokines, suppression of neutrophils accumulation and cytoprotection by overexpression of heat shock proteins. This is consistent with Iwaya et al (207) whom reported that marginal zinc deficiency exacerbated colitis by modulating the immune response through the impairment of TNFα production and TNFR1 expression, rather than through the impairment of epithelial barrier function. Another potential mechanism of action of zinc in ulcerative colitis has been suggested by Luk et al. (208) by reducing inflammation, inhibiting mast cell degranulation and histamine release. In addition, high dose of zinc has been shown to improve tight-junction permeability (209). A novel zinc compound, Z-103, a chelate compound consisting of zinc ion and L-carnosine, was utilized to assess the protective effect against colonic damage induced by TNBS in rats (210). The authors demonstrated that treatment with Z-103 reduced he inflammatory responses induced by TNBS, suggesting Z-103 may be as effective against TNBS-induced colitis.

Metallothioneins (MTs) are zinc-binding proteins whose overexpression may lead to sequestration of zinc ions. We have shown that the absence of MT was beneficial in the suppression of colitis in MT knockout ($MT^{-/-}$) mice receiving DSS, suggesting that the presence of MT may have promoted the induction of colitis. Similarly, as indicated by the histological severity scores, MT wildtype mice appeared more susceptible to DSS-induced colitis compared to $MT^{-/-}$ animals (204). Furthermore, Bruewer et al. (211) reported that MT overexpression may represent an important early step in the development of carcinogenesis of ulcerative colitis independent of p53 expression. This should be further investigated in the long term as an independent cancer risk factor in ulcerative colitis.

Human studies

The only double-blind controlled trial of oral zinc sulphate as adjuvant treatment in idiopathic ulcerative colitis or proctitis in relapse was reported by Dronfield et al. (212). In this trial, 51 patients were treated with zinc and the clinical and sigmoidoscopic improvement was similar in the treated and placebo group. Furthermore, it has been shown that zinc administration decreased peripheral blood natural killer cell activity in 13 inflammatory bowel disease patients, with stable disease and mild-moderate disease activity, in a double-blind randomized cross-over trial (213).

9. Conclusions

Animal models of acute and chronic intestinal inflammation are indispensable for our understanding of the pathogenesis of ulcerative colitis and Crohn's disease, even though the etiology of inflammatory bowel disease remains unclear. In conclusion, administration of the above novel therapies have potential benefits in suppressing clinical features, histological pathology scores and inflammatory indicators in colitis in experimental models. There are four types of experimental animal models of colitis; spontaneous colitis models, inducible colitis models with normal immune system, adoptive transfer models in immuno-compromised hosts, and genetically engineered models (knockout and transgenic mice). There is not one single experimental model of colitis that incorporates all the clinical and histopathological characteristics of human inflammatory bowel disease, however, information gained from studies using these different types of colitis models has revealed three fundamental underlying principles. Firstly, chronic intestinal inflammation is mainly mediated by T cells. Secondly, commensal enteric bacteria are required to initiate and achieve intestinal inflammation and finally, the genetic background of the animal is a pivotal factor of disease onset and severity (84). Using these different models of colitis, *in vitro* and *in vivo* studies have shown a variety of novel therapies including, pre- and probiotics, n-3 fatty acids, plant bioactives (resveratrol, black raspberries, ginseng, ginkgo) and helminthes which have potential benefits in suppressing clinical features, histological pathology scores and inflammatory indicators. These novel therapies act on specific mechanisms of action such as intestinal barrier function, mucosal immune function and intestinal microbiota, however, there are no single therapies that have a multifunctional mechanism of action to prevent and treat ulcerative colitis. Newer therapies which use a combination of agents to restore gut homeostasis should be more promising and closer to achieving long-term remission of ulcerative colitis. Thus, further studies are warranted to determine the mechanism of action by which these agents are able to protect against ulcerative colitis and to explore whether combination therapy could produce synergistic effects.

10. Acknowledgement

CDT was a recipient of the MS McLeod Post-Doctoral Fellowship funded by the Women's and Children's Hospital Foundation.

11. References

[1] Smith PD, Ochsenbauer-Jambor C, Smythies LE. Intestinal macrophages: unique effector cells of the innate immune system. Immunol Rev 2005;206:149-59.

[2] Rugtveit J, Brandtzaeg P, Halstensen TS, Fausa O, Scott H. Increased macrophage subset in inflammatory bowel disease: apparent recruitment from peripheral blood monocytes. Gut 1994;35(5):669-74.

[3] Rugtveit J, Nilsen EM, Bakka A, Carlsen H, Brandtzaeg P, Scott H. Cytokine profiles differ in newly recruited and resident subsets of mucosal macrophages from inflammatory bowel disease. Gastroenterol 1997;112(5):1493-505.

[4] Kamada N, Hisamatsu T, Okamoto S, Chinen H, Kobayashi T, Sato T, Sakuraba A, Kitazume MT, Sugita A, Koganei K, Akagawa KS, Hibi T. Unique CD14 intestinal macrophages contribute to the pathogenesis of Crohn's disease via IL-23/IFN-gamma axis. J Clin Invest 2008;118(6):2269-80.

[5] Rescigno M, Di Sabatino A. Dendritic cells in intestinal homeostasis and disease. J Clin Invest 2009;119(9):2441-50.

[6] Bilsborough J, Viney JL. Gastrointestinal dendritic cells play a role in immunity, tolerance, and disease. Gastroenterol 2004;127(1):300-9.

[7] Hart AL, Al-Hassi HO, Rigby RJ, Bell SJ, Emmanuel AV, Knight SC, Kamm MA, Stagg AJ. Characteristics of intestinal dendritic cells in inflammatory bowel diseases. Gastroenterol 2005;129(1):50-65.

[8] MacDermott RP, Nash GS, Bertovich MJ, Seiden MV, Bragdon MJ, Beale MG. Alterations of IgM, IgG, and IgA Synthesis and secretion by peripheral blood and intestinal mononuclear cells from patients with ulcerative colitis and Crohn's disease. Gastroenterol 1981;81(5):844-52.

[9] Scott MG, Nahm MH, Macke K, Nash GS, Bertovich MJ, MacDermott RP. Spontaneous secretion of IgG subclasses by intestinal mononuclear cells: differences between ulcerative colitis, Crohn's disease, and controls. Clin Exp Immunol 1986;66(1):209-15

[10] Mosmann TR, Cherwinski H, Bond MW, Giedlin MA, Coffman RL. Two types of murine helper T cell clone. I. Definition according to profiles of lymphokine activities and secreted proteins. J Immunol 1986;136(7):2348-57.

[11] Romagnani S. Human TH1 and TH2 subsets: regulation of differentiation and role in protection and immunopathology. Int Arch Allergy Immunol 1992;98(4):279-85.

[12] Annunziato F, Romagnani S. Do studies in humans better depict Th17 cells? Blood 2009;114(11):2213-9.

[13] Annunziato F, Cosmi L, Santarlasci V, Maggi L, Liotta F, Mazzinghi B, Parente E, Filì L, Ferri S, Frosali F, Giudici F, Romagnani P, Parronchi P, Tonelli F, Maggi E, Romagnani S. Phenotypic and functional features of human Th17 cells. J Exp Med 2007;204(8):1849-61.
[14] Annunziato F, Romagnani S. Heterogeneity of human effector CD4+ T cells. Arthritis Res Ther 2009;11(6):257.
[15] Cosmi L, Maggi L, Santarlasci V, Capone M, Cardilicchia E, Frosali F, Querci V, Angeli R, Matucci A, Fambrini M, Liotta F, Parronchi P, Maggi E, Romagnani S, Annunziato F. Identification of a novel subset of human circulating memory CD4(+) T cells that produce both IL-17A and IL-4. J Allergy Clin Immunol 2010;125(1):222-30.
[16] Jiang H, Chess L. An integrated view of suppressor T cell subsets in immunoregulation. J Clin Invest 2004;114(9):1198-208.
[17] Feuerer M, Hill JA, Mathis D, Benoist C. Foxp3+ regulatory T cells: differentiation, specification, subphenotypes. Nat Immunol 2009;10(7):689-95.
[18] Weaver CT, Harrington LE, Mangan PR, Gavrieli M, Murphy KM. Th17: an effector CD4 T cell lineage with regulatory T cell ties. Immunity 2006;24(6):677-88.
[19] Weaver CT, Hatton RD. Interplay between the TH17 and TReg cell lineages: a (co-)evolutionary perspective. Nat Rev Immunol 2009;9(12):883-9.
[20] Sakaguchi, S. Naturally arising Foxp3-expressing CD25+CD4+ regulatory T cells in immunological tolerance to self and non-self. Nat Immunol 2005; 6: 345-52.
[21] Fontenot JD, Gavin MA, Rudensky AY. Foxp3 programs the development and function of CD4+CD25+ regulatory T cells. Nat Immunol 2003;4: 330-36.
[22] Korn T, Oukka M, Kuchroo V, et al. Th17 cells: effector T cells with inflammatory properties. Sem Immuno 2007;19: 362-71.
[23] Parronchi P, Romagnani P, Annunziato F, Sampognaro S, Becchio A, Giannarini L, Maggi E, Pupilli C, Tonelli F, Romagnani S. Type 1 T-helper cell predominance and interleukin-12 expression in the gut of patients with Crohn's disease. Am J Pathol 1997;150(3):823-32.
[24] Monteleone G, Biancone L, Marasco R, Morrone G, Marasco O, Luzza F, Pallone F. Interleukin 12 is expressed and actively released by Crohn's disease intestinal lamina propria mononuclear cells. Gastroenterol 1997;112(4):1169-78.
[25] Fujino S, Andoh A, Bamba S, Ogawa A, Hata K, Araki Y, Bamba T, Fujiyama Y. Increased expression of interleukin 17 in inflammatory bowel disease. Gut 2003;52(1):65-70.
[26] Fuss IJ, Heller F, Boirivant M, Leon F, Yoshida M, Fichtner-Feigl S, Yang Z, Exley M, Kitani A, Blumberg RS, Mannon P, Strober W. Nonclassical CD1d-restricted NK T cells that produce IL-13 characterize an atypical Th2 response in ulcerative colitis. J Clin Invest 2004;113(10):1490-7.
[27] Heller F, Florian P, Bojarski C, Richter J, Christ M, Hillenbrand B, Mankertz J, Gitter AH, Bürgel N, Fromm M, Zeitz M, Fuss I, Strober W, Schulzke JD. Interleukin-13 is the key effector Th2 cytokine in ulcerative colitis that affects epithelial tight junctions, apoptosis, and cell restitution. Gastroenterol 2005;129(2):550-64.
[28] Cotran RS, Kumar V, Collins T. Pathologic Basis of Disease (6th edition). W.B. Saunders Company, USA; 1999.

[29] Xavier RJ, Podolsky DK. Unravelling the pathogenesis of inflammatory bowel disease. Nature 2007;448:427-34.
[30] Geier MS, Butler RN, Giffard PM, Howarth GS. Lactobacillus fermentum BR11, a potential new probiotic, alleviates symptoms of colitis induced by dextran sulfate sodium (DSS) in rats. Int J Food Microbiol 2007;114(3):267-74.
[31] Ishioka T, Kuwabara N, Oohashi Y, Wakabayashi K. Induction of colorectal tumors in rats by sulfated polysaccharides. Crit Rev Toxicol 1987;17(3):215-44.
[32] Geier MS TD, Yazbeck R, McCaughan GW, Abbott CA, Howarth GS. Development and resolution of experimental colitis in mice with targeted deletion of dipeptidyl peptidase IV. J Cell Physiol 2005;204:687-92.
[33] Vowinkel T KT, Mori M, Krieglstein CF, Granger DN. Impact of dextran sulfate sodium load on the severity of inflammation in experimental colitis. Dig Dis Sci 2004;49:556-64.
[34] Whittem CG, Williams AD, Williams CS. Murine Colitis modeling using Dextran Sulfate Sodium (DSS). J Vis Exp 2010;(35).
[35] Huang TC, Tsai SS, Liu LF, Liu YL, Liu HJ, Chuang KP. Effect of Arctium lappa L. in the dextran sulfate sodium colitis mouse model. World J Gastroenterol 2010;16(33):4193-9.
[36] Ni J, Chen SF, Hollander D. Effects of dextran sulphate sodium on intestinal epithelial cells and intestinal lymphocytes. Gut 1996;39(2):234-41.
[37] Sartor RB. Microbial influences in inflammatory bowel diseases. Gastroenterol 2008;134(2):577-94.
[38] Poritz LS, Garver KI, Green C, Fitzpatrick L, Ruggiero F, Koltun WA. Loss of the tight junction protein ZO-1 in dextran sulfate sodium induced colitis. J Surg Res 2007;140(1):12-9.
[39] Kitajima S, Takuma S, Morimoto M. Histological analysis of murine colitis induced by dextran sulfate sodium of different molecular weights. Exp Anim 2000;49(1):9-15.
[40] Okayasu I, Hatakeyama S, Yamada M, Ohkusa T, Inagaki Y, Nakaya R. A novel method in the induction of reliable experimental acute and chronic ulcerative colitis in mice. Gastroenterol 1990;98(3):694-702.
[41] Melgar S, Karlsson A, Michaëlsson E. Acute colitis induced by dextran sulfate sodium progresses to chronicity in C57BL/6 but not in BALB/c mice: correlation between symptoms and inflammation. Am J Physiol Gastrointest Liver Physiol 2005;288(6):G1328-38.
[42] Hirono I, Kuhara K, Hosaka S, Tomizawa S, Golberg L. Induction of intestinal tumors in rats by dextran sulfate sodium. J Natl Cancer Inst 1981;66(3):579-83.
[43] Parronchi P, Romagnani P, Annunziato F, Sampognaro S, Becchio A, Giannarini L, Maggi E, Pupilli C, Tonelli F, Romagnani S. Type 1 T-helper cell predominance and interleukin-12 expression in the gut of patients with Crohn's disease. Am J Pathol 1997;150(3):823-32.
[44] Neurath MF, Fuss I, Kelsall B, Meyer zum Büschenfelde KH, Strober W. Effect of IL-12 and antibodies to IL-12 on established granulomatous colitis in mice. Ann N Y Acad Sci 1996;795:368-70.
[45] Fuss IJ, Marth T, Neurath MF, Pearlstein GR, Jain A, Strober W. Anti-interleukin 12 treatment regulates apoptosis of Th1 T cells in experimental colitis in mice. Gastroenterol 1999;117(5):1078-88.

[46] Neurath MF, Fuss I, Kelsall BL, Stüber E, Strober W. Antibodies to interleukin 12 abrogate established experimental colitis in mice. J Exp Med 1995;182(5):1281-90.
[47] Neurath M, Fuss I, Strober W. TNBS-colitis. Int Rev Immunol 2000;19(1):51-62.
[48] Scheiffele F, Fuss IJ. Induction of TNBS colitis in mice. Curr Protoc Immunol 2002;Chapter 15:Unit 15.19.
[49] Kazi HA, Qian Z. Crocetin reduces TNBS-induced experimental colitis in mice by downregulation of NFkB. Saudi J Gastroenterol 2009;15(3):181-7.
[50] Yamada Y, Marshall S, Specian RD, Grisham MB. A comparative analysis of two models of colitis in rats. Gastroenterol 1992;102(5):1524-34.
[51] Ekström GM. Oxazolone-induced colitis in rats: effects of budesonide, cyclosporin A, and 5-aminosalicylic acid. Scand J Gastroenterol 1998;33(2):174-9.
[52] te Velde AA, Verstege MI, Hommes DW. Critical appraisal of the current practice in murine TNBS-induced colitis. Inflamm Bowel Dis 2006;12(10):995-9.
[53] Morris GP, Beck PL, Herridge MS, Depew WT, Szewczuk MR, Wallace JL. Hapten-induced model of chronic inflammation and ulceration in the rat colon. Gastroenterol 1989;96(3):795-803.
[54] Allgayer H, Deschryver K, Stenson WF. Treatment with 16,16'-dimethyl prostaglandin E2 before and after induction of colitis with trinitrobenzenesulfonic acid in rats decreases inflammation. Gastroenterol 1989;96(5 Pt 1):1290-300.
[55] Teh HS, Phillips RA, Miller RG. Quantitative studies on the precursors of cytotoxic lymphocytes. V. The cellular basis for the cross-reactivity of TNP-specific clones. J Immunol 1978;121(5):1711-7.
[56] Kunin S, Gallily R. Recognition and lysis of altered-self cells by macrophages. I. Modification of target cells by 2,4,6-trinitrobenzene sulphonic acid. Immunol 1983;48(2):265-72.
[57] Grisham MB, Volkmer C, Tso P, Yamada T. Metabolism of trinitrobenzene sulfonic acid by the rat colon produces reactive oxygen species. Gastroenterol 1991;101(2):540-7.
[58] MacNaughton WK, Wallace JL. A role for dopamine as an endogenous protective factor in the rat stomach. Gastroenterol 1989;96(4):972-80.
[59] Vilaseca J, Salas A, Guarner F, Rodriguez R, Malagelada JR. Participation of thromboxane and other eicosanoid synthesis in the course of experimental inflammatory colitis. Gastroenterol 1990;98(2):269-77.
[60] Wallace JL. Release of platelet-activating factor (PAF) and accelerated healing induced by a PAF antagonist in an animal model of chronic colitis. Can J Physiol Pharmacol 1988;66(4):422-5.
[61] Hawkins JV, Emmel EL, Feuer JJ, Nedelman MA, Harvey CJ, Klein HJ, Rozmiarek H, Kennedy AR, Lichtenstein GR, Billings PC. Protease activity in a hapten-induced model of ulcerative colitis in rats. Dig Dis Sci 1997;42(9):1969-80.
[62] Mazzon E, Puzzolo D, Caputi AP, Cuzzocrea S. Role of IL-10 in hepatocyte tight junction alteration in mouse model of experimental colitis. Mol Med 2002;8(7):353-66.
[63] Zingarelli B, Cuzzocrea S, Szabo' C, Salzman AL. Mercaptoethylguanidine, a combined inhibitor of nitric oxide synthase and peroxynitrite scavenger, reduces trinitrobenzene sulfonic acid-induced colon damage in rats. J Pharmacol Exp Ther 1998;287: 1048-1055.

[64] Zingarelli B, Szaboá C, Salzman AL. Reduced oxidative and nitrosative damage in murine experimental colitis in the absence of inducible nitric oxide synthase. 1999 Gut 45: 199-209.
[65] Qui BS, Vallance BA,. Blennerhassett PA, Collins SM. The role of CD4 lymphocytes in the susceptibility of mice to stress-induced reactivation of experimental colitis. Nat Med 1999;5:1178–1182.
[66] Wang X, Ouyang Q, Luo WJ. Oxazolone-induced murine model of ulcerative colitis. Chin J Dig Dis 2004;5(4):165-8.
[67] Kojima R, Kuroda S, Ohkishi T, Nakamaru K, Hatakeyama S. Oxazolone-induced colitis in BALB/C mice: a new method to evaluate the efficacy of therapeutic agents for ulcerative colitis. J Pharmacol Sci 2004;96(3):307-13.
[68] Schiechl G, Bauer B, Fuss I, Lang SA, Moser C, Ruemmele P, Rose-John S, Neurath MF, Geissler EK, Schlitt HJ, Strober W, Fichtner-Feigl S. Tumor development in murine ulcerative colitis depends on MyD88 signaling of colonic F4/80+CD11b(high)Gr1(low) macrophages. J Clin Invest 2011;121(5):1692-708.
[69] Schiechl G, Bauer B, Fuss I, Lang SA, Moser C, Ruemmele P, Rose-John S, Neurath MF, Geissler EK, Schlitt HJ, Strober W, Fichtner-Feigl S. Tumor development in murine ulcerative colitis depends on MyD88 signaling of colonic F4/80+CD11b(high)Gr1(low) macrophages. J Clin Invest 2011;121(5):1692-708.
[70] Heller F, Fuss IJ, Nieuwenhuis EE, Blumberg RS, Strober W: Oxazolone colitis, a Th2 colitis model resembling ulcerative colitis, is mediated by IL-13 producing NK-T cells. Immunity 2002; 17:629–638.
[71] Borthakur A, Bhattacharyya S, Dudeja PK, Tobacman JK. Carrageenan induces interleukin-8 production through distinct Bcl10 pathway in normal human colonic epithelial cells. Am J Physiol Gastrointest Liver Physiol 2007;292(3):G829-38.
[72] Tobacman JK. Review of harmful gastrointestinal effects of carrageenan in animal experiments. Environ Health Perspect 109: 983–994, 2001.
[73] Tobacman JK. Toxic considerations related to ingestion of carrageenan. In: Reviews in Food and Nutrition Toxicity, edited by Preedy VR and Watson RR. New York: Taylor & Francis, 2003, p. 204–229.
[74] Langman JM, Rowland R, Vernon-Roberts B. Carrageenan colitis in the guinea pig: pathological changes and the importance of ascorbic acid deficiency in disease induction. Aust J Exp Biol Med Sci 1985;63 (Pt 5):545-53.
[75] Fath RB Jr, Deschner EE, Winawer SJ, Dworkin BM. Degraded carrageenan-induced colitis in CF1 mice. A clinical, histopathological and kinetic analysis. Digestion 1984;29(4):197-203.
[76] Jobin C, Sartor RB. The I kappa B/NF-kappa B system: a key determinant of mucosalinflammation and protection. Am J Physiol Cell Physiol 2000;278(3):C451-62.
[77] Ruland J, Duncan GS, Elia A, del Barco Barrantes I, Nguyen L, Plyte S, Millar DG, Bouchard D, Wakeham A, Ohashi PS, Mak TW. Bcl10 is a positive regulator of antigen receptor-induced activation of NF-kappaB and neural tube closure. Cell 2001;104(1):33-42.
[78] Willerford DM, Chen J, Ferry JA, Davidson L, Ma A, Alt FW. Interleukin-2 receptor alpha chain regulates the size and content of the peripheral lymphoid compartment. Immunit. 1995;3(4):521-30.

[79] Rudolph U, Finegold MJ, Rich SS, Harriman GR, Srinivasan Y, Brabet P, Boulay G, Bradley A, Birnbaumer L. Ulcerative colitis and adenocarcinoma of the colon in G alpha i2-deficient mice. Nat Genet 1995;10(2):143-50.
[80] Sadlack B, Merz H, Schorle H, Schimpl A, Feller AC, Horak I. Ulcerative colitis-like disease in mice with a disrupted interleukin-2 gene. Cell 1993;75(2):253-61.
[81] Ehrhardt RO, Ludviksson B. Induction of colitis in IL2-deficient-mice: the role of thymic and peripheral dysregulation in the generation of autoreactive T cells. Res Immunol 1997;148(8-9):582-8.
[82] Contractor NV, Bassiri H, Reya T, Park AY, Baumgart DC, Wasik MA, Emerson SG, Carding SR. Lymphoid hyperplasia, autoimmunity, and compromised intestinal intraepithelial lymphocyte development in colitis-free gnotobiotic IL-2-deficient mice. J Immunol 1998;160(1):385-94.
[83] Baumgart DC, Olivier WA, Reya T, Peritt D, Rombeau JL, Carding SR. Mechanisms of intestinal epithelial cell injury and colitis in interleukin 2 (IL2)-deficient mice. Cell Immunol 1998;187(1):52-66.
[84] Ostanin DV, Bao J, Koboziev I, Gray L, Robinson-Jackson SA, Kosloski-Davidson M, Price VH, Grisham MB. T cell transfer model of chronic colitis: concepts, considerations, and tricks of the trade. Am J Physiol Gastrointest Liver Physiol 2009;296(2):G135-46.
[85] Berg DJ, Davidson N, Kühn R, Müller W, Menon S, Holland G, Thompson-Snipes L, Leach MW, Rennick D. Enterocolitis and colon cancer in interleukin-10-deficient mice are associated with aberrant cytokine production and CD4(+) TH1-like responses. J Clin Invest 1996;98(4):1010-20.
[86] Kühn R, Löhler J, Rennick D, Rajewsky K, Müller W. Interleukin-10-deficient mice develop chronic enterocolitis. Cell 1993;75(2):263-74.
[87] Davidson NJ, Fort MM, Müller W, Leach MW, Rennick DM. Chronic colitis in IL-10-/- mice: insufficient counter regulation of a Th1 response. Int Rev Immunol 2000;19(1):91-121.
[88] Knoch B, Nones K, Barnett MP, McNabb WC, Roy NC. Diversity of caecal bacteria is altered in interleukin-10 gene-deficient mice before and after colitis onset and when fed polyunsaturated fatty acids. Microbiol 2010;156(Pt 11):3306-16.
[89] Thomas ML. The leukocyte common antigen family. Annu Rev Immunol. 1989;7:339-69.
[90] Leach MW, Bean AG, Mauze S, Coffman RL, Powrie F. Inflammatory bowel disease in C.B-17 scid mice reconstituted with the CD45RBhigh subset of CD4+ T cells. Am J Pathol 1996;148(5):1503-15.
[91] Powrie F, Leach MW, Mauze S, Caddle LB, Coffman RL. Phenotypically distinct subsets of CD4+ T cells induce or protect from chronic intestinal inflammation in C. B-17 scid mice. Int Immunol 1993;5(11):1461-71.
[92] Read S, Malmström V, Powrie F. Cytotoxic T lymphocyte-associated antigen 4 plays an essential role in the function of CD25(+)CD4(+) regulatory cells that control intestinal inflammation. J Exp Med 2000;192(2):295-302.
[93] Asseman C, Mauze S, Leach MW, Coffman RL, Powrie F. An essential role for interleukin 10 in the function of regulatory T cells that inhibit intestinal inflammation. J Exp Med 1999;190(7):995-1004.
[94] Hendrickson BA GR, Cho JH. Clinical aspects and pathophysiology of inflammatory bowel disease. Clin Microbiol Rev 2002;15(79-94).

[95] Pithadia AB, Jain S. Treatment of inflammatory bowel disease (IBD). Pharmacol Rep 2011;63(3):629-42.
[96] Toruner M, Loftus EV, Harmsen WS, Zinsmeister AR, Orenstein R, Sandborn WJ, Colombel JF, Egan LJ. Risk factors for opportunistic infections in inflammatory bowel diseases: a case control study. Gastroenterology 2008; 134: 929-36.
[97] Sartor RB. Current concepts of the etiology and pathogenesis of ulcerative colitis and Crohn's disease. Gastroenterol Clin North Am 1995;24(3):475-507.
[98] Sartor RB: Micrbial factors in the pathogenesis of Crohn's disease, ulcerative colitis and experimental intestinal inflammation. In: Inflammatory Bowel Disease. 5th edn., Eds Kirsner JB, Hanauer S, Saunders, Philadelphia, 1999, 153-178.
[99] Uehara T, Kato K, Ohkusa T, Sugitani M, Ishii Y, Nemoto N, Moriyama M. Efficacy of antibiotic combination therapy in patients with active ulcerative colitis, including refractory or steroid-dependent cases. J Gastroenterol Hepatol 2010;25 Suppl 1:S62-6.
[100] Ohkusa T, Kato K, Terao S, Chiba T, Mabe K, Murakami K, Mizokami Y, Sugiyama T, Yanaka A, Takeuchi Y, Yamato S, Yokoyama T, Okayasu I, Watanabe S, Tajiri H, Sato N; Japan UC Antibiotic Therapy Study Group. Newly developed antibiotic combination therapy for ulcerative colitis: a double-blind placebo-controlled multicenter trial. Am J Gastroenterol 2010;105(8):1820-9.
[101] Turner D, Shah PS, Steinhart AH, Zlotkin S, Griffiths AM. Maintenance of remission in inflammatory bowel disease using omega-3 fatty acids (fish oil): a systematic review and meta-analyses. Inflamm Bowel Dis 2011;17:336-345.
[102] Hilsden RJ, Verhoef MJ, Best A, Pocobelli G. Complementary and alternative medicine use by Canadian patients with inflammatory bowel disease: results from a national survey. Am J Gastroenterol 2003;98(7):1563-8.
[103] Head K, Jurenka JS. Inflammatory bowel disease. Part II: Crohn's disease--pathophysiology and conventional and alternative treatment options. Altern Med Rev 2004;9(4):360-401.
[104] Korzenik JR, Podolsky DK. Evolving knowledge and therapy of inflammatory bowel disease. Nat Rev Drug Discov 2006;5(3):197-209.
[105] Rutgeerts P, Vermeire S, Van Assche G. Biological therapies for inflammatory bowel diseases. Gastroenterol 2009;136(4):1182-97.
[106] Akabas SR, Deckelbaum RJ. Summary of a workshop on n-3 fatty acids: current status of recommendations and future directions. Am J Clin Nutr. 2006;83:1536S-1538S.
[107] Ergas D, Eilat E, Mendlovic S, Sthoeger ZM. n-3 fatty acids and the immune system in autoimmunity. Isr Med Assoc J. 2002;4:34-38.
[108] Hooper L, Thompson RL, Harrison RA, Summerbell CD, Moore H, Worthington HV, Durrington PN, Ness AR, Capps NE, Davey Smith G, Riemersma RA, Ebrahim SB. Omega-3 fatty acids for prevention and treatment of cardiovascular disease [Systematic Review]. Cochrane Database Syst Rev. 2004;CD003177.
[109] Ruxton CH, Reed SC, Simpson MJ, Millington KJ. The health benefits of omega-3 polyunsaturated fatty acids: a review of the evidence. J Hum Nutr Diet 2004;17(5):449-59.
[110] Simopoulos AP. Omega-3 fatty acids in inflammation and autoimmune diseases. J Am Coll Nutr.2002;21:495-505.

[111] Mayer K, Seeger W. Fish oil in critical illness. Curr Opin Vlin Nutr Metab Care. 2008;11:121-127.
[112] James MJ, Gibson RA, Cleland LG. Dietary polyunsaturated fatty acids and inflammatory mediator production. Am J Clin Nutr 2000;71(suppl):343S-8S.
[113] MacLean CH, Mojica, WA, Newberry SJ, Pencharz J, Garland RH, Tu W, Hilton LG, Gralnek IM, Rhodes S, Khanna P, Morton SC. Systematic review of the effects of n-3 fatty acids in inflammatory bowel disease. Am J Clin Nutr 2005;82:611-9.
[114] Whiting CV, Bland P, Tarlton JF. Dietary n-3 polyunsaturated fatty acids reduce disease and colonic proinflammatory cytokines in a mouse model of colitis. Inflamm Bowel Dis 2005;11:340-349.
[115] Li Q, Zhang Q, Zhang M, Wang C, Zhu Z, Li N, Li J. Effect of n-3 polyunsaturated fatty acids on membrane microdomain localization of tight junction proteins in experimental colitis.
[116] Nishihara T, Matsuda M, Araki H, Oshima K, Kihara S, Funahashi T, Shimomura I. Effect of adiponectin on murine colitis induced by dextran sulfate sodium. Gastroenterol 2006;131(3):853-61.
[117] Fayad R, Pini M, Sennello JA, Cabay RJ, Chan L, Xu A, Fantuzzi G. Adiponectin deficiency protects mice from chemically induced colonic inflammation. Gastroenterol 2007;132(2):601-14.
[118] Yamamoto K, Kiyohara T, Murayama Y, Kihara S, Okamoto Y, Funahashi T, Ito T, Nezu R, Tsutsui S, Miyagawa JI, Tamura S, Matsuzawa Y, Shimomura I, Shinomura Y. Production of adiponectin, an anti-inflammatory protein, in mesenteric adipose tissue in Crohn's disease. Gut 2005;54(6):789-96.
[119] Matsunaga H, Hokari R, Kurihara C, Okada Y, Takebayashi K, Okudaira K, Watanabe C, Komoto S, Nakamura M, Tsuzuki Y, Kawaguchi A, Nagao S, Itoh K, Miura S. Omega-3 fatty acids exacerbate DSS-induced colitis through decreased adiponectin in colonic subepithelial myofibroblasts. Inflamm Bowel Dis 2008;14(10):1348-57.
[120] Hillier K, Jewell R, Dorrell L, Smith CL. Incorporation of fatty acids from fish oil and olive oil into colonic mucosal lipids and effects upon eicosanoid synthesis in inflammatory bowel disease. Gut. 1991;32:1151-1155.
[121] McCall TB, O'Leary D, Bloomfield J, O'Morain CA. Therapeutic potential of fish oil in the traetment of ulcerative colitis. Ailment Pharmacol Ther.1989;3 ;415-424.
[122] Almallah YZ, Richardson S, O'Hanrahan T, Mowat NA, Brunt PW, Sinclair TS, Ewen S, Heys SD, Eremin O. Distal procto-colitis, natural cytotoxicity, and essential fatty acids. Am J Gastroenterol 1998;93:804-9.
[123] Varghese TJ, Coomansingh D. Clinical response of ulcerative colitis with dietary omega-3 fatty acids: a double-blind randomized study. Br J Surg 2000;87(suppl):73 (abstr).
[124] Hawthorne AB, Daneshmend TK, Hawkey CJ, Belluzzi A, Everitt SJ, Holmes GK, Malkinson C, Shaheen MZ, Willars JE. Treatment of ulcerative colitis with fish oil supplementation: a prospective 12 month randomised controlled trial. Gut 1992;33(7):922-8.
[125] Greenfield SM, Green AT, Teare JP, Jenkins AP, Punchard NA, Ainley CC, Thompson RP. A randomized controlled study of evening primrose oil and fish oil in ulcerative colitis. Aliment Pharmacol Ther. 1993;7(2):159-66.

[126] Loeschke K, Ueberschaer B, Pietsch A, Gruber E, Ewe K, Wiebecke B, Heldwein W, Lorenz R. n-3 fatty acids only delay early relapse of ulcerative colitis in remission. Dig Dis Sci. 1996 ;41(10):2087-94.
[127] Mantzaris GJ, Archavlis E, Zografos C, Petraki K, Spiliades C, Triantafyllou G. A prospective, randomized, placebo-controlled study of fish oil in ulcerative colitis. Hellen J Gastroenterol 1996;9:138-141.
[128] Middleton SJ, Naylor S, Woolner J, Hunter JO. A double-blind, randomized, placebo-controlled trial of essential fatty acid supplementation in the maintenance of remission of ulcerative colitis. Aliment Pharmacol Ther 2002;16(6):1131-5.
[129] Hawthorne AB, Daneshmend TK, Hawkey CJ et al. Fish oil in ulcerative colitis: final results of a controlled clinical trial. Gastroenterol 1990;98:A174(abstr).
[130] Belluzzi A, Brignola C, Campieri M, Camporesi EP, Gionchetti P, Rizzello F, Belloli C, De Simone G, Boschi S, Miglioli M, et al. Effects of new fish oil derivative on fatty acid phospholipid-membrane pattern in a group of Crohn's disease patients. Dig Dis Sci. 1994;39:2589-2594.
[131] Seril DN, Liao J, Yang GY, Yang CS. Oxidative stress and ulcerative colitis-associated carcinogenesis: studies in humans and animal models. Carcinogenesis 2003;24(3):353-62.
[132] Sánchez-Fidalgo S, Cárdeno A, Villegas I, Talero E, de la Lastra CA. Dietary supplementation of resveratrol attenuates chronic colonic inflammation in mice. Eur J Pharmacol. 2010;633(1-3):78-84.
[133] Cui X, Jin Y, Hofseth AB, Pena E, Habiger J, Chumanevich A, Poudyal D, Nagarkatti M, Nagarkatti PS, Singh UP, Hofseth LJ. Resveratrol suppresses colitis and colon cancer associated with colitis. Cancer Prev Res (Phila) 2010;3(4):549-59.
[134] Tang T, Targan SR, Li ZS, Xu C, Byers VS, Sandborn WJ. Randomised clinical trial: herbal extract HMPL-004 in active ulcerative colitis - a double-blind comparison with sustained release mesalazine. Aliment Pharmacol Ther 2011;33(2):194-202.
[135] Afaq F, Saleem M, Krueger CG, Reed JD, Mukhtar H. Anthocyanin- and hydrolyzable tannin-rich pomegranate fruit extract modulates MAPK and NF-kappaB pathways and inhibits skin tumorigenesis in CD-1 mice. Int J Cancer 2005;113(3):423-33.
[136] Reddy MK, Alexander-Lindo RL, Nair MG. Relative inhibition of lipid peroxidation, cyclooxygenase enzymes, and human tumor cell proliferation by natural food colors. J Agric Food Chem 2005;53(23):9268-73.
[137] Rodrigo KA, Rawal Y, Renner RJ, Schwartz SJ, Tian Q, Larsen PE, Mallery SR. Suppression of the tumorigenic phenotype in human oral squamous cell carcinoma cells by an ethanol extract derived from freeze-dried black raspberries. Nutr Cancer 2006;54(1):58-68.
[138] Daniel E. Extraction, stability and quantitation of ellagic acid in various fruits and nuts. J Food Comp Anal 1989; 2:338-349.
[139] Wada L, Ou B. Antioxidant activity and phenolic content of Oregon caneberries. J Agric Food Chem 2002;50(12):3495-500.
[140] Olsson ME, Gustavsson KE, Andersson S, Nilsson A, Duan RD. Inhibition of cancer cell proliferation in vitro by fruit and berry extracts and correlations with antioxidant levels. J Agric Food Chem 2004;52(24):7264-71.

[141] Parry J, Su L, Moore J, Cheng Z, Luther M, Rao JN, Wang JY, Yu LL. Chemical compositions, antioxidant capacities, and antiproliferative activities of selected fruit seed flours. J Agric Food Chem 2006;54(11):3773-8.
[142] Renis M, Calandra L, Scifo C, Tomasello B, Cardile V, Vanella L, Bei R, La Fauci L, Galvano F. Response of cell cycle/stress-related protein expression and DNA damage upon treatment of CaCo2 cells with anthocyanins. Br J Nutr 2008;100(1):27-35.
[143] Shih PH, Yeh CT, Yen GC. Anthocyanins induce the activation of phase II enzymes through the antioxidant response element pathway against oxidative stress-induced apoptosis. J Agric Food Chem 2007;55(23):9427-35.
[144] Montrose DC, Horelik NA, Madigan JP, Stoner GD, Wang LS, Bruno RS, Park HJ, Giardina C, Rosenberg DW. Anti-inflammatory effects of freeze-dried black raspberry powder in ulcerative colitis. Carcinogenesis 2011;32(3):343-50.
[145] Hofseth LJ. Ginseng and Cancer. Healthy Aging 2006:53-58.
[146] Hofseth LJ, Wargovich MJ. Inflammation, cancer, and targets of ginseng. J Nutr 2007;137(1 Suppl):183S-185S.
[147] Hofseth LJ. Nitric oxide as a target of complementary and alternative medicines to prevent and treat inflammation and cancer. Cancer Lett 2008;268(1):10-30.
[148] Jin Y, Kotakadi VS, Ying L, Hofseth AB, Cui X, Wood PA, Windust A, Matesic LE, Pena EA, Chiuzan C, Singh NP, Nagarkatti M, Nagarkatti PS, Wargovich MJ, Hofseth LJ. American ginseng suppresses inflammation and DNA damage associated with mouse colitis. Carcinogenesis 2008;29(12):2351-9.
[149] Jin Y, Hofseth AB, Cui X, Windust AJ, Poudyal D, Chumanevich AA, Matesic LE, Singh NP, Nagarkatti M, Nagarkatti PS, Hofseth LJ. American ginseng suppresses colitis through p53-mediated apoptosis of inflammatory cells. Cancer Prev Res (Phila) 2010;3(3):339-47.
[150] Pehlivan M, Dalbeler Y, Hazinedaroglu S, Arikan Y, Erkek AB, Günal O, Türkçapar N, Türkçapar AG. An assessment of the effect of Ginkgo Biloba EGb 761 on ischemia reperfusion injury of intestine. Hepatogastroenterol 2002;49(43):201-4.
[151] Maitra I, Marcocci L, Droy-Lefaix MT, Packer L. Peroxyl radical scavenging activity of Ginkgo biloba extract EGb 761. Biochem Pharmacol 1995;49(11):1649-55.
[152] Kusmic C, Basta G, Lazzerini G, Vesentini N, Barsacchi R. The effect of Ginkgo biloba in isolated ischemic/reperfused rat heart: a link between vitamin E preservation and prostaglandin biosynthesis. J Cardiovasc Pharmacol 2004;44(3):356-62.
[153] Zhou YH, Yu JP, Liu YF, Teng XJ, Ming M, Lv P, An P, Liu SQ, Yu HG. Effects of Ginkgo biloba extract on inflammatory mediators (SOD, MDA, TNF-alpha, NF-kappaBp65, IL-6) in TNBS-induced colitis in rats. Mediators Inflamm. 2006;2006(5):92642.
[154] Kotakadi VS, Jin Y, Hofseth AB, Ying L, Cui X, Volate S, Chumanevich A, Wood PA, Price RL, McNeal A, Singh UP, Singh NP, Nagarkatti M, Nagarkatti PS, Matesic LE, Auclair K, Wargovich MJ, Hofseth LJ. Ginkgo biloba extract EGb 761 has anti-inflammatory properties and ameliorates colitis in mice by driving effector T cell apoptosis. Carcinogenesis 2008;29(9):1799-806.
[155] Prasad KV, Prabhakar BS. Apoptosis and autoimmune disorders. Autoimmunity 2003;36(6-7):323-30.

[156] Anderson GP. Resolution of chronic inflammation by therapeutic induction of apoptosis. Trends Pharmacol Sci 1996;17(12):438-42.
[157] Abdullaev FI. Cancer chemopreventive and tumoricidal properties of saffron (Crocus sativus L.). Exp Biol Med (Maywood) 2002;227(1):20-5.
[158] Kazi HA, Qian Z. Crocetin reduces TNBS-induced experimental colitis in mice by downregulation of NFkB. Saudi J Gastroenterol 2009 ;15(3):181-7.
[159] Toklu HZ, Dumlu MU, Sehirli O, Ercan F, Gedik N, Gökmen V, Sener G. Pomegranate peel extract prevents liver fibrosis in biliary-obstructed rats. J Pharm Pharmacol 2007;59(9):1287-95.
[160] Kasai K, Yoshimura M, Koga T, Arii M, Kawasaki S. Effects of oral administration of ellagic acid-rich pomegranate extract on ultraviolet-induced pigmentation in the human skin. J Nutr Sci Vitaminol (Tokyo) 2006;52(5):383-8.
[161] Gracious Ross R, Selvasubramanian S, Jayasundar S. Immunomodulatory activity of Punica granatum in rabbits--a preliminary study. Ethnopharmacol 2001;78(1):85-7.
[162] Aviram M, Dornfeld L. 2003. Methods of using pomegranate extracts for causing regression in lesions due to arteriosclerosis in humans. US patent. 6: 641, 850.
[163] Huang TH, Peng G, Kota BP, Li GQ, Yamahara J, Roufogalis BD, Li Y. Anti-diabetic action of Punica granatum flower extract: activation of PPAR-gamma and identification of an active component. Toxicol Appl Pharmacol 2005;207(2):160-9.
[164] Singh K, Jaggi AS, Singh N. Exploring the ameliorative potential of Punica granatum in dextran sulfate sodium induced ulcerative colitis in mice. Phytother Res 2009;23(11):1565-74.
[165] Marshall JK, Irvine EJ. Ketotifen treatment of active colitis in patients with 5-aminosalicylate intolerance. Can J Gastroenterol 1998;12(4):273-5.
[166] Elliott DE, Summers RW, Weinstock JV. Helminths as governors of immune-mediated inflammation. Int J Parasitol 2007;37(5):457-64.
[167] van den Biggelaar AH, Rodrigues LC, van Ree R, van der Zee JS, Hoeksma-Kruize YC, Souverijn JH, Missinou MA, Borrmann S, Kremsner PG, Yazdanbakhsh M. Long-term treatment of intestinal helminths increases mite skin-test reactivity in Gabonese schoolchildren. J Infect Dis 2004;189(5):892-900.
[168] Araújo MI, Hoppe BS, Medeiros M Jr, Carvalho EM. Schistosoma mansoni infection modulates the immune response against allergic and auto-immune diseases. Mem Inst Oswaldo Cruz 2004;99(5 Suppl 1):27-32.
[169] van den Biggelaar AH, van Ree R, Rodrigues LC, Lell B, Deelder AM, Kremsner PG, Yazdanbakhsh M. Decreased atopy in children infected with Schistosoma haematobium: a role for parasite-induced interleukin-10. Lancet 2000;356(9243):1723-7.
[170] Melon A, Wang A, Phan V, McKay DM. Infection with Hymenolepis diminuta is more effective than daily corticosteroids in blocking chemically induced colitis in mice. J Biomed Biotechnol 2010;2010:384523, 1-7.
[171] Khan WI, Blennerhasset PA, Varghese AK, Chowdhury SK, Omsted P, Deng Y, Collins SM. Intestinal nematode infection ameliorates experimental colitis in mice. Infect Immun. 2002;70(11):5931-7.
[172] Wang A, Fernando M, Leung G, Phan V, Smyth D, McKay DM. Exacerbation of oxazolone colitis by infection with the helminth Hymenolepis diminuta: involvement of IL-5 and eosinophils. Am J Pathol 2010;177(6):2850-9.

[173] Summers RW, Elliott DE, Urban JF Jr, Thompson RA, Weinstock JV. Trichuris suis therapy for active ulcerative colitis: a randomized controlled trial. Gastroenterol 2005;128(4):825-32.
[174] Guarner F, Malagelada JR. Gut flora in health and disease. Lancet 2003;361:512-9.
[175] Cummings JH, Antoine JM, Azpiroz F, Bourdet-Sicard R, Brandtzaeg P, Calder PC, Gibson GR, Guarner F, Isolauri E, Pannemans D, Shortt C, Tuijtelaars S, Watzl B. PASSCLAIM--gut health and immunity. Eur J Nutr 2004;43 Suppl 2:II118-II173.
[176] Gibson GR, Probert HM, Loo JV, Rastall RA, Roberfroid MB. Dietary modulation of the human colonic microbiota: updating the concept of prebiotics. Nutr Res Rev 2004;17:259-75.
[177] Guarner F. Prebiotics in inflammatory bowel diseases. Br J Nutr 2007;98 Suppl 1:S85-9.
[178] Marteau P. Probiotics, prebiotics, synbiotics: ecological treatment for inflammatory bowel disease? Gut 2006;55:1692-3.
[179] Videla S, Vilaseca J, Antolin M, Garcia-Lafuente A, Guarner F, Crespo E, Casalots J, Salas A, Malagelada JR. Dietary inulin improves distal colitis induced by dextran sodium sulfate in the rat. Am J Gastroenterol 2001;96:1486-93.
[180] Cherbut C, Michel C, Lecannu G. The prebiotic characteristics of fructooligosaccharides are necessary for reduction of TNBS-induced colitis in rats. J Nutr 2003;133:21-7.
[181] Madsen KL, Doyle JS, Jewell LD, Tavernini MM, Fedorak RN. Lactobacillus species prevents colitis in interleukin 10 gene-deficient mice. Gastroenterology 1999;116:1107-14.
[182] Rumi G, Tsubouchi R, Okayama M, Kato S, Mozsik G, Takeuchi K. Protective effect of lactulose on dextran sulfate sodium-induced colonic inflammation in rats. Dig Dis Sci 2004;49:1466-72.
[183] Camuesco D, Peran L, Comalada M, Nieto A, Di Stasi LC, Rodriguez-Cabezas ME, Concha A, Zarzuelo A, Galvez J. Preventative effects of lactulose in the trinitrobenzenesulphonic acid model of rat colitis. Inflamm Bowel Dis 2005;11:265-71.
[184] Casellas F, Borruel N, Torrejon A, Varela E, Antolin M, Guarner F, Malagelada JR. Oral oligofructose-enriched inulin supplementation in acute ulcerative colitis is well tolerated and associated with lowered faecal calprotectin. Aliment Pharmacol Ther 2007;25:1061-7.
[185] Sartor RB. Therapeutic manipulation of the enteric microflora in inflammatory bowel diseases: antibiotics, probiotics, and prebiotics. Gastroenterology 2004;126:1620-33.
[186] Borchers AT, Selmi C, Meyers FJ, Keen CL, Gershwin ME. Probiotics and immunity. J Gastroenterol 2009;44:26-46.
[187] Schlee M, Harder J, Koten B, Stange EF, Wehkamp J, Fellermann K. Probiotic lactobacilli and VSL#3 induce enterocyte beta-defensin 2. Clin Exp Immunol 2008;151:528-35.
[188] Zyrek AA, Cichon C, Helms S, Enders C, Sonnenborn U, Schmidt MA. Molecular mechanisms underlying the probiotic effects of Escherichia coli Nissle 1917 involve ZO-2 and PKCzeta redistribution resulting in tight junction and epithelial barrier repair. Cell Microbiol 2007;9:804-16.
[189] Kamada N, Maeda K, Inoue N, Hisamatsu T, Okamoto S, Hong KS, Yamada T, Watanabe N, Tsuchimoto K, Ogata H, Hibi T. Nonpathogenic Escherichia coli

strain Nissle 1917 inhibits signal transduction in intestinal epithelial cells. Infect Immun 2008;76:214-20.

[190] Dunne C, Murphy L, Flynn S, O'Mahony L, O'Halloran S, Feeney M, Morrissey D, Thornton G, Fitzgerald G, Daly C, Kiely B, Quigley EM, O'Sullivan GC, Shanahan F, Collins JK. Probiotics: from myth to reality. Demonstration of functionality in animal models of disease and in human clinical trials. Antonie Van Leeuwenhoek 1999;76:279-92.

[191] Ukena SN, Singh A, Dringenberg U, Engelhardt R, Seidler U, Hansen W, Bleich A, Bruder D, Franzke A, Rogler G, Suerbaum S, Buer J, Gunzer F, Westendorf AM. Probiotic Escherichia coli Nissle 1917 inhibits leaky gut by enhancing mucosal integrity. PLoS One 2007;2:e1308.

[192] Schultz M, Lindstrom AL. Rationale for probiotic treatment strategies in inflammatory bowel disease. Expert Rev Gastroenterol Hepatol 2008;2:337-55.

[193] Grabig A, Paclik D, Guzy C, Dankof A, Baumgart DC, Erckenbrecht J, Raupach B, Sonnenborn U, Eckert J, Schumann RR, Wiedenmann B, Dignass AU, Sturm A. Escherichia coli strain Nissle 1917 ameliorates experimental colitis via toll-like receptor 2- and toll-like receptor 4-dependent pathways. Infect Immun 2006;74:4075-82.

[194] Lee HS, Han SY, Bae EA, Huh CS, Ahn YT, Lee JH, Kim DH. Lactic acid bacteria inhibit proinflammatory cytokine expression and bacterial glycosaminoglycan degradation activity in dextran sulfate sodium-induced colitic mice. Int Immunopharmacol 2008;8:574-80.

[195] Schultz M, Veltkamp C, Dieleman LA, Grenther WB, Wyrick PB, Tonkonogy SL, Sartor RB. Lactobacillus plantarum 299V in the treatment and prevention of spontaneous colitis in interleukin-10-deficient mice. Inflamm Bowel Dis 2002;8:71-80.

[196] Peran L, Camuesco D, Comalada M, Bailon E, Henriksson A, Xaus J, Zarzuelo A, Galvez J. A comparative study of the preventative effects exerted by three probiotics, Bifidobacterium lactis, Lactobacillus casei and Lactobacillus acidophilus, in the TNBS model of rat colitis. J Appl Microbiol 2007;103:836-44.

[197] Menard O, Butel MJ, Gaboriau-Routhiau V, Waligora-Dupriet AJ. Gnotobiotic mouse immune response induced by Bifidobacterium sp. strains isolated from infants. Appl Environ Microbiol 2008;74:660-6.

[198] Hedin C, Whelan K, Lindsay JO. Evidence for the use of probiotics and prebiotics in inflammatory bowel disease: a review of clinical trials. Proc Nutr Soc 2007;66:307-15.

[199] Tsuda Y, Yoshimatsu Y, Aoki H, Nakamura K, Irie M, Fukuda K, Hosoe N, Takada N, Shirai K, Suzuki Y. Clinical effectiveness of probiotics therapy (BIO-THREE) in patients with ulcerative colitis refractory to conventional therapy. Scand J Gastroenterol 2007;42:1306-11.

[200] Vallee BL, Falchuk KH. The biochemical basis of zinc physiology. Physiol Rev 1993;73(1):79-118.

[201] MacDonald RS. The role of zinc in growth and cell proliferation. J Nutr. 2000;130(5S Suppl):1500S-8S.

[202] Chesters JK. Biochemical functions of zinc in animals. World Rev Nutr Diet. 1978;32:135-64.

[203] Zalewski PD, Forbes IJ, Seamark RF, Borlinghaus R, Betts WH, Lincoln SF, Ward AD. Flux of intracellular labile zinc during apoptosis (gene-directed cell death) revealed by a specific chemical probe, Zinquin. Chem Biol. 1994;1(3):153-61.

[204] Tran CD, Ball JM, Sundar S, Coyle P, Howarth GS. The role of zinc and metallothionein in the dextran sulfate sodium-induced colitis mouse model. Dig Dis Sci. 2007;52(9):2113-21.

[205] Ohkawara T, Takeda H, Kato K, Miyashita K, Kato M, Iwanaga T, Asaka M. Polaprezinc (N-(3-aminopropionyl)-L-histidinato zinc) ameliorates dextran sulfate sodium-induced colitis in mice. Scand J Gastroenterol 2005;40(11):1321-7.

[206] Chen BW, Wang HH, Liu JX, Liu XG. Zinc sulphate solution enema decreases inflammation in experimental colitis in rats. J Gastroenterol Hepatol 1999;14(11):1088-92.

[207] Iwaya H, Kashiwaya M, Shinoki A, Lee JS, Hayashi K, Hara H, Ishizuka S. Marginal zinc deficiency exacerbates experimental colitis induced by dextran sulfate sodium in rats. J Nutr 2011;141(6):1077-82.

[208] Luk HH, Ko JK, Fung HS, Cho CH. Delineation of the protective action of zinc sulfate on ulcerative colitis in rats. Eur J Pharmacol 2002;443(1-3):197-204.

[209] Sturniolo GC, Fries W, Mazzon E, Di Leo V, Barollo M, D'inca R. Effect of zinc supplementation on intestinal permeability in experimental colitis. J Lab Clin Med 2002;139(5):311-5.

[210] Yoshikawa T, Yamaguchi T, Yoshida N, Yamamoto H, Kitazumi S, Takahashi S, Naito Y, Kondo M. Effect of Z-103 on TNB-induced colitis in rats. Digestion 1997;58(5):464-8.

[211] Bruewer M, Schmid KW, Krieglstein CF, Senninger N, Schuermann G. Metallothionein: early marker in the carcinogenesis of ulcerative colitis-associated colorectal carcinoma. World J Surg 2002;26(6):726-31.

[212] Dronfield MW, Malone JD, Langman MJ. Zinc in ulcerative colitis: a therapeutic trial and report on plasma levels. Gut 1977;18(1):33-6.

[213] Van de Wal Y, Van der Sluys Veer A, Verspaget HW, Mulder TP, Griffioen G, Van Tol EA, Peña AS, Lamers CB. Effect of zinc therapy on natural killer cell activity in inflammatory bowel disease. Aliment Pharmacol Ther 1993;7(3):281-6.